Benefits of Resveratrol Supplementation

Benefits of Resveratrol Supplementation

Special Issue Editors

María P. Portillo
Alfredo Fernández-Quintela

MDPI • Basel • Beijing • Wuhan • Barcelona • Belgrade

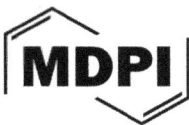

MDPI

Special Issue Editors
María P. Portillo
University of the Basque Country (UPV/EHU) Spain
Instituto de Salud Carlos III (CIBERobn)
Spain

Alfredo Fernández-Quintela
University of the Basque Country (UPV/EHU) Spain
Instituto de Salud Carlos III (CIBERobn)
Spain

Editorial Office
MDPI
St. Alban-Anlage 66
4052 Basel, Switzerland

This is a reprint of articles from the Special Issue published online in the open access journal *Nutrients* (ISSN 2072-6643) from 2018 to 2019 (available at: https://www.mdpi.com/journal/nutrients/ special_issues/Benefits_of_Resveratrol_Supplementation)

For citation purposes, cite each article independently as indicated on the article page online and as indicated below:

LastName, A.A.; LastName, B.B.; LastName, C.C. Article Title. *Journal Name* **Year**, *Article Number*, Page Range.

ISBN 978-3-03921-275-0 (Pbk)
ISBN 978-3-03921-276-7 (PDF)

Contents

About the Special Issue Editors

María P. Portillo completed her studies in Pharmacy at the University of Navarra (Spain). She then submitted her PhD thesis at the University of Navarra (Spain). After the PhD period, she continued at the Paul Sabatier University and Unit U377 INSERM in Toulouse (France). Following the postdoctoral period, Prof. Portillo was appointed Lecturer in the Department of Nutrition and Food Science at the University of the Basque Country (UPV/EHU) where, in 2010, she became a Professor. She leads the group "Nutrition and Obesity", one of the Basque Excellence Research Centers, and is also enrolled in CIBERobn, which is supported by Health Institute Carlos III. This group maintains scientific collaborations with several groups from the United States and Europe. She has participated as a collaborator in 17 competitive research projects and has led 30 projects supported by the Spanish Ministry, the Government of the Basque Country, and UPV/EHU. She has published 173 papers and several book chapters and supervised 12 PhD theses. Prof. Portillo's field of research covers the biological effects of different types of diets and biomolecules present in food on the prevention and treatment obesity, as well as on several obesity co-morbidities, such as insulin resistance and hepatic steatosis. In addition to her research activity, Prof. Portillo coordinates the bachelor's degree in "Nutrition and Dietetics", the master's program in "Nutrition and Health", and the doctorate program "Nutrigenomics and Personalized Nutrition" at UPV/EHU. She is President of the Spanish Nutrition Society, and a member of the Spanish Agency for Food Safety and the Editorial Board of both Nutrition and The British Journal of Nutrition.

Alfredo Fernández-Quintela is a graduate in Biology from the University of the Basque Country (UPV/EHU). Following his PhD degree, he conducted postdoctoral studies at the Rowett Research Institute (Aberdeen, Scotland). Thereafter, he was employed as an Associate Professor at the University of the Basque Country (UPV/EHU) in Vitoria (Spain) in 1994, where he is currently Lecturer in Human Nutrition and Food Sciences, and a Senior Researcher in the Department of Pharmacy and Food Sciences. His research focuses on the effects of bioactive molecules present in food (bioactive fatty acids, polyphenols) on obesity prevention and treatment, as well as on several of its co-morbidities (insulin resistance and hepatic steatosis). At present, he is also a Researcher at Health Institute Carlos III—CIBER Physiopathology of Obesity and Nutrition (CIBERobn). His translational research program spans from studying experimental models of disease to human studies. Dr Fernández-Quintela currently teaches the "Nutrition and Dietetics" course and supervises undergraduate, graduate student (PhD and MSc), and postdoctoral fellow research programs in Pharmacy and Human Nutrition as part of his research program.

Preface to "Benefits of Resveratrol Supplementation"

Resveratrol (3,5,4'-trihydroxy-trans-stilbene) is a phytoalexin that belongs to the group of stilbenes. Some plants produce resveratrol in response to infection, stress, injury, or ultraviolet radiation. Resveratrol is also found in grapes, wine, grape juice, peanuts, and some berries, such as blueberries, bilberries, and cranberries. Moreover, the glucosides of resveratrol are also widely reported to be beneficial to human health.Several of these positive effects have been compiled in this monograph, based on a Special Issue of Nutrients which contains 16 papers (4 reviews and 12 original publications). We, as Guest Editors, want to acknowledge the effort of the authors and to give the reader an overview of the current topics of research regarding the effects of resveratrol supplementation. Included are studies providing insights into the effects of resveratrol, some derivatives (ε-viniferin), or their metabolites, in promoting overall health and preventing or treating diseases such as inflammation, obesity, cardiovascular diseases, diabetes, and cancer.Interestingly, the final outcome of resveratrol supplementation depends on its bioavailability and pharmacokinetics. Several factors affect these two parameters: resveratrol formulation, ingested dose, food matrix, host gut microbiota, and circadian variation, amongst others. For example, the solid dispersion of resveratrol on magnesium dihydroxide increases its solubility and bioavailability and, therefore, this approach could enhance the biological properties of resveratrol.Inflammation or oxidative stress have been described as hallmarks of major diseases. Resveratrol, in combination with other polyphenols present in a red wine extract, has been involved in anti-inflammatory responses which are mediated by a strong decrease in IL-1 secretion and gene expression in macrophages which, in turn, occur through modulation of the expression of key proteins involved in the inflammasome complex. In addition, resveratrol improves kidney function, exerting protective effects on aging kidneys by mitigating oxidative stress and inflammation. The mechanisms underlying these effects are suppression of angiotensin II, involved in increased oxidative stress, and activation of the angiotensin 1-7/Mas receptor axis that counteracts the effects of angiotensin II.Regarding obesity, several mechanisms have been explored concerning the resveratrol-induced reduction of body fat accumulation. Thus, it has been demonstrated that resveratrol supplementation reverses the leptin resistance—caused by diet-induced obesity—in peripheral organs using tissue-specific mechanisms and in a dose-dependent manner. Resveratrol is also able to increase thermogenicity in interscapular brown adipose tissue (IBAT), and the oxidative capacities of both IBAT and skeletal muscle, contributing to the aforementioned anti-obesity action of the phenolic compound. However, a combination of resveratrol with energy restriction did not increase these effects.In addition, resveratrol has been reported to show positive effects on cardiovascular diseases. Thus, it has been proposed as a promising drug for slowing down atherosclerosis as part of the treatment of cardiovascular conditions, due to the resveratrol-mediated moderation of free radical generation and proinflammatory response diminishment. In addition, clinical studies have shown an association between resveratrol and vascular protection. Sirtuin-1 plays an important role in vascular biology and regulates some aspects of age-dependent atherosclerosis. Sirtuin-1 promotes vascular vasodilation, endothelium regeneration, and cardiomyocyte protection under stress conditions, including cellular toxicity as a result of reactive oxygen species activity. Resveratrol supplementation has been demonstrated to induce increased serum concentrations of Sirtuin-1, mirroring the effects of caloric restriction.Cardiovascular complications are the prime cause of morbidity and mortality in type 2 diabetic patients, particularly in women. Most antidiabetic treatments fail to decrease cardiovascular risk. Consequently, dietary supplements, in combination with antidiabetic medication, could potentially improve cardiovascular outcomes in diabetic patients, and resveratrol shows great promise for protecting the heart of type 2 diabetic women against myocardial infarction. Other complications linked to diabetes mellitus are oxidative stress and cataract formation. Long-term hyperglycemia leads to the overproduction of reactive oxygen species (ROS) in mitochondria which, in turn, causes an imbalance between ROS and endogenous defense mechanisms, leading to increased protein oxidation in the lens and, consequently, accumulation of insoluble aggregates and lens opacity. Resveratrol has demonstrated antioxidative activity in the lens of diabetic rats, reducing oxidative stress and possibly providing indirect benefits against cataract formation. Metabolic syndrome is a constellation of metabolic alterations such as insulin resistance, hypertension, and dyslipidemia. This Special Issue covers some of the interesting approaches used to study the effects of resveratrol on metabolic syndrome and its associated conditions, either through resveratrol itself or through the changes mediated in gut microbiota which, in turn, promote the changes associated with a healthy phenotype either directly or through the action of byproducts. Polyphenols constitute an important group of phytochemicals that have been gaining increased research attention since it was discovered that they could possess both cancer preventive and anticancer activities. Pharmacological approaches are a key tool in cancer treatment. Cisplatin is an anticancer drug used in the treatment of various types of cancer, including human breast cancer. However, resistance to cisplatin is a major cause of treatment failure. Resveratrol has been proposed as a chemosensitizer agent based on in vitro studies and, therefore, may help to improve the treatment of human breast cancer. A grape seed extract rich in stilbenes also demonstrated anticancer effects in prostate cancer cell lines.Finally, resveratrol has been postulated to aid in exercise performance. Indeed, in a preclinical study, resveratrol supplementation alone, or in combination with resistance exercise, effectively induced synergistic increases not only in terms of anaerobic performance and endurance but also in exercise-induced lactate production for better physiological adaption, muscular hypertrophy, and glycogen content.When translating all these positive preclinical effects of resveratrol supplementation to humans, several discrepancies have been observed, probably due to human metabolism and biotransformation of resveratrol, as reviewed in this Special Issue. Therefore, more studies are needed to further investigate the effects of resveratrol, and its metabolites, on human health.

María P. Portillo, Alfredo Fernández-Quintela
Special Issue Editors

nutrients

MDPI

Article

Gene Expression of Sirtuin-1 and Endogenous Secretory Receptor for Advanced Glycation End Products in Healthy and Slightly Overweight Subjects after Caloric Restriction and Resveratrol Administration

Alessandra Roggerio, Célia M. Cassaro Strunz, Ana Paula Pacanaro, Dalila Pinheiro Leal, Julio Y. Takada, Solange D. Avakian and Antonio de Padua Mansur *

Instituto do Coração, Hospital das Clínicas—HCFMUSP, Faculdade de Medicina, Universidade de São Paulo, Av Dr Eneas de Carvalho Aguiar, 44. CEP 05403-900 São Paulo, SP, Brazil; alessandra.roggerio@incor.usp.br (A.R.); labcelia@incor.usp.br (C.M.C.S.); ana.pacanaro@incor.usp.br (A.P.P.); dalila.pinheiro.leal@hotmail.com (D.P.L.); jyt@bol.com.br (J.Y.T.); solange.avakian@incor.usp.br (S.D.A.)
* Correspondence: apmansur@usp.br

Received: 30 June 2018; Accepted: 19 July 2018; Published: 21 July 2018

Abstract: Sirtuin-1 (Sirt-1) and an endogenous secretory receptor for an advanced glycation end product (esRAGE) are associated with vascular protection. The purpose of this study was to examine the effects of resveratrol (RSV) and caloric restriction (CR) on gene expression of Sirt-1 and esRAGE on serum levels of Sirt1 and esRAGE in healthy and slightly overweight subjects. The study included 48 healthy subjects randomized to 30 days of RSV (500 mg/day) or CR (1000 cal/day). Waist circumference ($p = 0.011$), TC ($p = 0.007$), HDL ($p = 0.031$), non-HDL ($p = 0.025$), ApoA1 ($p = 0.011$), and ApoB ($p = 0.037$) decreased in the CR group. However, TC ($p = 0.030$), non-HDL ($p = 0.010$), ApoB ($p = 0.034$), and HOMA-IR ($p = 0.038$) increased in the RSV group. RSV and CR increased serum levels of Sirt-1, respectively, from 1.06 ± 0.71 ng/mL to 5.75 ± 2.98 ng/mL ($p < 0.0001$) and from 1.65 ± 1.81 ng/mL to 5.80 ± 2.23 ng/mL ($p < 0.0001$). esRAGE serum levels were similar in RSV ($p = $ NS) and CR ($p = $ NS) groups. Significant positive correlation was observed between gene expression changes of Sirt-1 and esRAGE in RSV ($r = 0.86$; $p < 0.0001$) and in CR ($r = 0.71$; $p < 0.0001$) groups, but not for the changes in serum concentrations. CR promoted increases in the gene expression of esRAGE (post/pre). Future long-term studies are needed to evaluate the impact of these outcomes on vascular health.

Keywords: resveratrol; caloric restriction; esRAGE; Sirt-1

1. Introduction

Sirtuin-1 (Sirt-1) and an endogenous secretory receptor for an advanced glycation end product (esRAGE) are associated with vascular protection. Sirt1 plays an important role in vascular biology and regulates aspects of age-dependent atherosclerosis. In mammals, there are seven sirtuin isoforms from Sirt-1 to Sirt7. Sirt1 is found predominantly in the cell nucleus and has a number of modulators such as polyphenolic activators (resveratrol). Animal models confer cardio-protection, reduce neurodegeneration, promote increased fatty acid oxidation and gluconeogenesis in the liver, reduce lipogenesis in the white adipose tissue, and increase insulin secretion in the pancreas and insulin sensitivity in the muscle [1]. Sirt1 through stimulation of nitric oxide synthase promotes vascular vasodilation, endothelium regeneration, and cardiomyocyte protection under stressful conditions and cellular toxicity to reactive oxygen species [2,3]. Caloric restriction (CR) and resveratrol (RSV) are two interventions associated with higher gene expression and serum concentrations of Sirt-1 in animal studies [4,5] and in humans [6,7]. Studies have shown that increased concentrations of Sirt-1 are associated with better vascular homeostasis and metabolic profile and protection against endothelial senescence [8,9]. The receptor for advanced glycation end-products (RAGE) is a multi-ligand receptor for the final products of non-enzymatic glycation termed advanced glycation end products (AGEs) and expressed in alveolar epithelial cells of the lung and in endothelial and smooth muscle vascular cells [10]. Overconsumption of dietary AGEs causes chronic high-oxidative stress and inflammation and induces diabetic vasculopathy [11]. Bacon, processed beef, chicken, oils (olive and peanut), and cheeses (parmesan, American, and feta) are primary dietary source of AGEs [12]. Overexpression of RAGE has been associated with atherosclerosis and diabetic vascular diseases [13]. In prediabetic patients, AGEs were associated with the down-regulation of Sirt-1 expression and enzyme activity [14]. RAGE undergoes extensive alternative splicing to produce a variety of transcripts from a single gene. Alternative splicing produces different RAGE protein isoforms with diverse functions. Two major splicing variants have been characterized. Membrane bound RAGE is also known as a full-length RAGE (flRAGE) and esRAGE is a circulating truncated variant of the RAGE isoform [15]. esRAGE acts as a soluble antagonist that competes with cell surface RAGE as a receptor scavenger for circulating AGEs and reducing their availability for RAGE receptors located in the cell membrane. This decreases the harmful effects on cells. Studies have shown that low plasma concentrations of esRAGE is associated with the risk of diabetes, coronary artery disease, and all-cause mortality [16,17]. The purpose of this study was to examine the effect of RSV consumption, CR on Sirt-1, RAGE expression, and serum concentration in healthy and slightly overweight subjects.

2. Materials and Methods

The trial design has been described elsewhere [7]. The trial was a prospective randomized trial conducted in 48 healthy subjects from 55 to 65 years of age. The subjects were sedentary or on light physical activity. The subjects were recruited consecutively based on their normal clinical history, physical examination, and normal resting electrocardiogram. After a period of washout of 15 days without the use of any medications or supplements, 24 men and 24 women after menopause (01 year of natural amenorrhea) were randomized to CR or RSV groups. Twenty-four subjects (12 women and 12 men) were prescribed a low-calorie diet (1000 calories/day) and the remaining 24 subjects (12 women and 12 men) received 500 mg of resveratrol (trial registration: http://www.ClinicalTrials.gov; identifier:NCT01668836). Exclusion criteria were BMI $\geq$ 30 kg/m^2, smokers, hypertension (using antihypertensive medication or diastolic blood pressure $\geq$ 90 mmHg), dyslipidemia (use of lipid-lowering medication or serum triglyceride levels $\geq$ 150 mg/dL or total cholesterol $\geq$ 240 mg/dL), fasting glucose $\geq$ 110 mg/dL or using hypoglycemic medication, hormone replacement therapy, premenopausal women, and any other self-reported history or treatment for chronic renal failure (serum creatinine $\geq$ 2.0 mg/dL), liver failure, or metabolic clinically significant endocrine, hematologic, and respiratory factors. Clinical characteristics and laboratory tests were obtained before the interventions and 30 days after the interventions. The main clinical features analyzed were age, sex, BMI, waist circumference, blood pressure, and heart rate. All participants provided written informed consent for study participation. The Ethics Committee of the University of São Paulo Medical School approved the study (CAAE:00788012.8.0000.0068).

2.1. Interventions

The CR dietary intervention was a standard diet of 1000 calories from our Department of Nutrition, which corresponded to a reduction of around 50% of the daily caloric intake of the study subjects. A food nutritional control diary was also used to analyze adherence to the proposed diet. Subjects were instructed to write down all ingested food on a day-by-day basis. A daily food record was not used in the RSV group. RSV was administered 500 mg/day (250 mg twice a day) to the RSV study group. The capsules were obtained from a manipulation pharmacy (Buenos Ayres Pharmacy, São Paulo, Brazil).

The purity of the product supplied was analyzed by capillary electrophoresis using the Proteome Lab PA800 from Beckman Coulter (Fullerton, CA, USA) in the Laboratory of Capillary Chromatography and Electrophoresis at the Chemistry Institute of the University of São Paulo. The samples of the manipulated capsules and the standards of RSV were performed in triplicate. The areas under the peak were compared. The purity obtained was $87 \pm 1.1\%$ on average (coefficient of variation 1.2%).

2.2. Laboratory Tests

Laboratory tests were performed with biological samples collected after a 12 h fast. Venous blood samples were collected to obtain serum samples for biochemical analysis and whole blood for RNA extraction. Total cholesterol, triglycerides, HDL-cholesterol, and glucose were obtained by commercial colorimetric-enzymatic methods. LDL cholesterol was calculated using the Friedewald equation. The measurements were performed using the automated equipment Dimension RxL from Siemens Healthcare Diagnostics Inc. (Newark, DE, USA) with dedicated reagents. Insulin was analyzed by a chemi-luminescence assay using automated equipment Immulite 2000 from Siemens Healthcare. HOMA-IR was calculated using insulin and glucose levels. Sirt-1 serum concentration was determined with the ELISA kit from Uscn Life Science, Inc. (Wuhan, Hubei, China). Sirt-1 samples before and after interventions were analyzed in duplicate and in the same ELISA plate (coefficient of variation of 12% according to the manufacturer). esRAGE concentration was determined using the ELISA kit from the B-Bridge International (Santa Clara, CA, USA) using the Multiscan FC plate reader (Thermo Fischer Scientific, Vantaa, Finland). All tests were performed according to the manufacturers' instructions.

2.3. Sirt-1 and RAGE Expression

Gene expression of Sirt-1 (Hs01009005_m1, Applied Biosystems; Foster City, CA, USA), flRAGE (00542592_G1), and esRAGE (HS00542584_G1, Applied Biosystems) [18] were evaluated pre-inclusion and postinclusion, according to the protocol. Total RNA was obtained using the TRIZOL reagent (Life Technologies, Waltham, MA, USA) from whole blood collected into an EDTA tube. cDNA synthesis was made with the Superscript II kit (Life Technologies) using 1ug from total RNA in a final volume of 20-µL reaction, according to the manufacturer's instructions. The housekeeping gene was glyceraldehyde 3-phosphate dehydrogenase (GAPDH) (Hs02758991_g1). The reaction mix was prepared using 5 µL of the Universal Master Mix (Life Technologies), 0.5 µL of primers and probes mix (20×), and 2.5 µL of cDNA diluted samples (1:5). The PCR reaction was performed according to the following protocol: enzymatic activation for 2 min at 50 °C, initial denaturation for 10 min at 95 °C followed by 40 cycles of denaturation for 15 s at 95 °C, and annealing for 20 s at 60 °C. The reactions were run in triplicate and relative expression levels were calculated by normalizing the targets to the endogenously expressed housekeeping GAPDH gene. The results included the ratio between pre-intervention and postintervention values expressed in arbitrary units (AU).

2.4. Statistical Analysis

The sample size of 48 patients with 24 subjects per treatment arm was determined to yield a power of 80% with a 5% significance level to detect a 30% difference in Sirt1 plasma concentrations. Eligible female and male subjects were randomly assigned in a 1:1 ratio with the use of computer-generated random numbers to receive either RSV or CR. Pre-intervention and post-intervention variables were summarized with the use of descriptive statistics. All variables were analyzed descriptively. For the continuous variables, data are expressed as mean $\pm$ standard deviation (SD). Student *t* tests for comparisons between pre-interventions and post-interventions were performed for variables with normal distribution, which was verified by the analysis of the equality of variances (Folded F). Depending on the result of this analysis, the Pooled method (variances with $p \geq 0.05$) or the Satterthwaite method (variances with $p < 0.05$) was used. The Spearman rank correlation method was used for correlations between variables. The level of significance was set at $p < 0.05$. The statistical software used was SAS version 9.3 (SAS Institute, Cary, NC, USA).

3. Results

Clinical features and laboratory data of participants before and after 30 days of intervention (CR and RSV groups) are shown in Table 1. For the RSV group, we observed increased serum concentrations of total cholesterol and non-HDL and HOMA-IR score. The other variables analyzed did not show any statistically significant differences after resveratrol administration. No side effects were reported. For the CR group, we observed that the average caloric intake for the 24 participants was 922.21 ± 27.37 kcal/day. Decreases occurred in weight, abdominal circumference, total cholesterol, HDL, non-HDL, and LDL. Serum concentration of Sirt1 was increased after both interventions, but showed no difference between study groups. The serum levels of esRAGE remained unaltered after interventions and no differences between groups were observed. Gene expression of Sirt1 was increased in both interventions without a difference between RSV and CR groups ($p = 0.64$). The relative expression of RAGE isoforms (post/pre) showed that esRAGE was increased after interventions, and flRAGE remained unchanged after interventions (Figure 1). esRAGE expression was about 57% higher than flRAGE in both groups but was statistically significant only in CR ($p = 0.02$). Positive correlations were observed between Sirt1, esRAGE, and flRAGE gene expressions in both groups. Sirt1 expression correlated with esRAGE expression ($r = 0.86$, $p < 0.0001$) and with flRAGE expression ($r = 0.57$, $p < 0.0001$) in the RSV group. In the CR group, Sirt-1 expression correlated with esRAGE expression ($r = 0.71$, $p < 0.0001$) and with flRAGE expression ($r = 0.57$; $p = 0.0001$). In the CR group, serum concentrations of esRAGE were correlated with esRAGE gene expression ($r = 0.33$, $p = 0.04$) and with Sirt1 gene expression ($r = 0.32$, $p = 0.05$). In the RSV group, serum concentrations of Sirt1 were negatively correlated with flRAGE expression ($r = -0.30$, $p = 0.04$).

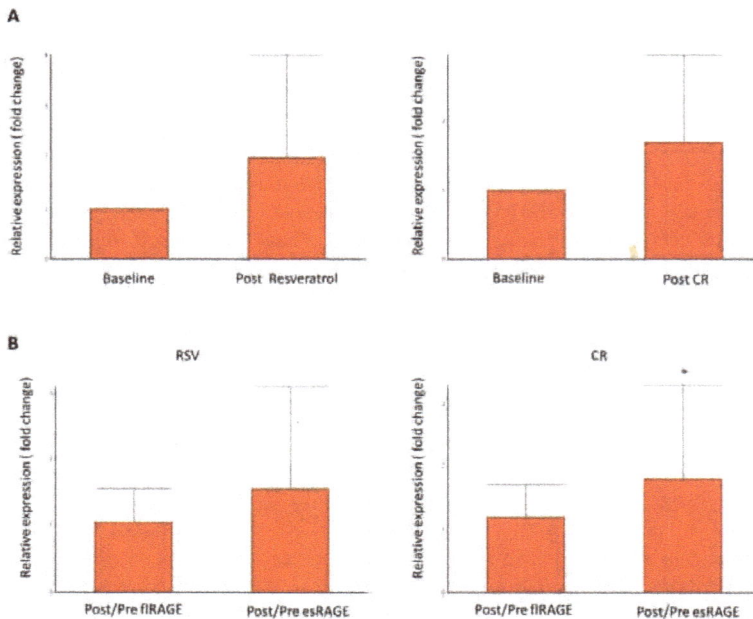

Figure 1. Real-time RT-PCR of Sirt-1 (**A**), esRAGE and flRAGE relation (**B**) after 30 days of caloric restriction or resveratrol intervention. Relative expressions (fold change) of mRNA transcripts were obtained by normalizing GAPDH gene. RSV: resveratrol, CR: caloric restriction. * $p < 0.05$.

Table 1. Clinical and laboratory characteristics of study participants before and after 30 days of resveratrol administration and caloric restriction.

	Resveratrol			Caloric Restriction		
	Baseline $n = 24$	30 days $n = 24$	p	Baseline $n = 24$	30 days $n = 24$	p
Age, years	58.46 ± 3.44			58.63 ± 3.65		
Weight, kg	83.01 ± 21.88	91.14 ± 17.77	0.328	69.13 ± 7.99	64.60 ± 7.30	0.002
Body mass index, kg/m^2	27.61 ± 4.24	27.79 ± 4.38	0.370	25.84 ± 3.22	25.50 ± 3.21	0.083
Waist circumference, cm	96.82 ± 12.08	96.90 ± 11.36	0.457	94.27 ± 7.50	91.82 ± 7.12	0.011
Heart rate, bpm	64.61 ± 8.46	65.65 ± 8.22	0.269	62.50 ± 9.60	62.32 ± 10.51	0.902
Systolic BP, mmHg	131.46 ± 15.48	128.95 ± 15.44	0.660	129.73 ± 15.65	124.23 ± 12.81	0.109
Diastolic BP, mmHg	81.21 ± 10.81	81.95 ± 9.22	0.612	82.86 ± 10.96	79.36 ± 9.92	0.070
Total cholesterol, mmol/L	5.38 ± 0.85	5.64 ± 1.14	0.030	5.60 ± 1.12	5.25 ± 1.01	0.007
HDL-cholesterol, mmol/L	1.27 ± 0.35	1,25 ± 0.35	0.260	1.43 ± 0.47	1.35 ± 0.42	0.008
LDL-cholesterol, mmol/L	3.43 ± 0.68	3.61 ± 1.03	0.089	3.59 ± 0.93	3.37 ± 0.85	0.031
Non-HDL cholesterol mmol/L	4.11 ± 0.77	4.39 ± 1.07	0.010	4.17 ± 1.04	3.90 ± 0.98	0.025
Triglycerides, mmol/L	1.40 ± 0.73	1.68 ± 1.03	0.075	1.26 ± 0.70	1.15 ± 0.67	0.234
Glucose, mmol/L	5.26 ± 0.74	5.41 ± 0.79	0.165	5.20 ± 0.58	5.03 ± 0.32	0.118
Insulin, µUI/mL	7.85 ± 5.57	8.52 ± 5.67	0.066	6.71 ± 4.37	6.13 ± 3.16	0.428
HOMA-IR	1.66 ± 1.55	1.87 ± 1.70	0.038	1.49 ± 1.27	1.25 ± 0.74	0.275
Sirtuin1, ng/mL	1.06 ± 0.71	5.75 ± 2.98	<0.001	1.65 ± 1.81	5.80 ± 2.23	<0.001
esRAGE, pg/mL	255.78 ± 128.87	246.96 ± 115.32	0.800	246.67 ± 111.62	253.33 ± 116.81	0.857

BP: blood pressure, hsCRP: high-sensitivity C-reactive protein, HOMA: homeostatic model assessment, RAGE: endogenous soluble receptor for advanced glycation end products, AU: arbitrary unity.

4. Discussion

In this study, we compared the 30-day effects of RSV supplementation and CR in healthy slightly overweight individuals on Sirt-1 and RAGE isoform expression and serum levels. The important finding of the present study is that both RSV supplementation and CR stimulated Sirt-1 serum concentrations and CR elevated esRAGE mRNA production.

The molecular mechanisms by which CR confers metabolic benefits are not entirely clear, but have been at least partly attributable to the regulation of energy homeostasis by Sirt-1 activation. Sirt-1 is an evolutionary conserved family of deacetylases and ADP-ribosyltransferases that directly regulates glucose and/or fat utilization in metabolically active tissues [19]. Howitz et al. [20] identified RSV as an activator of Sirt-1 and it has been suggested as a CR mimetic in the improvement of metabolic health [21]. Our results show that both interventions could directly induce increases in Sirt-1 expression at transcriptional and translational levels.

A transcriptional increase was also observed for esRAGE isoform after both interventions. RAGE is a multi-ligand receptor member of an immunoglobulin superfamily of cell-surface molecules. RAGE activation may be important for initializing and maintaining the pathological process that results in various diseases [22,23]. esRAGE has been the object of intense clinical research. The generation of soluble receptor isoforms represents an important mechanism to regulate aberrant receptor signaling in biological systems [24]. Soluble forms of RAGE seem to prevent ligands to interact with RAGE or other cell surface receptors [25]. esRAGE has an activity that neutralizes the AGE action and protects vascular cells against the activation of the cell-surface receptors and the AGE harmful positive loop of regulation [23,26]. Kierdorf et al. [27] have proposed that soluble RAGE does not act as a simple competitor but attenuates the activation of flRAGE by disturbing the preassembly of the receptor on the cell surface. Interactions between both RAGE molecules occur via the V and C1 domain, which enables the soluble RAGE to interact with membrane-bound flRAGE. The resulting hetero-multimers does not have competent signaling [27]. Decreased levels of esRAGE and/or increases in flRAGE are thought to enhance RAGE-mediated inflammation [18]. Prediabetic and diabetic patients exhibit lower esRAGE plasma levels and gene expression, which are inversely related to markers of inflammation and atherosclerotic risk [28]. Low levels of esRAGE have also been related to diastolic dysfunction [29]. Therefore, esRAGE could be a potential protective factor against the occurrence of cardiovascular disease. Our results show that esRAGE expression was approximately 57% higher than flRAGE expression after interventions. The relationship between CR or RSV and RAGE was previously demonstrated in experimental studies in which both significantly reduced RAGE mRNA transcripts [30,31]. However, little is known about CR and RSV interactions with esRAGE. In addition, the regulatory mechanism of the alternative splicing of esRAGE remains unknown. Alternative splicing is a regulated process that is mainly influenced by the activities of splicing regulators such as serine/arginine-rich proteins (SR proteins) or heterogeneous nuclear ribonucleoproteins (hnRNPs) [32]. Liu et al. [33] demonstrated the existence of hnRNP A1 in the splicing complex of RAGE and showed its involvement in the regulation of RAGE splicing. Splicing factor expression is known to be deregulated in senescent cells of multiple lineages and is a direct cause of multiple aspects of both aging and age-related disease in mammals [34]. Dietary restriction slows the accumulation of senescent cells [35]. Markus et al. [36] demonstrated that RSV could influence the splicing machinery. RSV had a selective effect on the levels of splicing factors inclusive of hnRNPA1. The increases in esRAGE expression may suggest a role for CR and RSV in the control of deleterious effects of the RAGE cascade. This increase of esRAGE stimulated by interventions may be supported by the positive correlation between esRAGE serum concentrations and Sirt-1 mRNA expression in CR and negative correlation of Sirt-1 serum levels and flRAGE gene expression in the RSV group. Serum levels of esRAGE remained unchanged, which may be due to the short follow-up time of 30 days. Despite the increase in gene expression, the steady-state protein levels in cells depend on the balance between their production and degradation. Protein ubiquitination is the central cellular process that directs protein degradation. Evankovich et al. identified that ubiquitin E3 ligase subunit F-box protein O10 (FBOX10), which mediates RAGE ubiquitination and degradation [37]. Possibly longer exposure to interventions could reverse the potential effect of ubiquitination on esRAGE proteins and increase serum levels of esRAGE.

Drugs like statins [38], methotrexate [39], metformin [40], and thiazolidinedione [41] were shown to increase soluble forms of RAGE. However, little is known about esRAGE alternative splicing induction by drugs and also about the increase of esRAGE in normal subjects. The elucidation of regulatory mechanisms of esRAGE is important from a clinical viewpoint and would provide a molecular basis for the development of drugs that can induce esRAGE and suppress cytotoxic effects of flRAGE.

The current study has some limitations, which include the small number of participants and the short follow-up period. However, in the literature, the studies citing esRAGE were obtained in patients with chronic degenerative disease.

This study was the first one in healthy or slightly overweight subjects that showed an increase in esRAGE expression after CR and RSV interventions. Long-term randomized trials are needed to evaluate the possible clinical benefits of increased esRAGE expression in cardiovascular disease prevention.

In conclusion, this study shows that CR and RSV could effectively stimulate the increase in esRAGE expression in healthy subjects.

Author Contributions: Conceptualization: A.R., C.M.C.S. and A.d.P.M. Methodology: A.R., C.M.C.S. and A.d.P.M. Validation: A.R., C.M.C.S. and A.d.P.M. Formal Analysis: A.R., C.M.C.S., A.d.P.M., D.P.L. and J.Y.T. Investigation: A.P.P. Writing—Original Draft Preparation: A.R., C.M.C.S. and A.d.P.M. Writing—Review & Editing: A.R., C.M.C.S., A.d.P.M., S.D.A., J.Y.T., D.P.L. and A.P.P.

Funding: This research was funded by Fundação de Amparo à Pesquisa do Estado de São Paulo, grant number: FAPESP-2012/01051-5.

Acknowledgments: We thank the staff of the Clinic Laboratory of the Instituto do Coração, Hospital das Clínicas—HCFMUSP.

Conflicts of Interest: The authors declare no conflict of interest.

References

1. Haigis, M.C.; Sinclair, D.A. Mammalian sirtuins: Biological insights and disease relevance. *Annu. Rev. Pathol.* **2010**, *5*, 253–295. [CrossRef] [PubMed]
2. Ristow, M.; Zarse, K. How increased oxidative stress promotes longevity and metabolic health: The concept of mitochondrial hormesis (mitohormesis). *Exp. Gerontol.* **2010**, *45*, 410–418. [CrossRef] [PubMed]
3. Nisoli, E.; Tonello, C.; Cardile, A.; Cozzi, V.; Bracale, R.; Tedesco, L.; Falcone, S.; Valerio, A.; Cantoni, O.; Clementi, E.; et al. Calorie restriction promotes mitochondrial biogenesis by inducing the expression of eNOS. *Science* **2005**, *310*, 314–317. [CrossRef] [PubMed]
4. Nemoto, S.; Fergusson, M.M.; Finkel, T. Nutrient availability regulates SIRT1 through a fork head dependent pathway. *Science* **2004**, *306*, 2105–2108. [CrossRef] [PubMed]
5. Lagouge, M.; Argmann, C.; Gerhart-Hines, Z.; Meziane, H.; Lerin, C.; Daussin, F.; Messadeq, N.; Milne, J.; Lambert, P.; Elliott, P.; et al. Resveratrol improves mitochondrial function and protects against metabolic disease by activating SIRT1 and PGC-1α. *Cell* **2006**, *127*, 1109–1122. [CrossRef] [PubMed]
6. Mariani, S.; Fiore, D.; Persichetti, A.; Basciani, S.; Lubrano, C.; Poggiogalle, E.; Genco, A.; Donini, L.M.; Gnessi, L. Circulating SIRT1 Increases After Intragastric Balloon Fat Loss in Obese Patients. *Obes. Surg.* **2016**, *26*, 1215–1220. [CrossRef] [PubMed]
7. Mansur, A.P.; Roggerio, A.; Goes, M.F.; Avakian, S.D.; Leal, D.P.; Maranhão, R.C.; Strunz, C.M. Serum concentrations and gene expression of sirtuin 1 in healthy and slightly overweight subjects after caloric restriction or resveratrol supplementation: A randomized trial. *Int. J. Cardiol.* **2017**, *15*, 788–794. [CrossRef] [PubMed]
8. Kitada, M.; Kume, S.; Takeda-Watanabe, A.; Tsuda, S.; Kanasaki, K.; Koya, D. Calorie restriction in overweight males ameliorates obesity-related metabolic alterations and cellular adaptations through anti-aging effects, possibly including AMPK and SIRT1 activation. *Biochim. Biophys. Acta* **2013**, *1830*, 4820–4827. [CrossRef] [PubMed]
9. Ota, H.; Akishita, M.; Eto, M.; Iijima, K.; Kaneki, M.; Ouchi, Y. Sirt1 modulates premature senescence-like phenotype in human endothelial cells. *J. Mol. Cell. Cardiol.* **2007**, *43*, 571–579. [CrossRef] [PubMed]
10. Brett, J.; Schmidt, A.M.; Yan, S.D.; Zou, Y.S.; Weidman, E.; Pinsky, D.; Nowygrod, R.; Neeper, M.; Przysiecki, C.; Shaw, A.; et al. Survey of the distribution of a newly characterized receptor for advanced glycation end products in tissues. *Am. J. Pathol.* **1993**, *143*, 1699–1712. [PubMed]
11. Vlassara, H.; Cai, W.; Crandall, J.; Goldberg, T.; Oberstein, R.; Dardaine, V.; Peppa, M.; Rayfield, E.J. Inflammatory mediators are induced by dietary glycotoxins, a major risk factor for diabetic angiopathy. *Proc. Natl. Acad. Sci. USA* **2002**, *99*, 15596–15601. [CrossRef] [PubMed]
12. Uribarri, J.; Woodruff, S.; Goodman, S.; Cai, W.; Chen, X.; Pyzik, R.; Yong, A.; Striker, G.E.; Vlassara, H. Advanced glycation end products in foods and a practical guide to their reduction in the diet. *J. Am. Diet. Assoc.* **2010**, *110*, 911–916. [CrossRef] [PubMed]
13. Schmidt, A.M.; Yan, S.D.; Wautier, J.L.; Stern, D. Activation of receptor for advanced glycation end products: A mechanism for chronic vascular dysfunction in diabetic vasculopathy and atherosclerosis. *Circ. Res.* **1999**, *84*, 489–497. [CrossRef] [PubMed]
14. De Kreutzenberg, S.V.; Ceolotto, G.; Papparella, I.; Bortoluzzi, A.; Semplicini, A.; Dalla Man, C.; Cobelli, C.; Fadini, G.P.; Avogaro, A. Downregulation of the longevity-associated protein SIRT1 in insulin resistance and metabolic syndrome. Potential biochemical mechanisms. *Diabetes* **2010**, *59*, 1006–1015. [CrossRef] [PubMed]
15. Hudson, B.I.; Carter, A.M.; Harja, E.; Kalea, A.Z.; Arriero, M.; Yang, H.; Grant, P.J.; Schmidt, A.M. Identification, classification, and expression of RAGE gene splice variants. *FASEB J. Off. Publ. Fed. Am. Soc. Exp. Biol.* **2008**, *22*, 1572–1580. [CrossRef] [PubMed]
16. Falcone, C.; Emanuele, E.; D'Angelo, A.; Buzzi, M.P.; Belvito, C.; Cuccia, M.; Geroldi, D. Plasma levels of soluble receptor for advanced glycation end products and coronary artery disease in non-diabetic men. *Arterioscler. Thromb. Vasc. Biol.* **2005**, *25*, 1032–1037. [CrossRef] [PubMed]
17. Selvin, E.; Halushka, M.K.; Rawlings, A.M.; Hoogeveen, R.C.; Ballantyne, C.M.; Coresh, J.; Astor, B.C. sRAGE and risk of diabetes, cardiovascular disease, and death. *Diabetes* **2013**, *62*, 2116–2121. [CrossRef] [PubMed]
18. Mulrennan, S.; Baltic, S.; Aggarwal, S.; Wood, J.; Miranda, A.; Frost, F.; Kaye, J.; Thompson, P.J. The role of receptor for advanced glycation end products in airway inflammation in CF and CF related diabetes. *Sci. Rep.* **2015**, *10*, 8931. [CrossRef] [PubMed]

19. Lan, Y.Y.; Peterson, C.M.; Ravussin, E. Resveratrol vs. calorie restriction: Data from rodents to humans. *Exp. Gerontol.* **2013**, *48*, 1018–1024. [CrossRef]
20. Howitz, K.T.; Bitterman, K.J.; Cohen, H.Y.; Lamming, D.W.; Lavu, S.; Wood, J.G.; Zipkin, R.E.; Chung, P.; Kisielewski, A.; Zhang, L.L.; et al. Small molecule activators of sirtuins extend *Saccharomyces cerevisiae* lifespan. *Nature* **2003**, *425*, 191–196. [CrossRef] [PubMed]
21. Barger, J.L. An adipocentric perspective of resveratrol as a calorie restriction mimetic. *Ann. N. Y. Acad. Sci.* **2013**, *1290*, 122–129. [CrossRef] [PubMed]
22. Park, S.; Yoon, S.J.; Tae, H.J.; Shin, C.Y. RAGE and cardiovascular disease. *Front. Biosci.* **2001**, *16*, 486–497.
23. Basta, G. Receptor of advanced glycation end products and atherosclerosis: From basis mechanisms to clinal implications. *Atherosclerosis* **2008**, *196*, 9–21. [CrossRef] [PubMed]
24. Kalea, A.Z.; See, F.; Harja, E.; Arriero, M.; Schmidt, A.M.; Hudson, B.I. Alternatively spliced RAGEv1 inhibits tumorigenesis through suppression of JNK signaling. *Cancer Res.* **2010**, *70*, 5628–5638. [CrossRef] [PubMed]
25. Bierhaus, A.; Humpert, P.M.; Morcos, M.; Wendt, T.; Chavakis, T.; Arnold, B.; Stern, D.M.; Nawroth, P.P. Understanding RAGE, the receptor for advanced glycation end products. *J. Mol. Med.* **2005**, *83*, 876–886. [CrossRef] [PubMed]
26. Yonekura, H.; Yamamoto, Y.; Sakurai, S.; Petrova, R.G.; Abedin, M.J.; Li, H.; Yasui, K.; Takeuchi, M.; Makita, Z.; Takasawa, S.; et al. Novel splice variants of the receptor for advanced glycation end-products expressed in human vascular endothelial cells and pericytes, and their putative roles in diabetes-induced vascular injury. *Biochem. J.* **2003**, *15*, 1097–1109. [CrossRef] [PubMed]
27. Kierdof, K.; Fritz, G. RAGE regulation and signaling in inflammation and beyond. *J. Leukoc. Biol.* **2013**, *94*, 55–68. [CrossRef] [PubMed]
28. Di Pino, A.; Urbano, F.; Zagami, R.M.; Filippello, A.; Di Mauro, S.; Piro, S.; Purrello, F.; Rabuazzo, A.M. Low endogenous secretory receptor for advanced glycation end-products levels are associated with inflammation and carotid atherosclerosis in prediabetes. *J. Clin. Endocrinol. Metab.* **2016**, *101*, 1701–1709. [CrossRef] [PubMed]
29. Di Pino, A.; Mangiafico, S.; Urbano, F.; Scicali, R.; Scandura, S.; D'Agate, V.; Piro, S.; Tamburino, C.; Purrello, F.; Rabuazzo, A.M. HbA1c Identifies Subjects with Prediabetes and Subclinical Left Ventricular Diastolic Dysfunction. *J. Clin. Endocrinol. Metab.* **2017**, *102*, 3756–3764. [CrossRef] [PubMed]
30. Aris, J.P.; Elios, M.C.; Bimstein, E.; Wallet, S.M.; Cha, S.; Lakshmyya, K.N.; Katz, J. Gingival RAGE expression in calorie-restricted versus ad libitum-fed rats. *J. Periodontol.* **2010**, *81*, 1481–1487. [CrossRef] [PubMed]
31. Moridi, H.; Karimi, J.; Sheikh, N.; Goodarzi, M.T.; Saidijam, M.; Yadegarazari, R.; Khazaei, M.; Khodadadi, I.; Tavilani, H.; Piri, H.; et al. Resveratrol-dependent down-regulation of receptor for advanced glycation end-products and oxidative stress in kidney of rats with diabetes. *Int. J. Endocrinol. Metab.* **2015**, *13*, e23542. [CrossRef] [PubMed]
32. Busch, A.; Hertel, K.J. Evolution of SR protein and hnRNP splicing regulatory factors. *Wiley Interdiscip. Rev. RNA* **2012**, *3*, 1–12. [CrossRef] [PubMed]
33. Liu, X.Y.; Li, H.L.; Su, J.B.; Ding, F.H.; Zhao, J.J.; Chai, F.; Li, Y.X.; Cui, S.C.; Sun, F.Y.; Wu, Z.Y.; et al. Regulation of RAGE splicing by hnRNP A1 and Tra2β-1 and its potential role in AD pathogenesis. *J. Neurochem.* **2015**, *133*, 187–198. [CrossRef] [PubMed]
34. Holly, A.C.; Melzer, D.; Pilling, L.C.; Fellows, A.C.; Tanaka, T.; Ferrucci, L.; Harries, L.W. Changes in splicing factor expression are associated with advancing age in man. *Mech. Ageing Dev.* **2013**, *134*, 356–366. [CrossRef] [PubMed]
35. Baker, D.J.; Childs, B.G.; Durik, M.; Wijers, M.E.; Sieben, C.J.; Zhong, J.; Saltness, R.A.; Jeganathan, K.B.; Verzosa, G.C.; Pezeshki, A.; et al. Naturally occurring p16(Ink4a)-positive cells shorten healthy lifespan. *Nature* **2016**, *530*, 184–189. [CrossRef] [PubMed]
36. Markus, M.A.; Marques, F.Z.; Morris, B.J. Resveratrol, by modulating RNA processing factor levels, can influence the alternative splicing of pre-mRNAs. *PLoS ONE* **2011**, *6*, e28926. [CrossRef] [PubMed]
37. Evankovich, J.; Lear, T.; Mckelvey, A.; Dunn, S.; Londino, J.; Liu, Y.; Chen, B.B.; Mallampalli, R.K. Receptor for advanced glycation end products is targeted by FBXO10 for ubiquitination and degradation. *FASEB J.* **2017**, *31*, 3894–3903. [CrossRef] [PubMed]
38. Quade-Lyssy, P.; Kanarek, A.M.; Baiersdörfer, M.; Postina, R.; Kojro, E. Statins stimulate the production of a soluble form of the receptor for advanced glycation end products. *J. Lipid Res.* **2013**, *54*, 3052–3061. [CrossRef] [PubMed]

39. Pullerits, R.; Bokarewa, M.; Dahlberg, L.; Tarkowski, A. Decreased levels of soluble receptor for advanced glycation end products in patients with rheumatoid arthritis indicating deficient inflammatory control. *Arthritis Res. Ther.* **2005**, *7*, R817–R824. [CrossRef] [PubMed]
40. Haddad, M.; Knani, I.; Bouzidi, H.; Berriche, O.; Hammami, M.; Kerkeni, M. Plasma Levels of Pentosidine, Carboxymethyl-Lysine, Soluble Receptor for Advanced Glycation End Products, and Metabolic Syndrome: The Metformin Effect. *Dis. Markers* **2016**, *2016*, 6248264. [CrossRef] [PubMed]
41. Koyama, H.; Tanaka, S.; Monden, M.; Shoji, T.; Morioka, T.; Fukumoto, S.; Mori, K.; Emoto, M.; Shoji, T.; Fukui, M.; et al. Comparison of effects of pioglitazone and glimepiride on plasma soluble RAGE and RAGE expression in peripheral mononuclear cells in type 2 diabetes: Randomized controlled trial (PioRAGE). *Atherosclerosis* **2014**, *234*, 329–334. [CrossRef] [PubMed]

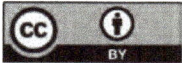

nutrients

MDPI

Article

Induction of p53 Phosphorylation at Serine 20 by Resveratrol Is Required to Activate p53 Target Genes, Restoring Apoptosis in MCF-7 Cells Resistant to Cisplatin

Jorge Hernandez-Valencia [1], Enrique Garcia-Villa [1], Aquetzalli Arenas-Hernandez [1], Jaime Garcia-Mena [1], Jose Diaz-Chavez [2,*] and Patricio Gariglio [1,*]

[1] Departamento de Genética y Biología Molecular, Centro de Investigación y de Estudios Avanzados (CINVESTAV-IPN), Av. IPN No. 2508, Gustavo A. Madero, Ciudad de México 07360, Mexico; jhernandezv@cinvestav.mx (J.H.-V.); liebre1963@yahoo.com (E.G.-V.); aquetzalliarenas@gmail.com (A.A.-H.); jgmena@cinvestav.mx (J.G.-M.)
[2] Unidad de Investigación Biomédica en Cáncer, Instituto de Investigaciones Biomédicas, UNAM/Instituto Nacional de Cancerología, Av. San Fernando No. 22, Sección XVI, Tlalpan, Ciudad de México 14080, Mexico
* Correspondence: jdiazchavez03@gmail.com (J.D.-C.); vidal@cinvestav.mx (P.G.); Tel.: +52-5628-0400 (ext. 62005) (J.D.-C.); +52-555-747-3337 (P.G.); Fax: +52-555-061-3931 (P.G.)

Received: 28 July 2018; Accepted: 20 August 2018; Published: 23 August 2018

Abstract: Resistance to cisplatin (CDDP) is a major cause of cancer treatment failure, including human breast cancer. The tumor suppressor protein p53 is a key factor in the induction of cell cycle arrest, DNA repair, and apoptosis in response to cellular stimuli. This protein is phosphorylated in serine 15 and serine 20 during DNA damage repair or in serine 46 to induce apoptosis. Resveratrol (Resv) is a natural compound representing a promising chemosensitizer for cancer treatment that has been shown to sensitize tumor cells through upregulation and phosphorylation of p53 and inhibition of RAD51. We developed a CDDP-resistant MCF-7 cell line variant (MCF-7$_R$) to investigate the effect of Resv in vitro in combination with CDDP over the role of p53 in overcoming CDDP resistance in MCF-7$_R$ cells. We have shown that Resv induces sensitivity to CDDP in MCF-7 and MCF-7$_R$ cells and that the downregulation of p53 protein expression and inhibition of p53 protein activity enhances resistance to CDDP in both cell lines. On the other hand, we found that Resv induces serine 20 (S20) phosphorylation in chemoresistant cells to activate p53 target genes such as *PUMA* and *BAX*, restoring apoptosis. It also changed the ratio between BCL-2 and BAX, where BCL-2 protein expression was decreased and at the same time BAX protein was increased. Interestingly, Resv attenuates CDDP-induced p53 phosphorylation in serine 15 (S15) and serine 46 (S46) probably through dephosphorylation and deactivation of ATM. It also activates different kinases, such as CK1, CHK2, and AMPK to induce phosphorylation of p53 in S20, suggesting a novel mechanism of p53 activation and chemosensitization to CDDP.

Keywords: breast cancer; cisplatin; p53; phosphorylation; resistance; resveratrol

1. Introduction

Cisplatin (CDDP) is an anticancer drug for the treatment of various types of cancer including human breast cancer. CDDP mediates its anticancer effect by inhibition of DNA synthesis or by saturation of the cellular capacity to repair platinum adducts of DNA. However, resistance to CDDP is a major cause of treatment failure, and the molecular mechanisms are poorly understood [1].

Due to this phenomenon, it is necessary to continue the search for effective chemosensitizers for cancer treatment. One promising possibility is the use of natural compounds like resveratrol

(Resv), which is a phytoalexin present in extracts of more than 70 plant species with a broad spectrum of beneficial health effects including anticancer functions. The reported anticancer activities of Resv are mediated through the modulation of several cell signaling molecules that regulate cell cycle progression, proliferation, apoptosis, invasion, metastasis, and angiogenesis of tumor cells. Although not fully understood, most of the activities of Resv are due to the presence of a phenol and m-hydroquinone moieties, especially the 4-hydroxyl group of the phenol ring which has been attributed with scavenging of free radicals, inhibition of proliferation, and genotoxic activity [2–5]. Resv can sensitize resistant cells to chemotherapeutic agents, including CDDP, by overcoming one or more mechanisms of chemoresistance [6,7]. Evidence suggests that the downregulation of the wild-type p53 tumor suppressor protein enhanced tumor cell survival, conferring a mechanism of chemoresistance [8]. However, in a few cases, Resv has been shown to sensitize tumor cells to chemotherapeutic agents through p53 dependent [9,10] or p53 independent pathways [11,12].

p53 is a key transcriptional factor in the induction of cycle arrest, DNA repair, and apoptosis in response to cellular stimuli. Promoter preference of target genes is determined by modification status of the p53 protein since it has two critical roles in the decision of cell fate, stopping the cell cycle to repair damaged DNA or the causing induction of apoptotic cell death [13]. Once cells are exposed to genotoxic agents, p53 is phosphorylated at the N-terminal transactivation domain by several kinases, resulting in an increment of expression. Serine 15 (S15) is phosphorylated by ATM at an earlier inductive phase (<24 h), followed by ATR at a later steady-state phase (>24 h) [14,15], and serine 20 (S20) is phosphorylated by CHK1/2. Both phosphorylations enable p53 to escape from MDM2-mediated ubiquitination and degradation. Stabilized p53 transactivates its target genes promoting cell cycle arrest (e.g., *P21*) followed by DNA repair. Under severe DNA damage (>24 h), serine 46 (S46) is also sequentially phosphorylated to maintain the level of S46 phosphorylation by ATM [15], and other kinases such as HIPK2 in response to UV irradiation [16], and DYRK2 in response to adriamycin and UV irradiation [13]. The phosphorylation of S46 is necessary to induce p53-mediated apoptosis-related genes such as *PUMA, NOXA, BAX*, and *PIG3* [17–19] and transcriptional repression of genes such as *BCL-2* [8].

It has been described that MCF-7 breast cancer cells have a surface integrin ($\alpha V\beta 3$) that works as a receptor for Resv. This receptor is linked to induction of ERK1/2 and phosphorylation of p53 in S15 and S20 by Resv leading to apoptosis [20,21]. Moreover, we previously reported that treatment of MCF-7 cells with Resv induces the downregulation of several genes related to mismatch repair, DNA replication, and homologous recombination, decreasing protein levels of the MRN complex (MRE11-NBS1-RAD50) which is part of the homologous recombination DNA repair pathway [22]. Indeed, we found that downregulation of RAD51 sensitizes MCF-7 cells to CDDP treatment [23]. However, it is of maximal importance to understand the molecular mechanisms by which Resv overcome chemoresistance in cancer cells, alone or in combination with chemotherapeutic agents (e.g., CDDP), to enhance treatment efficacy and reduce toxicity.

Considering the previously reported anticancer function of Resv and its chemosensitizer capacity as well as phosphorylation of p53 induced by Resv, in this work we developed a CDDP-resistant MCF-7 cell line variant (MCF-7$_R$) and investigated the effect of Resv in vitro in combination with CDDP in MCF-7 and MCF-7$_R$ cells, the role of p53 in CDDP resistance, the involvement of Resv in p53 phosphorylation, and the role of the p53 pathway for overcoming resistance in MCF-7$_R$ cells.

2. Materials and Methods

2.1. Reagents and Antibodies

Cisplatin (CDDP), resveratrol (Resv), 3-(4,5-dimethylthiazol-2-yl)-2,5-diphenyltetrazolium bromide (MTT), pifithrin-α, VP-16 and monoclonal anti-β-actin-HRP were purchased from Sigma-Aldrich (St. Louis, MO, USA). The AMPK inhibitor Compound C (or dorsomorphin), the CK1 inhibitor D4476, the Chk2 inhibitor, anti-rabbit and anti-mouse secondary antibodies, mouse monoclonal anti-phospho-ATM (S1981), rabbit polyclonal anti-ATM, monoclonal anti-p53-HRP (DO-1), and monoclonal anti-BCL-2 were purchased from Santa Cruz Biotechnology (San Diego, CA, USA). Rabbit monoclonal anti-BAX-HRP was purchased from Abcam (Cambridge, UK). Rabbit polyclonal anti-phospho-p53 (S15, S20 and S46) were from Cell Signaling Technology (Beverly, CA, USA).

2.2. Cell Lines and Cell Culture

The MCF-7 human breast cancer cells (ATCC) and MCF-7$_R$ cells were cultured in Dulbecco's modified Eagle's medium (DMEM) supplemented with 10% (*v/v*) fetal bovine serum, penicillin (100 U/mL), streptomycin (100 µg/mL), and amphotericin B (0.25 µ/mL) in a 5% CO_2 incubator at 37 °C. Additionally, MCF-7$_R$ cells were continuously cultured with 5.5 µM of CDDP. Resv and CDDP stock solutions were prepared at a concentration of 80 mM in absolute ethanol and DMSO, respectively. Both compounds were diluted in culture medium at the final concentration indicated in each experiment.

2.3. Generation of the CDDP-Resistant MCF-7 Cell Line Variant (MCF-7$_R$)

The MCF-7 human breast cancer cells were cultured with an initial treatment of 2 µM of CDDP and maintained at this concentration for 45 days until the monolayer density of the surviving cells was ~85%. Cells were harvested and plated 24 h before the second treatment with 4 µM of CDDP. After 33 days under treatment the surviving cells' monolayer density reached ~85%. Finally, cells were harvested and plated 24 h before the third treatment with 6 µM of CDDP. After 13 days under treatment the surviving cells monolayer density was ~85%. At concentrations >6.5 µM of CDDP the cells died or formed clusters that prevented the formation of a cell monolayer. To create a MCF-7$_R$ cell bank, cells were seeded at a density of 2×10^5 cells/dish in p100 cell culture dishes and were continuously cultured with 5.5 µM of CDDP until the cell monolayer density was ~85%. Cells were frozen at a density of 2×10^6 cells/cryovial and stored in liquid nitrogen. At the same time, the parental cell line was grown, so that the passages necessary to create the resistant cell line variant were equal for both cell lines.

2.4. Silencing of p53 Expression in MCF-7 and MCF-7$_R$ Cells by shRNA

The SureSilencing shRNA Plasmid Kit (SABiosciences Qiagen, Frederick, MD, USA) was used to create stable MCF-7 and MCF-7$_R$ cell lines with a down-regulated expression of p53 (MCF-7 p53-shRNA and MCF-7$_R$ p53-shRNA). Control cells received a non-effective scrambled sequence (MCF-7 Ctrl-shRNA and MCF-7$_R$ Ctrl-shRNA). Lipofectamine 2000 (Invitrogen, Gaithersburg, MD, USA) was used for transfections according to the manufacturer's protocol. Additionally, for obtaining stable clones, cells were selected post transfection using Geneticin (G418, Thermo Fisher Scientific, Somerset, NJ, USA). Cell clones were expanded, and p53 contents were tested by Western blot.

2.5. Cell Viability Assay

Cells were plated at a density of 2×10^5 cells/dish in p60 cell culture dishes 24 h before the assay. Cells were treated with different concentrations of CDDP (5, 10, 20, 30, 40 and 50 µM) with or without Resv (100 µM) for 48h. At the end of the treatment period, the cells were incubated with MTT (0.5 mg/mL) for 30 min. The medium was removed and the synthesized formazan dye crystals were solubilized with 500 µL of acid isopropanol, and absorbance was measured at a 570-nm wavelength (Tecan's Sunrise absorbance microplate reader, Tecan Group Ltd., Männedorf, Switzerland). The growth percentage was calculated using the number of control cells with vehicle as 100% at 48 h.

2.6. Western Blot

Cells were seeded at a density of 2×10^5 cells/dish in p60 cell culture dishes 24 h before the treatment. After the corresponding treatment, cells were lysed with RIPA lysis buffer (150 mM NaCl, 0.5% sodium deoxycholate, 0.1% SDS, 50 mM Tris, pH 7.4), $1 \times$ Complete Mini Protease Inhibitor Cocktail (Roche Diagnostics, Branchburg, NJ, USA) and $1 \times$ Phosphatase Inhibitor Cocktail C (Santa Cruz Biotechnology, Dallas, TX, USA). The cell suspension was sonicated and the supernatants were collected by centrifugation. Briefly, equal amount protein was resolved on a SDS-10% (w/v) polyacrylamide gel (for ATM and BCL-2 proteins values were 6% and 16% w/v, respectively). Proteins were transferred to a nitrocellulose membrane (GE Healthcare, Madison, WI, USA). Membranes were blocked (room temperature, 1 h) with Tween 20 (0.05%, v/v; TBS-Tween 20) containing bovine serum albumin (5%; w/v), then incubated overnight at 4 °C with the corresponding primary antibodies, followed by 1 h incubation with secondary antibodies conjugated to horse radish peroxidase (HRP). Protein was detected by Super Signal West Pico Chemiluminescent Substrate (Thermo Fisher Scientific, Somerset, NJ, USA). Signal intensity was determined densitometrically using Image Lab software, version 5.1 from Bio-Rad Laboratories (Hercules, CA, USA). All quantified Western blot data were corrected for loading using the anti-α-actin blots. Western blot figures are representative of at least three independent experiments.

2.7. Real-Time RT-PCR

Cells were plated at a density of 2×10^5 cells/dish in p60 cell culture dishes 24 h before the treatment. After the corresponding treatment, total RNA was isolated using TRIzol reagent (Invitrogen Life Technologies) as described elsewhere. Integrity of RNA was determined by agarose gel analysis and quantified using a NanoDrop instrument (Thermo Scientific NanoDrop One/One, Waltham, MA, USA). Reverse transcription of total RNA was performed using the First Strand cDNA Synthesis Kit (Thermo Fisher Scientific, Somerset, NJ, USA). Real-time RT-PCR was performed using SYBR Green master mix (Thermo Fisher Scientific, Somerset, NJ, USA) in a 7300 Real Time PCR System instrument (Applied Biosystems, Foster City, CA, USA). The specificity of each PCR was examined by the melting temperature profiles of the final products. Reactions were conducted in triplicate, and relative amounts of gene were normalized to Beta-2 microglobulin (B2M). The relative gene expression data were analyzed by the comparative CT method ($2^{-\Delta\Delta CT}$ method). Primers: *P21*, *PUMA*, *NOXA*, *BAX*, *PIG3*, and *B2M* were purchased from Integrated DNA Technologies (IDT, Skokie, IL, USA) and forward and reverse sequences are presented in Table S1.

2.8. Apoptosis Analysis

Cells were plated at a density of 2×10^5 cells/dish in p60 cell culture dishes 24 h before the treatment. After treatment, apoptosis analysis was performed using the Alexa Fluor 488 AnnexinV/Dead Cell Apoptosis Kit (Invitrogen V13245). Briefly, the cells were harvested, washed with cold PBS, and resuspended in 100 µL of Annexin binding buffer (ABB). Cells then were centrifuged and resuspended again in ABB supplemented with Alexa Fluor 488 Annexin V and 1 µg/mL of propidium iodide (PI). Cells then were incubated at room temperature for 15 min and finally, resuspended in 400 µL of ABB. Cells were analyzed by flow cytometry at 530 nm and 575 nm in a FACSCalibur instrument. Data analysis was performed on 20,000 events with the Summit Software Version 4.3. (Beckman Coulter Inc., Fullerton, CA, USA).

2.9. Statistical Analysis

Results are expressed as the mean $\pm$ SD of at least three independent experiments. The IC$_{50}$ values for CDDP were calculated by nonlinear regression (curve fit) by log[CDDP] vs. normalized response–variable slope. Statistical analysis was carried out by one-way ANOVA followed by Dunnett's Multiple Comparison test (compare the mean of each column with the mean of a control column) or Turkey's Multiple Comparison test (compare the mean of each column with the mean of every other column). All statistical analysis was carried out using PRISM Software (Version 6.0; GraphPad, San Diego, CA, USA). *p* values $p < 0.05$, 0.01 and 0.001 were considered to be significant.

3. Results

3.1. Resv Induces Sensitivity to CDDP in MCF-7$_R$ Cells

To determine the effect of Resv in inducing chemosensitivity to MCF-7 and the CDDP-resistant cell line variant (MCF-7$_R$); both cells were treated with different CDDP concentrations (5, 10, 20, 30, 40, 50 μM) with or without Resv (100 μM) for 48 h. As shown in Figure 1, we found that the IC$_{50}$ of CDDP was decreased by Resv in both cell lines; in MCF-7 cells the IC$_{50}$ for CDDP was reduced by ~38-fold, from 4.95 μM to 0.13 μM. On the other hand, in MCF-7$_R$ cells the IC$_{50}$ of CDDP was decreased by ~53-fold, from 9.57 μM to 0.18 μM. These results suggest that Resv significantly reduced the concentration necessary of CDDP to reach the IC$_{50}$ in both MCF-7 and MCF-7$_R$ cells and increases the sensibility to CDDP.

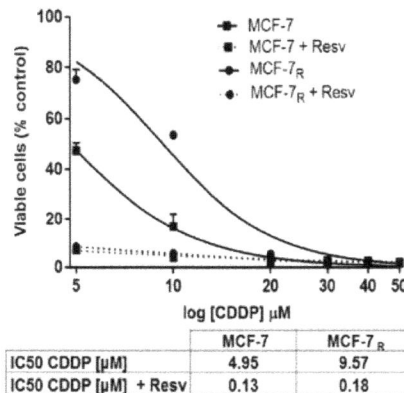

	MCF-7	MCF-7$_R$
IC50 CDDP [μM]	4.95	9.57
IC50 CDDP [μM] + Resv	0.13	0.18

Figure 1. Resveratrol (Resv) induces sensitivity to cisplatin (CDDP) in MCF-7$_R$ cells. MCF-7 and MCF-7$_R$ cells were treated with different concentrations of CDDP (5, 10, 20, 30, 40, and 50 μM) with or without Resv (100 μM) for 48 h. Cell viability was tested by 3-(4,5-dimethylthiazol-2-yl)-2,5-diphenyltetrazolium bromide (MTT) assay. Each data point is the mean of four independent experiments ± SD. The IC$_{50}$ values for CDDP were calculated and shown in the box.

3.2. Down-Regulation of p53 Expression and Inhibition of the p53 Protein Activity Enhances Resistance to CDDP and Resv in MCF-7 and MCF-7$_R$ Cells

To evaluate the role of p53 in CDDP resistance, MCF-7 and MCF-7$_R$ cells were transfected with shRNA targeting p53 (p53-shRNA) or control (Ctrl-shRNA). Stably transfected cells were treated with CDDP (6 μM; 48 h) to stimulate p53 expression. In the presence of p53-shRNA, p53 induction in CDDP treated MCF-7$_R$ cells decreased to 40.5% ± 2.3%, when compared to control transfected MCF-7$_R$ cells (Supplementary Figure S1A,B, lane 3, *** $p < 0.001$), and the inhibition of p53 induction was higher for MCF-7 p53-shRNA cells (19.7% ± 1.18%), compared to control transfected MCF-7 cells (Supplementary Figure S1A,B lane 5, *** $p < 0.001$).

To analyze the effect of p53 down-regulation on CDDP and CDDP + Resv treatments, MCF-7 and MCF-7$_R$ cells containing p53-shRNA were treated for 48 h with different CDDP concentrations (5, 10, 20, 30, 40, 50 μM) with or without Resv (100 μM). We found an increase in the IC$_{50}$ of CDDP in both treatments and in both cell lines. For MCF-7 p53-shRNA the IC$_{50}$ = 13.45 μM (CDDP) increased ~3-fold; and IC$_{50}$ = 0.92 μM (CDDP + Resv) increased ~7-fold, compared with non-transfected MCF-7 cells

(Figure 2A,C). On the other hand, in MCF-7$_R$ p53-shRNA the IC$_{50}$ = 12.38 μM (CDDP) increased ~1.3-fold; while IC$_{50}$ = 5.58 μM (CDDP + Resv) increased ~31-fold, compared with non-transfected MCF-7$_R$ cells (Figure 2A,C). Interestingly, the increase of IC$_{50}$ for both cell lines was more significant when the CDDP + Resv treatment was used, suggesting that p53 expression plays a more important role in this treatment. Unexpectedly, we found a decrease in the IC$_{50}$ for CDDP of the MCF-7 Ctrl-shRNA and MCF-7$_R$ Ctrl-shRNA cells in both treatments (Supplementary Figure S2), compared with non-transfected cells (Figure 1).

To examine the role of p53 transactivation activity in CDDP resistance, MCF-7 and MCF-7$_R$ cells were cultured in the presence of pifithrin-α (Pifi-α), an inhibitor of the p53 gene transcription activity. The cells were pretreated for 24 h with 10 μM of Pifi-α and then treated with different CDDP concentrations (5, 10, 20, 30, 40, 50 μM) with or without Resv (100 μM) for 48 h. As shown in Figure 2B,C, a significant increase in the IC$_{50}$ of CDDP was observed in both treatments and in both cell lines. In MCF-7 cells the IC$_{50}$ of CDDP was 19.20 μM (~4-fold increased), and 4.34 μM (CDDP + Resv, ~33-fold increased) compared with MCF-7 cells without pifithrin-α (Figure 2B,C). On the other hand, in MCF-7$_R$ cells the IC$_{50}$ of CDDP was 18.60 μM (~2-fold increased), and 9.43 μM (CDDP + Resv, ~52-fold increased), compared with MCF-7$_R$ cells without pifithrin-α (Figure 2B,C). Indeed, pifithrin-α enhanced CDDP and CDDP + Resv resistance, probably because inhibition of p53 transactivation activity was more efficient than completely down-regulating p53 expression. Taken together, these results demonstrate that down-regulation of p53 expression or inhibition of p53-dependent gene transcription enhanced chemoresistance to CDDP in MCF-7 and MCF-7$_R$ cells under both treatments, suggesting a key role of p53 in overcoming the chemoresistance of MCF-7$_R$ cells.

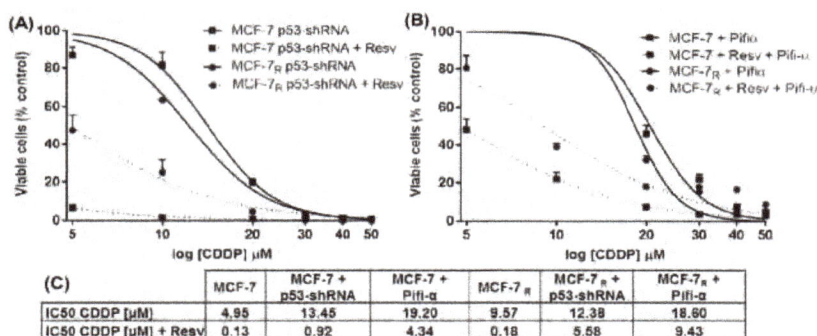

(C)	MCF-7	MCF-7 + p53-shRNA	MCF-7 + Pifi-α	MCF-7$_R$	MCF-7$_R$ + p53-shRNA	MCF-7$_R$ + Pifi-α
IC50 CDDP [μM]	4.95	13.45	19.20	9.57	12.38	18.60
IC50 CDDP [μM] + Resv	0.13	0.92	4.34	0.18	5.58	9.43

Figure 2. Down-regulation of p53 expression and inhibition of the p53 protein activity enhances resistance to CDDP and Resv in MCF-7 and MCF-7$_R$ cells. (A) p53-shRNA transfected cells and (B) MCF-7 and MCF-7$_R$ cells were pretreated with 10 μM of pifithrin-α (Pifi-α) for 24 h; both were treated for 48 h with indicated CDDP concentrations with or without Resv (100 μM). Cell viability was tested by MTT assay. Each data point is the mean of three independent experiments ± SD. (C) A summary of the IC$_{50}$ values for CDDP that were calculated by nonlinear regression (curve fit) by log[CDDP] vs. normalized response–variable slope.

3.3. Resv Induces S20 Phosphorylation and Attenuates Phosphorylation of p53 in S15 and S46 in CDDP-Treated MCF-7$_R$ Cells

We next evaluate the hypothesis that phosphorylation of p53, which is required for p53-mediated apoptosis, is reduced in response to CDDP [24] in chemoresistant cells, and that Resv activates p53-mediated apoptosis through restoring phosphorylation of p53 in S15 (p53–pS15), S20 (p53–pS20) and S46 (p53–pS46) to chemosensitize MCF-7$_R$ cells. We treated MCF-7 and MCF-7$_R$ cells with CDDP (6 μM) with or without Resv (100 μM) or Resv alone (100 μM) for 6, 12, and 24 h to analyze p53 phosphorylation status in S15, S20, and S46. In Figure 3A,B, we found that in MCF-7 cells, p53–pS15 phosphorylation after CDDP had its highest peak at 6 h and then gradually diminished (but not completely) at 12 and 24 h; however, for Resv and CDDP + Resv, p53–pS15 phosphorylation was maintained at 6 to 12 h and has highest peak at 24 h. p53–pS20 phosphorylation in CDDP started at 6 h although the highest point was at 12 h. Resv induced S20 phosphorylation at 6 h and diminished at 12 h, with a little increase at 24 h. CDDP + Resv induced a similar behavior than Resv with a moderate rise at 24 h. p53–pS46 phosphorylation was very similar for the three treatments being induced at 6 h and having its highest peak at 24 h. However, in MCF-7$_R$ cells, contrary to what we hypothesized, CDDP showed activation of S15 and S46, although it was delayed until 12 h and 24 h, respectively. On the other hand, phosphorylated p53–pS20 was not increased by CDDP treatment as compared with the control (without treatment). Interestingly, CDDP + Resv and Resv treatments showed a converse pattern of p53 phosphorylation by CDDP, phosphorylating S20 at 6 h and 12 h and inhibiting S15 and S46 phosphorylation, suggesting that phosphorylation at S20 is an important event for CDDP resistance and Resv restoration of sensibility. We used VP-16 treatment as positive phosphorylation control for MCF-7-sensitive cells. Interestingly, when used VP-16 treatment in MCF-7$_R$ cells we found the same effect as in the treatment with Resv, suggesting the possibility that both have a similar signaling pathway to induce p53 phosphorylation at S20.

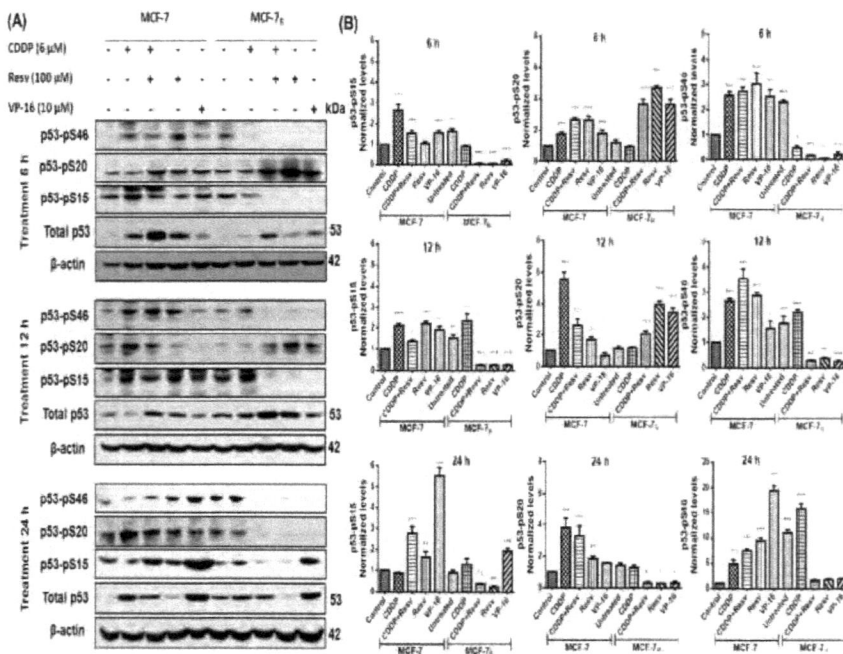

Figure 3. Resv induces serine 20 (S20) phosphorylation and attenuates phosphorylation of p53 in serine 15 (S15) and serine 46 (S46) in CDDP-treated MCF-7$_R$ cells. (**A**) MCF-7 and MCF-7$_R$ cells were treated with DMSO-ethanol vehicle as control or CDDP (6 μM) with or without Resv (100 μM) for 6, 12, and 24 h. Total and phospho-p53 contents were assessed by Western blot using antibodies directed against total p53 (DO-1) or against specific phosphorylated residues on p53, as indicated. VP-16 (10 μM) treated cells was used as positive control of p53 phosphorylation. (**B**) Densitometric analysis of phospho-p53 after β-actin normalization. One-way ANOVA followed by Dunnett's Multiple Comparison test were used to compare untreated MCF-7 cells (used as control group) with all the other groups of data at each time point. Results are presented as mean of three independent experiments $\pm$ SD. * $p < 0.05$; ** $p < 0.01$; *** $p < 0.001$.

3.4. Early Phosphorylation of p53 in S20 Induced by Resv Is Sufficient to Activate p53-Dependent Gene Transcription in MCF-7$_R$ Cells

Stabilized p53 transactivates its target genes promoting cell cycle arrest (e.g., *P21*), DNA repair [9], and apoptosis under severe DNA damage (*PUMA, NOXA, BAX* and *PIG3*) [17–19]. We observed that the only phosphorylation of p53 in MCF-7$_R$ induced by Resv was at S20, so we treated MCF-7 and MCF-7$_R$ cells with CDDP (6 μM) with or without Resv (100 μM) or Resv alone (100 μM) for 6 and 12 h to evaluate whether this phosphorylation is sufficient to activate p53-dependent gene transcription in MCF-7$_R$ cells. RT-qPCR was used to determine the mRNA level of the mentioned genes. As shown in Figure 4, expression of all genes was triggered at 6 h. *P21* and *PUMA* genes were highly up-regulated by all conditions of treatment (CDDP with or without Resv or Resv alone). *NOXA* was elevated by CDDP and CDDP + Resv, although activation by the combination was lower and the maximum peak was at 12 h. Perhaps in combination Resv hinders CDDP activation, since Resv alone does not induce *NOXA*. On the other hand, *PIG3* barely responded to Resv alone (nearly 4-fold after Resv treatment in MCF-7$_R$ cells) suggesting null participation of this gene. Unexpectedly, there does not seem to be a synergy between the treatments, since activation of all genes in the combination treatment always was lower than in CDDP or Resv alone, suggesting that just one of them is responsible for the activation of a particular gene. Interestingly, *BAX*, one of the main apoptotic effectors, is only activated by Resv, indicating this could be a key event for the induction of apoptosis in MCF-7$_R$ cells.

Taken together, these data suggest that early phosphorylation of p53 in S20 induced by Resv in MCF-7$_R$ cells is sufficient to activate p53-dependent gene transcription of selected genes and does not require phosphorylation of p53 in S15 and S46.

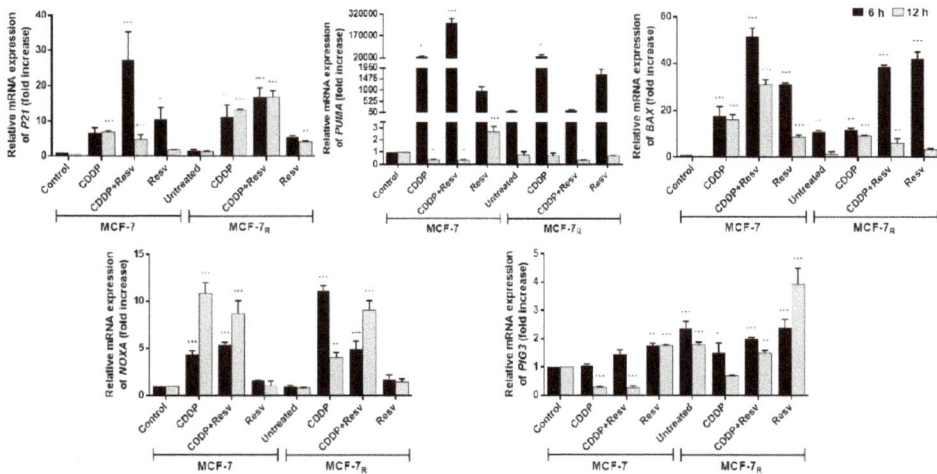

Figure 4. Early phosphorylation of p53 in S20 induced by Resv is sufficient to activate p53-dependent gene transcription in MCF-7$_R$ cells. Total RNA extracted from cells treated with DMSO-ethanol vehicle as control or CDDP (6 μM) with or without Resv (100 μM) for 6 and 12 h was assessed for expression levels of *P21, BAX, NOXA, PUMA* and *PIG3* by RT-PCR. The mRNA level of genes was normalized to the *B2M* housekeeping gene. One-way ANOVA followed by Dunnett's Multiple Comparison test were used to compare untreated MCF-7 cells (used as control group) with all the other groups of data at each time point. Results are presented as mean of three independent experiments ± SD. * $p < 0.05$; ** $p < 0.01$; *** $p < 0.001$.

3.5. Resv Overcome CDDP-Resistance and Induces Apoptosis in MCF-7$_R$ Cells

We evaluated the induction of apoptosis triggered by Resv by flow cytometry using Annexin V/PI in MCF-7 and MCF-7$_R$ cells treated with CDDP (6 µM) with or without Resv (100 µM) for 48 h. Figure 5A shows the percentage of total apoptosis (early and late apoptosis) for MCF-7 cells (left panel) with CDDP treatment was 82.02% ± 1.79%, for CDDP + Resv it was 76.55% ± 11.16%, and for Resv alone it was 60.52% ± 5.57% (Figure 5B, *p* < 0.001, left graph). As expected, MCF-7$_R$ cells (right panel) treated with CDDP did not show apoptosis; however, with CDDP + Resv treatment showed 77.89% ± 13.80% and Resv alone 59.61% ± 10.16% total apoptotic cells, similar to their chemosensitive counterpart (Figure 5B, *p* < 0.001, right graph). These data suggest that Resv with or without CDDP induces apoptosis in chemoresistant MCF-7$_R$ cells.

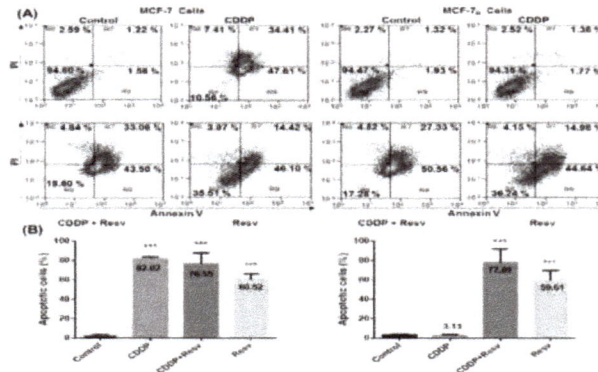

Figure 5. Resv overcome CDDP-resistance and induces apoptosis in MCF-7$_R$ cells. (**A**) MCF-7 and MCF-7$_R$ cells were treated with a DMSO–ethanol vehicle as control or CDDP (6 µM) with or without Resv (100 µM) for 48 h and were double-stained with Annexin V and propidium iodide (PI) followed by flow cytometry analysis to determine apoptotic cells. The viable cells are located in the lower left quadrant (double negative with Annexin V−/PI−). Apoptotic cells (Annexin V+/PI−) appear in the lower right (early apoptosis) and upper right (late apoptosis) quadrant of data plots. Data are presented as percentage of the cell population. (**B**) The combined results of three independent cytometry analyses depicting the mean levels of total apoptotic cells are shown. Results are presented as the means ± SD. *** *p* < 0.001 by one-way ANOVA followed by Dunnett's Multiple Comparison test.

3.6. Early Phosphorylation of p53 in S20 Induced by Resv Is Necessary for p53-Stability in MCF-7$_R$ Cells

It has been reported that CK1, CHK2, and AMPK can induce p53-pS20 phosphorylation in response to various types of stress such as CK1 in virus infection (DNA virus HHV-6B) [25], ionizing radiation for CHK2 [26], and metabolic stress for AMPK [27]. To elucidate which activation signal is induced by Resv to phosphorylate S20, we treated MCF-7$_R$ cells with CDDP (6 µM) with or without Resv (100 µM) in the presence of specific p53–pS20 kinase inhibitors: CK1 inhibitor D4476 (60 µM), CHK2 inhibitor (25 µM), or AMPK inhibitor compound C (40 µM) during 6 h. As shown in Figure 6A, inhibition of S20 phosphorylation by CK1 and CHK2 inhibitors only take place in Resv treatment; while inhibition of AMPK impeded S20 phosphorylation in both CDDP and Resv treatments. We found that in CDDP treated cells only the AMPK inhibitor blocks S20 phosphorylation but unexpectedly all three inhibitors block p53-pS20 phosphorylation in Resv-treated cells. Furthermore, in the CDDP treatment with AMPK inhibitor the p53 stability was unaffected given that in MCF-7$_R$ cells treated with CDDP, p53 was also phosphorylated on S15 and S46 (see Figures 3A and 6A). However, Resv treatment inhibits p53–pS15 and p53–pS46 phosphorylation in MCF-7$_R$ cells (see Figure 3A), consequently loss of S20 phosphorylation by AMPK and CK1 inhibitors resulted in a complete impairment of p53 stability (Figure 6A). On the other hand, with the CHK2 inhibitor, p53 stability was not affected, suggesting that in the presence of Resv another post-translational modification in p53 is involved in an attenuation of the effect of p53–pS20 loss.

In order to compare the effect of the inhibitors with their chemosensitive counterpart, we also treated MCF-7 cells with Resv (100 µM) and with specific p53–pS20 site kinase inhibitors for 6 h. As shown in Figure 6B, CK1, CHK2 and AMPK inhibitors suppress p53–pS20 phosphorylation without degradation of p53 since p53–pS15 and p53–S46 phosphorylations are induced by Resv (see Figures 3A and 6A). All together these data suggest that in MCF-7$_R$ cells the early phosphorylation of p53 in S20 induced by Resv is sufficient for p53 stabilization and their transactivation function and that its inhibition induces p53 degradation compared with their chemosensitive counterpart where p53 is still stable after the inhibition of p53–pS20, probably because it contains phosphorylation in S15 and S46 induced by Resv.

To investigate the effect that the inhibitors had in p53-induced apoptosis, we treated MCF-7$_R$ cells with CDDP (6 µM) + Resv (100 µM) and with specific p53–pS20 kinase inhibitors for 48 h and evaluated the induction of apoptosis with Annexin V/PI and flow cytometry. As shown in Figure 6C, the MCF-7$_R$ cells treated with CK1 and AMPK inhibitors (degraded p53) had 59.25% $\pm$ 4.27 and 70.91% $\pm$ 3.43% total apoptotic cells, respectively, suggesting a p53-independent apoptosis. On the other hand, the MCF-7$_R$ cells in the presence of CHK2 inhibitor (low p53 level) showed a significant reduction of apoptotic cells with 20.95% $\pm$ 1.43% vs. 68.44% $\pm$ 8.94% of apoptotic cells without inhibitor (Figure 6D, *** $p < 0.001$), suggesting that the presence of a non-functional p53 form in MCF-7$_R$ cells (without phosphorylation in S15, S20 and S46) can hamper the induction of apoptosis.

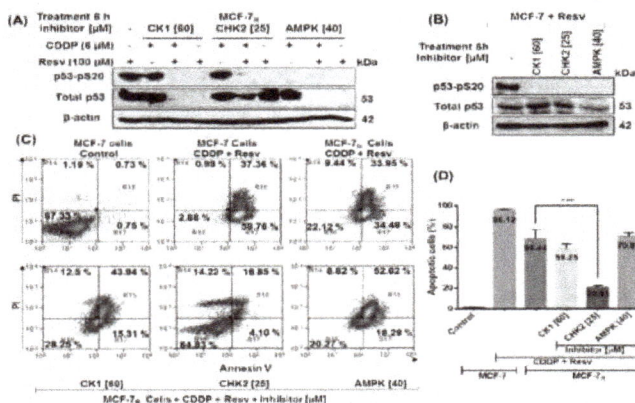

Figure 6. Early phosphorylation of p53 in S20 induced by Resv is necessary for p53-stability in MCF-7$_R$ cells. (**A**) MCF-7$_R$ cells were treated with CDDP (6 µM) with or without Resv (100 µM) and (**B**) MCF-7 cells were treated with Resv (100 µM); both cell cultures were treated for 6 h with specific p53-pS20 site kinase inhibitors: CK1 (60 µM), CHK2 (25 µM) or AMPK (40 µM). Total and phospho-p53 contents are assessed by Western blot using antibodies directed against total p53 (DO-1) or against the specific phosphorylated residue on S20, as indicated. (**C**) MCF-7 and MCF-7$_R$ cells were treated with a DMSO–ethanol vehicle as control or CDDP (6 µM) with resveratrol (100 µM) and cultured in combination with CK1 (60 µM), CHK2 (25 µM) or AMPK (40 µM) inhibitors for 48 h and were double-stained with Annexin V and propidium iodide (PI) followed by flow cytometry analysis to determine apoptotic cells. The viable cells are located in the lower left quadrant (double negative with Annexin V–/PI–). Apoptotic cells (Annexin V+/PI–) appear in the lower right (early apoptosis) and upper right (late apoptosis) quadrant of data plots. Data are presented as a percentage of the cell population. (**D**) The combined results of three independent cytometry analyses depicting the mean levels of total apoptotic cells are shown. Results are presented as the means $\pm$ SD. *** $p < 0.001$ by one-way ANOVA followed by Turkey's Multiple Comparison test.

3.7. Resv Promotes Early Dephosphorylation of ATM, Inhibition of BCL-2, and Upregulation of BAX

It has been reported that S15 of p53 is phosphorylated by activated ATM (S1981-phosphorylated ATM) at an earlier inductive phase after DNA damage [14,15]. S46 is also sequentially phosphorylated by ATM [15]; supporting these observations, we found that the treatment of MCF-7$_R$ cells with Resv with or without CDDP for 6 h promotes early deactivation of ATM by dephosphorylation in S1981 regardless of the total ATM level (Figure 7A), so it is possible that the decrease in p53 phosphorylation in S15 and S46 MCF-7$_R$ cells (see Figure 3A) could be due to dephosphorylation of ATM by Resv. On the other hand, to investigate the blockade of apoptosis in MCF-7$_R$ cells treated with CDDP, we analyzed the ratio of anti-apoptotic BCL-2 and proapoptotic BAX proteins, finding that BCL-2 was elevated while BAX was decreased after 6 h treatment with CDDP. On the other hand, in cells treated with CDDP + Resv or only Resv, BCL-2 protein expression was decreased while at the same time BAX was increased (Figure 7B–E). This result suggests that elevated BCL-2 in CDDP treatment blocked apoptosis and that Resv partly induces apoptosis by changing the ratio between BCL-2 and BAX proteins.

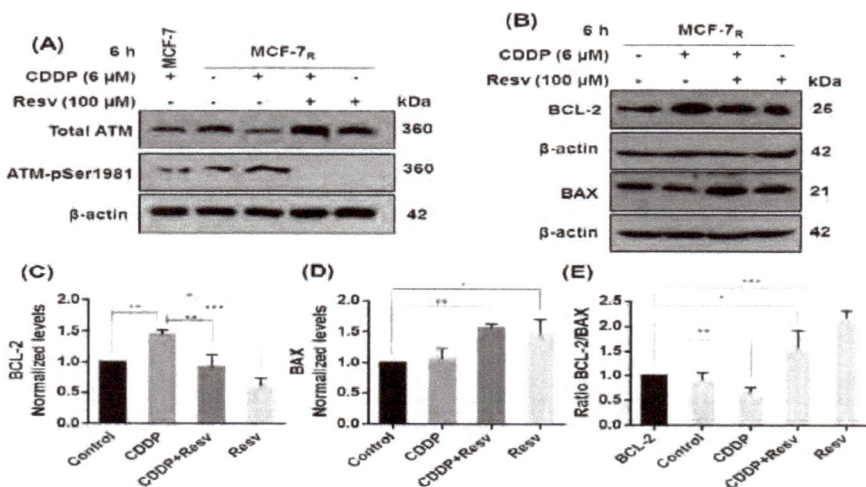

Figure 7. Resv promotes early dephosphorylation of ATM, inhibition of BCL-2, and upregulation of BAX. MCF-7$_R$ cells were treated with CDDP (6 µM) with or without Resv (100 µM) for 6 h. (**A**) Total and phospho-ATM and (**B**) BCL-2 and BAX proteins were assessed by Western blot using antibodies directed against total ATM, a specific phosphorylated residue on S1981 of ATM, BCL-2, or BAX. MCF-7 cells with CDPP were used as positive control of ATM phosphorylation. (**C**) Densitometric analysis of BCL-2 and (**D**) BAX after β-actin normalization. (**E**) Ratio between BCL-2/BAX by *t* test. All results are presented as mean of three independent experiments ± SD. * $p < 0.05$; ** $p < 0.01$; *** $p < 0.001$ by one-way ANOVA followed by Turkey's or Dunnett's Multiple Comparison test.

4. Discussion and Conclusions

CDDP is one of the most widely used anticancer drugs in the treatment of various types of cancer, including human breast cancer [28], but its use commonly results in adverse effects and toxicities affecting healthy systems, with resistance a major cause of treatment failure [1,29]. Therefore, it is of interest to continue searching for effective chemosensitizers. Resv is known to be an anticancer and protective agent which has the potential for preventing CDDP-related toxicity; it can sensitize chemoresistant cells by overcoming mechanisms of chemoresistance, including the upregulation of p53 [7,9,10]. Considering the chemosensitizer capacity of Resv, we developed a CDDP-resistant MCF-7$_R$ cell line variant employing only 6 µM of CDDP because at higher concentrations (>6.5 µM) the cells died or formed clusters into the medium that prevented the formation of cell monolayers; a similar effect was previously described in other CDDP-resistant cancer cells [30,31]. Our results showed that Resv induces CDDP sensitivity, decreasing the IC_{50} of CDDP in MCF-7 and our MCF-7_R cells.

The contribution of p53 to chemosensitivity and chemoresistance remains partly unclear. It has been reported that acquisition of resistance to chemotherapeutic drugs including CDDP also occurs in cancer cells expressing p53 wt. One mechanism proposed to explain this phenomenon is that this p53 protein becomes inactive. p53 could be activated by phosphorylation in response to various cell stress signals, protecting p53 from MDM2-mediated ubiquitination and proteasomal degradation. Phosphorylation of p53 in S15 and S20 is required to perform DNA repair [14,15], and under severe DNA damage, S46 is also sequentially phosphorylated for p53-induced apoptosis [13,16]. We think that resistance of MCF-7 cells to CDDP could be related to the lack of phosphorylation in these specific sites of the p53 protein as was described previously in CDDP-resistant ovarian cancer cells [24]. We treated MCF-7 and MCF-7_R cells with 6 µM of CDDP (maximal concentration for the survival of chemoresistant cells) to compare the effect in both cell lines. Our data showed that the inhibition of p53 expression (p53 shRNA) or its transactivation activity (pifithrin-α) enhances the resistance of both cell lines to CDDP and CDDP + Resv, suggesting the active participation of p53 after drug treatment. This effect was also observed in other reports that show that the downregulation of p53 enhances CDDP resistance [32,33] and importantly, Resv also has been reported to induce apoptosis through a p53-dependent pathway [9,10]. CDDP treatment induced p53 phosphorylation of S15, S20, and S46 in MCF-7 cells; in MCF-7_R cells S15 and S46, also appeared to be constitutively phosphorylated even without treatment, but these cells survive. Interestingly, S20 phosphorylation was inhibited in CDDP-treated MCF-7_R cells while at the same time was strongly enhanced in CDDP + Resv and Resv treatments, suggesting that S20 phosphorylation could be key for p53 to activate target genes, specifically *BAX*, to overcome CDDP resistance in MCF-7_R cells. Furthermore, the importance of this site is highlighted by the fact that the treatment with CDDP in combination with Resv or Resv alone attenuated p53 phosphorylation at S15 and S46 but promoted apoptosis. However, we do not discard the possible phosphorylation of p53 in other sites that collaborate with S20 to induce apoptosis. Interestingly, we found the same effect observed for Resv in chemoresistant cells treated with VP-16, suggesting that both compounds have a similar signaling pathway to induce p53 phosphorylation in S20. Regarding the inhibition of phosphorylation in S15 and S46 in MCF-7_R cells, it is most probably related to the loss of ATM activation in CDDP + Resv and Resv treatments, consistent with our results (Figure 7) and reports that describe that S15 of p53 is phosphorylated by activated ATM at an early phase after DNA damage [14,15], and then S46 is sequentially phosphorylated by ATM [20]. Furthermore, since ATM activity is a key regulator of DNA damage response that is related to genotoxic resistance, the inhibition of ATM activity [34,35] could also contribute to the chemosensitivity of MCF-7_R cells. Previously, it was reported that Resv induced phosphorylation of p53 in S15 and S20 in MCF-7 cells [20,21], but to our knowledge this is the first time that it has been shown that Resv also induces phosphorylation in S46. Our results are consistent with reports in MCF-7 cells and in several chemosensitive and chemoresistant cancers indicating that Resv increases p53-dependent transcriptional activity including increase of mRNA levels of *BAX*, *BAK*, and *PUMA* [36,37].

In order to elucidate which kinase pathway is responsible for p53–pS20 activation in MCF-7_R cells, we used three known specific inhibitors of kinases that phosphorylate p53 in S20 which include the DNA damage pathway (CHK2 inhibitor), oncogene activation (CK1 inhibitor), and metabolic stress (AMPK inhibitor). We observed that the low continuous phosphorylation of S20 in CDDP treated MCF-7_R cells is induced by AMPK since it was sensitive to the AMPK inhibitor. Activation of AMPK by CDDP has been previously reported, and it was related to apoptosis inhibition and acquired resistance [38,39]. It is very interesting that the kinase responsible for S20 phosphorylation by CDDP is the same that could be responsible for apoptosis inhibition. Surprisingly, when we used the three inhibitors in CDDP + Resv and Resv treated MCF-7_R cells, all of them blocked S20 phosphorylation, suggesting that Resv activates the three kinases to phosphorylate p53. At this point we cannot explain the codependence of the three kinases to phosphorylate S20 but it is possible that Resv activates the three kinases to assure or maintain phosphorylation for a longer time. Under this scenario, we think that there could be a fluid dynamic between the three enzymes for the interaction in the docking site for S20 and the hampering of any of the enzymes could block the site for the other two. There is also the possibility of an unknown cross-talk between them or that the interaction of the three kinases in the docking sites of Box-V domain of p53 was also important for allowing S20 phosphorylation. Nevertheless, this interesting result should be analyzed further in future works. Additionally, the inhibition of S20 phosphorylation by CK1 and AMPK kinase inhibitors in MCF-7$_R$ results in loss of p53 stability, while the inhibition of CHK2 conserves some of the p53 total protein expression in the presence of Resv, suggesting that other phosphorylation sites for CHK2 along the p53 protein could be essential to maintain p53 stability. Although the three kinases were necessary in phosphorylating p53–S20, we performed apoptosis assays in the presence of each of the three inhibitors to elucidate if one of the kinases is key or more important for the activation of apoptosis. Unfortunately, complete loss of p53 stability with CK1 and AMPK inhibitors produced an elevated induction of apoptosis, masking the object of the experiment. Although the result was unsought, there have been some works describing the same phenomenon in MCF-7 cells. For example, in a study in MCF-7 cells, disruption of p53 with a plasmid expressing the E6 oncoprotein sensitizes them to CDDP [40]. In the same manner, Mendez and Lupu silenced p53 to elucidate if the apoptosis induced in MCF-7 cells by the inhibition of FASN was through the p53 pathway; unexpectedly, they found an elevation of 300% in apoptosis [41]. Also, specific down-regulation of p53 showed an increase in apoptosis via SMAD4 [42]. Finally, using a RNAi for p53 also sensitized MCF-7 cells to apoptosis induced by ceramide [43]. These observations could partially explain our results since the treatments we used were CDDP and Resv, which are known to induce apoptosis also by ceramide induction. However, another interesting observation was that with the CHK2 inhibitor some of the total but probably inactive p53 protein was conserved; the induction of apoptosis was strongly diminished, suggesting that inactive p53 protein not only diminished the induction of apoptosis but also blocked it. Finally, we also observed another important difference in BCL2–*BAX* balance between CDDP and CDDP + Resv treated MCF-7$_R$ cells. First, RT-qPCR results show that pro-apoptotic *BAX* gene expression was highly elevated in CDDP + Resv and Resv treatments, while in the CDDP treatment it was slightly decreased. On the other hand, anti-apoptotic BCL-2 protein was elevated in CDDP treatment, while in CDDP + Resv and Resv treatments the BCL-2 protein expression was diminished. As previously reported, the balance between BCL-2 and BAX is a key regulatory element [44] and could be an additional mechanism explaining the induction of apoptosis in MCF-7$_R$ cells in the presence of Resv or CDDP + Resv. Our results suggest a new model of chemosensitization by Resv in MCF-7$_R$ cells, involving phosphorylation in p53–pS20. This model is in accord with our previous observation of Resv sensitizing MCF-7 cells by downregulation of RAD51 since p53 could repress RAD51 mRNA and protein expression [23,45].

Our results show that Resv reduces the IC$_{50}$ of CDDP necessary to induce apoptosis in chemosensitive and in CDDP-resistant MCF-7 cell line variant, increasing the capability to arrest, delay or reverse carcinogenesis in an adjuvant CDDP therapy. This study provides evidence on the role of p53 for a potential CDDP acquired resistance model and the molecular mechanism of Resv to chemosensitize resistant breast cancer cells to CDDP. We demonstrated for a resistant cell line variant that down-regulation of p53 and inhibition of p53-dependent gene transcription enhanced chemoresistance to CDDP in chemosensitive and chemoresistant cells, suggesting that the chemosensitization to CDDP by Resv is mainly p53-dependent. Moreover, in chemoresistant cells Resv induces early phosphorylation of p53 in S20 and attenuates CDDP-induced p53 phosphorylation in S15 and S46 residues, probably through dephosphorylation and deactivation of ATM. This phosphorylation in p53–pS20 is sufficient to activate p53-dependent gene transcription including *PUMA* and *BAX* genes restoring apoptosis in MCF-7$_R$ cells. Resv activates different kinases, such as CK1, CHK2, and AMPK to induce phosphorylation of p53 in S20, suggesting a novel mechanism of p53 activation and chemosensitization to CDDP. At the same time, Resv downregulates BCL-2 expression, a key player in apoptosis inhibition. On the other hand, CDDP induces p53 phosphorylation in chemoresistant cells but the apoptosis is probably blocked downstream at least in part by the up-regulation of BCL-2 protein despite the up-regulation of *PUMA* and *NOXA* (see model in Figure 8). A more thorough understanding of the molecular mechanism underlying this particular chemoresistance and the chemosensitization by Resv in this resistant cell variant may ultimately help for improvement in the treatment of human breast cancer.

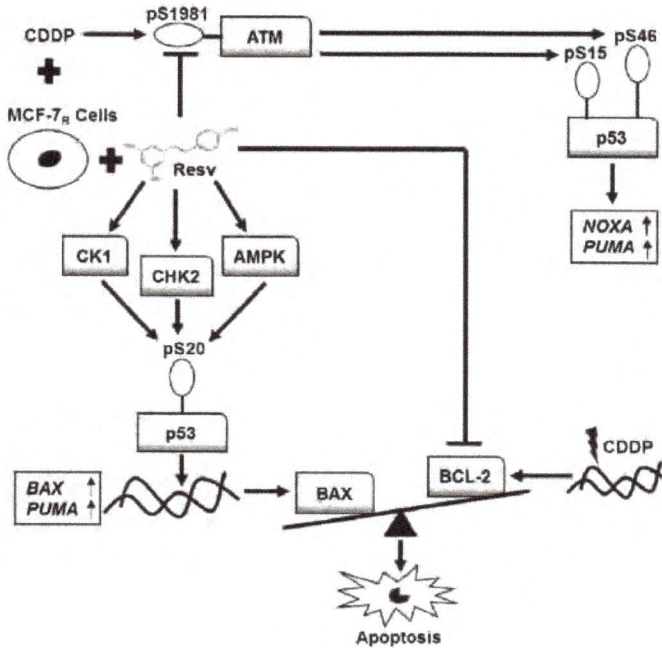

Figure 8. In the MCF-7 resistant cell variant (MCF-7$_R$), Resv attenuates phosphorylation in S15 and S46 of p53 by dephosphorylation and deactivation of ATM. However, it activates kinases CK1, CHK2, and AMPK to induce phosphorylation of p53 in S20 (which is required to activate p53 in order to upregulate *BAX* and *PUMA* genes) and modifies the ratio between BCL-2/BAX expression. The BAX protein was increased while BCL-2 protein was decreased, restoring apoptosis and overcoming chemoresistance. On the other hand, the overexpression of BCL-2 in MCF-7$_R$ cells after CDDP treatment maintains the chemoresistance and blocks apoptosis despite the phosphorylation of p53 in S15 and S46 and the upregulation of *NOXA* and *PUMA*.

Supplementary Materials: The following are available online at http://www.mdpi.com/2072-6643/10/9/1148/s1, Figure S1: Down-regulation of p53 in MCF-7 and MCF-7$_R$ cells by shRNA; Figure S2: Transfected cells with Ctrl-shRNA are sensitive to Resv; Table S1: Primers for RT-qPCR p53 target gene analysis.

Author Contributions: Conceptualization, J.H.-V. and E.G.-V.; Data curation, J.H.-V. and E.G.-V.; Formal analysis, J.H.-V. and E.G.-V.; Funding acquisition, J.D.-C. and P.G.; Investigation, J.H.-V. and E.G.-V.; Methodology, J.H.-V., E.G.-V., and A.A.-H.; Project administration, J.D.-C. and P.G.; Resources, J.G.-M., J.D.-C., and P.G.; Supervision, E.G.-V. and J.D.-C.; Validation, J.G.-M., J.D.-C., and P.G.; Visualization, J.H.-V.; Writing—original draft, J.H.-V.; Writing—review and editing, E.G.-V., J.G.-M., J.D.-C., and P.G.

Funding: This research was funded by Consejo Nacional de Ciencia y Tecnología, Mexico, grant number (236767). The funder had no role in study design, data collection and analysis, decision to publish, or preparation of the manuscript.

Acknowledgments: The authors would like to thank to Elizabeth Álvarez-Ríos, Rodolfo Ocádiz-Delgado, Lauro Macias-González and ML Bazán-Tejeda for technical support. Special thanks to RM Bermúdez-Cruz for the donation of the anti-ATM antibody.

Conflicts of Interest: The authors declare no conflict of interest.

References

1. Brabec, V.; Kasparkova, J. Modifications of DNA by platinum complexes. Relation to resistance of tumors to platinum antitumor drugs. *Drug Resist. Updat.* **2005**, *8*, 131–146. [CrossRef] [PubMed]

2. Kaur, G.; Verma, N. Nature curing cancer—Review on structural modification studies with natural active compounds having anti-tumor efficiency. *Biotechnol. Rep. (Amst.)* **2015**, *6*, 64–78. [CrossRef] [PubMed]

3. Fulda, S. Resveratrol and derivatives for the prevention and treatment of cancer. *Drug Discov. Today* **2010**, *15*, 757–765. [CrossRef] [PubMed]

4. Fabris, S.; Momo, F.; Ravagnan, G.; Stevanato, R. Antioxidant properties of resveratrol and piceid on lipid peroxidation in micelles and monolamellar liposomes. *Biophys. Chem.* **2008**, *135*, 76–83. [CrossRef] [PubMed]

5. Caruso, F.; Tanski, J.; Villegas-Estrada, A.; Rossi, M. Structural basis for antioxidant activity of trans-resveratrol: Ab initio calculations and crystal and molecular structure. *J. Agric. Food Chem.* **2004**, *52*, 7279–7285. [CrossRef] [PubMed]

6. Aggarwal, B.B.; Bhardwaj, A.; Aggarwal, R.S.; Seeram, N.P.; Shishodia, S.; Takada, Y. Role of resveratrol in prevention and therapy of cancer: Preclinical and clinical studies. *Anticancer Res.* **2004**, *24*, 2783–2840. [PubMed]

7. Gupta, S.C.; Kannappan, R.; Reuter, S.; Kim, J.H.; Aggarwal, B.B. Chemosensitization of tumors by resveratrol. *Ann. N. Y. Acad. Sci.* **2011**, *1215*, 150–160. [CrossRef] [PubMed]

8. Miyashita, T.; Krajewski, S.; Krajewska, M.; Wang, H.G.; Lin, H.K.; Liebermann, D.A.; Hoffman, B.; Reed, J.C. Tumor suppressor p53 is a regulator of bcl-2 and bax gene expression in vitro and in vivo. *Oncogene* **1994**, *9*, 1799–1805. [PubMed]

9. Ferraz da Costa, D.C.; Casanova, F.A.; Quarti, J.; Malheiros, M.S.; Sanches, D.; Dos Santos, P.S.; Fialho, E.; Silva, J.L. Transient transfection of a wild-type p53 gene triggers resveratrol-induced apoptosis in cancer cells. *PLoS ONE* **2012**, *7*, e48746. [CrossRef] [PubMed]

10. Huang, C.; Ma, W.Y.; Goranson, A.; Dong, Z. Resveratrol suppresses cell transformation and induces apoptosis through a p53-dependent pathway. *Carcinogenesis* **1999**, *20*, 237–242. [CrossRef] [PubMed]

11. Gogada, R.; Prabhu, V.; Amadori, M.; Scott, R.; Hashmi, S.; Chandra, D. Resveratrol induces p53-independent, x-linked inhibitor of apoptosis protein (xiap)-mediated bax protein oligomerization on mitochondria to initiate cytochrome c release and caspase activation. *J. Biol. Chem.* **2011**, *286*, 28749–28760. [CrossRef] [PubMed]

12. Prabhu, V.; Srivastava, P.; Yadav, N.; Amadori, M.; Schneider, A.; Seshadri, A.; Pitarresi, J.; Scott, R.; Zhang, H.; Koochekpour, S.; et al. Resveratrol depletes mitochondrial DNA and inhibition of autophagy enhances resveratrol-induced caspase activation. *Mitochondrion* **2013**, *13*, 493–499. [CrossRef] [PubMed]

13. Taira, N.; Nihira, K.; Yamaguchi, T.; Miki, Y.; Yoshida, K. Dyrk2 is targeted to the nucleus and controls p53 via ser46 phosphorylation in the apoptotic response to DNA damage. *Mol. Cell* **2007**, *25*, 725–738. [CrossRef] [PubMed]

14. Shieh, S.Y.; Ikeda, M.; Taya, Y.; Prives, C. DNA damage-induced phosphorylation of p53 alleviates inhibition by mdm2. *Cell* **1997**, *91*, 325–334. [CrossRef]

15. Kodama, M.; Otsubo, C.; Hirota, T.; Yokota, J.; Enari, M.; Taya, Y. Requirement of ATM for rapid p53 phosphorylation at Ser46 without ser/thr-gln sequences. *Mol. Cell. Biol.* **2010**, *30*, 1620–1633. [CrossRef] [PubMed]

16. D'Orazi, G.; Cecchinelli, B.; Bruno, T.; Manni, I.; Higashimoto, Y.; Saito, S.; Gostissa, M.; Coen, S.; Marchetti, A.; Del Sal, G.; et al. Homeodomain-interacting protein kinase-2 phosphorylates p53 at Ser 46 and mediates apoptosis. *Nat. Cell Biol.* **2002**, *4*, 11–19. [CrossRef] [PubMed]

17. Villunger, A.; Michalak, E.M.; Coultas, L.; Mullauer, F.; Bock, G.; Ausserlechner, M.J.; Adams, J.M.; Strasser, A. P53- and drug-induced apoptotic responses mediated by bh3-only proteins puma and noxa. *Science* **2003**, *302*, 1036–1038. [CrossRef] [PubMed]

18. Kong, W.; Jiang, X.; Mercer, W.E. Downregulation of wip-1 phosphatase expression in mcf-7 breast cancer cells enhances doxorubicin-induced apoptosis through p53-mediated transcriptional activation of bax. *Cancer Biol. Ther.* **2009**, *8*, 555–563. [CrossRef] [PubMed]

19. Zhang, W.; Luo, J.; Chen, F.; Yang, F.; Song, W.; Zhu, A.; Guan, X. Brca1 regulates pig3-mediated apoptosis in a p53-dependent manner. *Oncotarget* **2015**, *6*, 7608–7618. [CrossRef] [PubMed]

20. Hsieh, T.C.; Wong, C.; John Bennett, D.; Wu, J.M. Regulation of p53 and cell proliferation by resveratrol and its derivatives in breast cancer cells: An in silico and biochemical approach targeting integrin alphavbeta3. *Int. J. Cancer* **2011**, *129*, 2732–2743. [CrossRef] [PubMed]

21. Zhang, S.; Cao, H.J.; Davis, F.B.; Tang, H.Y.; Davis, P.J.; Lin, H.Y. Oestrogen inhibits resveratrol-induced post-translational modification of p53 and apoptosis in breast cancer cells. *Br. J. Cancer* **2004**, *91*, 178–185. [CrossRef] [PubMed]

22. Leon-Galicia, I.; Diaz-Chavez, J.; Garcia-Villa, E.; Uribe-Figueroa, L.; Hidalgo-Miranda, A.; Herrera, L.A.; Alvarez-Rios, E.; Garcia-Mena, J.; Gariglio, P. Resveratrol induces downregulation of DNA repair genes in mcf-7 human breast cancer cells. *Eur. J. Cancer Prev.* **2013**, *22*, 11–20. [CrossRef] [PubMed]

23. Leon-Galicia, I.; Diaz-Chavez, J.; Albino-Sanchez, M.E.; Garcia-Villa, E.; Bermudez-Cruz, R.; Garcia-Mena, J.; Herrera, L.A.; Garcia-Carranca, A.; Gariglio, P. Resveratrol decreases rad51 expression and sensitizes cisplatinresistant mcf7 breast cancer cells. *Oncol. Rep.* **2018**, *39*, 3025–3033. [PubMed]

24. Fraser, M.; Bai, T.; Tsang, B.K. Akt promotes cisplatin resistance in human ovarian cancer cells through inhibition of p53 phosphorylation and nuclear function. *Int. J. Cancer* **2008**, *122*, 534–546. [CrossRef] [PubMed]

25. MacLaine, N.J.; Oster, B.; Bundgaard, B.; Fraser, J.A.; Buckner, C.; Lazo, P.A.; Meek, D.W.; Hollsberg, P.; Hupp, T.R. A central role for ck1 in catalyzing phosphorylation of the p53 transactivation domain at serine 20 after hhv-6b viral infection. *J. Biol. Chem.* **2008**, *283*, 28563–28573. [CrossRef] [PubMed]

26. Craig, A.; Scott, M.; Burch, L.; Smith, G.; Ball, K.; Hupp, T. Allosteric effects mediate chk2 phosphorylation of the p53 transactivation domain. *EMBO Rep.* **2003**, *4*, 787–792. [CrossRef] [PubMed]

27. Hawley, S.A.; Boudeau, J.; Reid, J.L.; Mustard, K.J.; Udd, L.; Makela, T.P.; Alessi, D.R.; Hardie, D.G. Complexes between the lkb1 tumor suppressor, strad alpha/beta and mo25 alpha/beta are upstream kinases in the amp-activated protein kinase cascade. *J. Biol.* **2003**, *2*, 28. [CrossRef] [PubMed]

28. Zhang, J.; Wang, L.; Xing, Z.; Liu, D.; Sun, J.; Li, X.; Zhang, Y. Status of bi- and multi-nuclear platinum anticancer drug development. *Anticancer Agents Med. Chem.* **2010**, *10*, 272–282. [CrossRef] [PubMed]

29. Tsang, R.Y.; Al-Fayea, T.; Au, H.J. Cisplatin overdose: Toxicities and management. *Drug Saf.* **2009**, *32*, 1109–1122. [CrossRef] [PubMed]

30. Maubant, S.; Staedel, C.; Gauduchon, P. Integrins, cell response to anti-tumor agents and chemoresistance. *Bull. Cancer* **2002**, *89*, 923–934. [PubMed]

31. Nista, A.; Leonetti, C.; Bernardini, G.; Mattioni, M.; Santoni, A. Functional role of alpha4beta1 and alpha5beta1 integrin fibronectin receptors expressed on adriamycin-resistant mcf-7 human mammary carcinoma cells. *Int. J. Cancer* **1997**, *72*, 133–141. [CrossRef]

32. Nadkarni, A.; Rajesh, P.; Ruch, R.J.; Pittman, D.L. Cisplatin resistance conferred by the rad51d (e233g) genetic variant is dependent upon p53 status in human breast carcinoma cell lines. *Mol. Carcinog.* **2009**, *48*, 586–591. [CrossRef] [PubMed]

33. Jiang, M.; Yi, X.; Hsu, S.; Wang, C.Y.; Dong, Z. Role of p53 in cisplatin-induced tubular cell apoptosis: Dependence on p53 transcriptional activity. *Am. J. Physiol. Ren. Physiol.* **2004**, *287*, F1140–F1147. [CrossRef] [PubMed]

34. Weber, A.M.; Ryan, A.J. ATM and ATR as therapeutic targets in cancer. *Pharmacol. Ther.* **2015**, *149*, 124–138. [CrossRef] [PubMed]

35. Luong, K.V.; Wang, L.; Roberts, B.J.; Wahl, J.K., 3rd; Peng, A. Cell fate determination in cisplatin resistance and chemosensitization. *Oncotarget* **2016**, *7*, 23383–23394. [CrossRef] [PubMed]

36. Sakamoto, T.; Horiguchi, H.; Oguma, E.; Kayama, F. Effects of diverse dietary phytoestrogens on cell growth, cell cycle and apoptosis in estrogen-receptor-positive breast cancer cells. *J. Nutr. Biochem.* **2010**, *21*, 856–864. [CrossRef] [PubMed]

37. Shankar, S.; Chen, Q.; Siddiqui, I.; Sarva, K.; Srivastava, R.K. Sensitization of trail-resistant lncap cells by resveratrol (3, 4′, 5 tri-hydroxystilbene): Molecular mechanisms and therapeutic potential. *J. Mol. Signal.* **2007**, *2*, 7. [CrossRef] [PubMed]

38. Kim, H.S.; Hwang, J.T.; Yun, H.; Chi, S.G.; Lee, S.J.; Kang, I.; Yoon, K.S.; Choe, W.J.; Kim, S.S.; Ha, J. Inhibition of amp-activated protein kinase sensitizes cancer cells to cisplatin-induced apoptosis via hyper-induction of p53. *J. Biol. Chem.* **2008**, *283*, 3731–3742. [CrossRef] [PubMed]

39. Harhaji-Trajkovic, L.; Vilimanovich, U.; Kravic-Stevovic, T.; Bumbasirevic, V.; Trajkovic, V. Ampk-mediated autophagy inhibits apoptosis in cisplatin-treated tumour cells. *J. Cell. Mol. Med.* **2009**, *13*, 3644–3654. [CrossRef] [PubMed]

40. Fan, S.; Smith, M.L.; Rivet, D.J., 2nd; Duba, D.; Zhan, Q.; Kohn, K.W.; Fornace, A.J., Jr.; O'Connor, P.M. Disruption of p53 function sensitizes breast cancer mcf-7 cells to cisplatin and pentoxifylline. *Cancer Res.* **1995**, *55*, 1649–1654. [PubMed]

41. Menendez, J.A.; Lupu, R. RNA interference-mediated silencing of the p53 tumor-suppressor protein drastically increases apoptosis after inhibition of endogenous fatty acid metabolism in breast cancer cells. *Int. J. Mol. Med.* **2005**, *15*, 33–40. [CrossRef] [PubMed]

42. Wu, B.; Li, W.; Qian, C.; Zhou, Z.; Xu, W.; Wu, J. Down-regulated p53 by sirna increases smad4's activity in promoting cell apoptosis in mcf-7 cells. *Eur. Rev. Med. Pharmacol. Sci.* **2012**, *16*, 1243–1248. [PubMed]

43. Struckhoff, A.P.; Patel, B.; Beckman, B.S. Inhibition of p53 sensitizes mcf-7 cells to ceramide treatment. *Int. J. Oncol.* **2010**, *37*, 21–30. [PubMed]

44. Delbridge, A.R.; Grabow, S.; Strasser, A.; Vaux, D.L. Thirty years of bcl-2: Translating cell death discoveries into novel cancer therapies. *Nat. Rev. Cancer* **2016**, *16*, 99–109. [CrossRef] [PubMed]

45. Arias-Lopez, C.; Lazaro-Trueba, I.; Kerr, P.; Lord, C.J.; Dexter, T.; Iravani, M.; Ashworth, A.; Silva, A. P53 modulates homologous recombination by transcriptional regulation of the rad51 gene. *EMBO Rep.* **2006**, *7*, 219–224. [CrossRef] [PubMed]

nutrients

MDPI

Article

The Synergistic Effects of Resveratrol combined with Resistant Training on Exercise Performance and Physiological Adaption

Nai-Wen Kan [1], Mon-Chien Lee [2,†], Yu-Tang Tung [3,4,†], Chien-Chao Chiu [2], Chi-Chang Huang [2,*] and Wen-Ching Huang [5,*]

[1] Center for General Education, Taipei Medical University, Taipei 11031, Taiwan; kevinkan@tmu.edu.tw
[2] Graduate Institute of Sports Science, National Taiwan Sport University, Taoyuan 33301, Taiwan; 1061304@ntsu.edu.tw (M.-C.L.); chiu2295@yahoo.com.tw (C.-C.C.)
[3] Graduate Institute of Metabolism and Obesity Sciences, Taipei Medical University, Taipei City 11031, Taiwan; f91625059@tmu.edu.tw
[4] Nutrition Research Center, Taipei Medical University Hospital, Taipei 11031, Taiwan
[5] Department of Exercise and Health Science, National Taipei University of Nursing and Health Sciences, Taipei 11219, Taiwan
* Correspondence: john5523@ntsu.edu.tw (C.-C.H.); wenching@ntunhs.edu.tw (W.-C.H.); Tel.: +886-3-328-3201 (ext. 2409) (C.-C.H.); +886-2-2822-7101 (ext. 7721) (W.-C.H.)
† These authors contributed equally to this work.

Received: 29 July 2018; Accepted: 20 September 2018; Published: 22 September 2018

Abstract: The comprehensive studies done on resveratrol (RES) support that this polyphenol has multiple bioactivities and is widely accepted for dietary supplementation. Furthermore, regular exercise is known to have benefits on health and is considered as a form of preventive medicine. Although the vast majority of prior studies emphasize the efficacy of aerobic exercise in promoting physiological adaptions, other types of exercise, such as resistance exercise and high-intensity interval training (HIIT), may achieve similar or different physiological outcomes. Few studies have looked into the effectiveness of a combinational, synergistic approach to exercise using a weight-loading ladder climbing animal platform. In this study, ICR mice were allocated randomly to the RES and training groups using a two-way ANOVA (RES × Training) design. Exercise capacities, including grip strength, aerobic performance, and anaerobic performance, were assessed and the physiological adaptions were evaluated using fatigue-associated indexes that were implemented immediately after the exercise intervention. In addition, glycogen levels, muscular characteristics, and safety issues, including body composition, histopathology, and biochemistry, were further elucidated. Synergistic effects were observed on grip strength, anaerobic capacities, and exercise lactate, with significant interaction effects. Moreover, the training or RES may have contributed significantly to elevating aerobic capacity, tissue glycogen, and muscle hypertrophy. Toxic and other deleterious effects were also considered to evaluate the safety of the intervention. Resistance exercise in combination with resveratrol supplementation may be applied in the general population to achieve better physiological benefits, promote overall health, and promote participation in regular physical activities.

Keywords: resveratrol; resistance exercise; hypertrophy; physiological adaption; performance

1. Introduction

Resveratrol (trans-3,4′,5-trihydroxystilbene, RES), a stilbenoid, is a natural polyphenol that has be widely investigated for its bioactivity and potential therapeutic applications. RES occurs naturally in a wide variety of plant species, including grapes, blueberries, raspberries, and mulberries [1]. Moreover, RES is a phytoalexin, which is a class of compounds produced by many plants in response to infection by pathogens or to physical injury due to, for example, cutting, crushing, or ultraviolet radiation [2]. Both cis- and trans-resveratrol are fat-soluble and bound to a glucose molecule, also called piceid [3]. One theory to explain the "French Paradox", a term used to describe the phenomenon of the French people having a relatively low incidence of coronary heart disease (CHD) despite their relatively high consumption of high-fat foods, focuses on the positive impact of dietary behaviors such as a high consumption of red wine and food diversity [4]. Since the confirmation of its presence in red wine in the early 1990s, the effects of resveratrol on health-related issues have been widely studied by the scientific community. Previous studies have reported on the positive effects of RES in the realms of cancer prevention [5], cardiovascular disease prevention [6], glucose homeostasis [7], neurodegenerative diseases [8], and longevity due to its anti-oxidation, anti-inflammation, and calorie restriction mimetic qualities [9]. Resistance exercise (weight training) is a form of exercise that improves muscular strength/endurance by using the practitioner's bodyweight, weighted barbells, dumbbells and elastic bands as resistance for muscles.

Resistance exercise contributes many factors, including mechanical tension, muscle damage, and metabolic stress to mediate the hypertrophic process in exercise-induced muscle growth/hypertrophy [10]. Age-related muscle loss is an important health issue. Individuals lose an average of 3% to 8% of their muscle mass per decade, and this rate increases significantly after 70 years of age [11,12]. However, although the literature has emphasized the beneficial effects of aerobic activity, little encouragement has been offered for resistance training. Recently, resistance exercise has been shown to have positive effects on functional improvements and disease prevention, including muscle growth, resting metabolism recharging, body compositions, elderly physical function, chronic metabolic disease, and mental health [13,14]. Athletes in different activity areas were asked to incorporate resistance exercise into their regular training regimens and the before-after effects on performance and injury incidence were evaluated [15]. A position statement on resistance training in a youth population addressing technical skill and competency was developed that promoted the performance of a variety of resistance training exercises at appropriate intensities and volumes while providing youth an opportunity to participate in programs that are safe and effective [16].

A previous study by the present authors elucidated the beneficial effects of RES on aerobic-exercise-induced peripheral fatigue through improving physiological adaption and energy content [17]. Another report also demonstrated that RES, in combination with aerobic exercise, significantly elevated not only muscle hypertrophy but also muscle torque and power in an elderly population [18]. However, the dual effect of RES antioxidant supplementation in human studies is a well-known issue. Free radical production during exercise might be a necessary trigger for adaptations to exercise stimuli leading to the well-known improvements in exercise performance or exercise-induced positive effects on the metabolism. Correspondingly, reducing the increase in production of exercise-induced oxidative stress by using antioxidant supplements is now being discussed as being counterproductive and even preventing health-promoting effects of exercise [19]. Based on the above, RES is a widely accepted dietary supplement and resistance exercise is an increasingly accepted form of exercise with health-promotion and functional benefits. However, few studies have addressed the effects of RES supplementation in combination with anaerobic exercise and resistance training. Thus, the purpose of this study was to determine the effects of a 4-week resistance exercise program combined with RES on functional performance, physiological adaption, muscular hypertrophy, and safety.

2. Materials and Methods

2.1. Materials

The nutraceutical ingredient trans-resveratrol (>98%) used in this study was purchased from Vitacost (Boca Raton, FL, USA), shown in Figure 1A, and the resistance exercise program used was adapted from a program used in a previous study [20]. The exercise equipment was about 100 cm in height with variable angles (30–85 degrees) to adjust the intensity of protocol. The ladder was modified to use a 1 cm^2 stainless net in order to avoid climbing arrest if a load became stuck into the ladder gaps, shown in Figure 1B, and a screw washer was used to increase the load according to the bodyweight of each animal for appropriate adjustment of intensity.

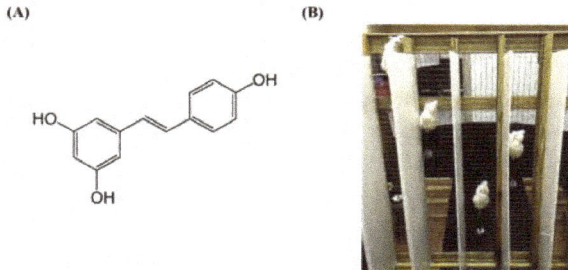

Figure 1. The structure of resveratrol (**A**) and the climbing device (**B**) for resistance training.

2.2. Animals and Experiment Design

Male ICR mice (6 weeks old, SPF grade) from BioLASCO Taiwan (Yi-Lan, Taiwan) were used in this animal study. These mice were familiarized with the ladder equipment and acclimatized to the environment and dietary differences during the 1-week period immediately prior to the training protocol. All animals were given a standard laboratory diet #5001 (PMI Nutrition International, MO, USA) and distilled water ad libitum, and maintained in stable photoperiod, temperature, and humidity conditions (12-h light/12-h dark cycle, 24 ± 2 °C, and 55–65%, respectively) during the experiment. The Institutional Animal Care and Use Committee (IACUC) of National Taiwan Sport University inspected all of the animal experiments in this study and the study conformed to the IACUC-10604 protocol guidelines approved by the IACUC ethics committee.

The recommended resveratrol dosage of 25 mg/kg bodyweight, which was applied to our previous exercise fatigue study [17], was administrated by oral gavage for 4 consecutive weeks. The two-way experiment (Training × Resveratrol) was designed for 4 groups (*n* = 10/group) to figure out the main effects and interactions on physiological assessments. The detailed experimental procedure is illustrated in Figure 2A. The weight, dietary, and social behaviors were monitored during the supplementation period and the daily training and interventions began at a regular time. Physical fitness was assessed using direct forelimb grip strength, aerobic endurance, and anaerobic performance, including assessments of ladder-climbing time and time taken to reach exhaustion for strength and endurance parameters, respectively. The exercise-related biochemistries were immediately assessed after a fixed exercise time/intensity for physiological adaption.

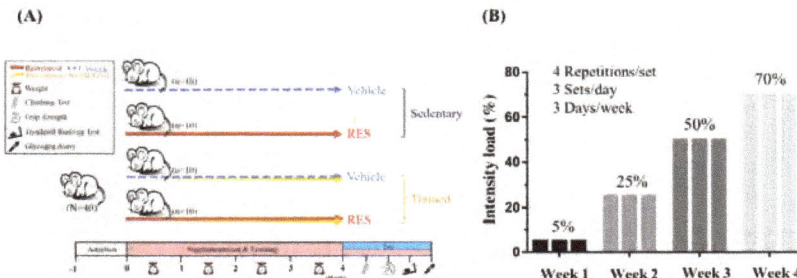

Figure 2. The experimental procedure to evaluate the effects of progressive resistance exercise and resveratrol on aerobic capacity, anaerobic capacity, physiological adaption, and safety (**A**). The incremental loading intensity applied to current training protocol (**B**).

2.3. Anaerobic Exercise Training and Capacity Test

The resistance training protocol was performed 3 days/week for 4 weeks and the indicated intensity load was adjusted by individual animal weight using the protocol, as seen in Figure 2B. In resistance training, the climbing procedures used 4 repetitions/set and 3 sets/day, with 2 min of rest provided between sets. The equipment was set into water of 5 cm in depth to provide negative stimulation in order to increase climbing motivation. Performance was evaluated as the climbing time, and the number of climbs until exhaustion was reached was used to evaluate the anaerobic performance.

2.4. Aerobic Exercise Endurance Performance Test

A motor-driven treadmill that was designed for rodents (model MK-680, Muromachi Kikai, Tokyo, Japan) was used to evaluate aerobic endurance and the electric shock grid was used to increase test motivation with veterinarian surveillance. All of the mice were initially acclimated to running on a motorized treadmill at 10 m/min, 5% grade, for 5 min/day during the week prior to the exhaustive exercise. The mice were run on the treadmill at an initial speed of 15 m/min and grade 15% for 2 min, and then every subsequent 2 min the speed was increased by 3 m/min until exhaustion [21]. Exhaustion was defined as the point at which mice maintained continuous contact with the shock grid for 5 s. Aerobic endurance capacity was expressed as time-to-exhaustion (min).

2.5. Forelimb Grip Strength

A low-force testing system (Model-RX-5, Aikoh Engineering, Nagoya, Japan) was applied to measure grip strength, as described previously [22].

2.6. Fatigue-Associated Biochemical Variables

The effect on fatigue-associated biochemical indexes, based on our previous reports [23], were slightly modified to accurately reflect the actual physiological status. The blood was sampled by submandibular blood collection immediately after 15 min of acute exercise with constant intensity, and was tested to measure glucose, lactate, blood urine nitrogen (BUN), creatine kinase (CK), and ammonia levels. The blood samples were centrifuged at $1000 \times g$ and 4 °C for 15 min after complete clotting for serum separation and analyzed using an autoanalyzer (Hitachi 7060, Hitachi, Tokyo, Japan).

2.7. Clinical Biochemical Profiles

All of the mice were euthanatized by 95% CO_2 asphyxiation one hour after the last treatment and their blood was immediately sampled via cardiac puncture. Serum was separated using centrifugation, with clinical biochemical variables, including aspartate aminotransferase (AST), alanine transaminase (ALT), creatine kinase (CK), glucose (GLU), lactate dehydrogenase (LDH), blood urea nitrogen (BUN), creatinine (CREA), uric acid (UA), albumin (ALB), triglycerides (TG), and total protein (TP), measured using an autoanalyzer (Hitachi 7060).

2.8. Body Composition and Glycogen Content Analysis

The important visceral organs, including liver, kidney, heart, lung, muscle (gastrocnemius), MT (thigh muscle), EPF (epididymal fat pad) and BAT (brown adipocyte tissue) were accurately excised and weighed after sacrifice. Then, the organs were preserved in 10% formalin for further histopathology and immunohistochemistry procedures. Part of the muscle samples were kept in liquid nitrogen for glycogen content analysis, as described previously [24].

2.9. Immunohistochemical Staining

The muscle tissues (gastrocnemius) embedded in paraffin were further analyzed to study the effects of training and resveratrol supplementation on type I and type II fibers. The primary antibodies of myosin-heavy chain fast (WB-MHCf) and myosin-heavy chain slow (WB-MHCs) were purchased from Novocastra (Leica Biosystem, Wetzlar, Germany) and applied in order to distinguish the fiber types. The epitope of MHCf and MHCs was retrieved using ER2 retrieval solution (AR9640, Leica Biosystem, Wetzlar, Germany), followed by primary incubation. The detection kits (Bond Polymer Refine Detection & Bond Polymer Refine Red Detection) used an automated BondMax double staining system. Finally, the results were examined by a veterinary pathologist under a light microscope that was equipped with a CCD camera (BX-51, Olympus, Tokyo, Japan).

2.10. Histopathology

The visceral organs preserved in 10% formalin were trimmed to provide tissue sections of 4 µm thickness, which were then embedded in paraffin. Tissue sections were further stained with hematoxylin and eosin (H&E) and examined by a veterinary pathologist under the abovementioned CCD-camera-enabled light microscope (BX-51, Olympus, Tokyo, Japan).

2.11. Statistical Analysis

The data were represented as mean $\pm$ standard error of mean (SEM). Two-way analysis of variance (resistance training $\times$ resveratrol supplementation) was used to analyze the statistical differences among the groups in terms of physical activity, biochemistry, body composition, diet, and glycogen content to verify the main and interaction effects by SPSS v19.0 analysis. Eta-square (η^2) is an effect size measurement for the analysis of variance (ANOVA). It measures the strength of the effect on a continuous field. Data were considered statistically significant when the probability of a type I error was <0.05.

3. Results

3.1. The Effects of Climb Training and Resveratrol on Grip Strength

In terms of forelimb absolute grip strength, as seen in Figure 3A, the climb training (Trained) + vehicle (Veh) and Trained + Res groups increased grip strength, as compared to the untrained groups, (Sedentary, Sed) + Veh and Sed + RES, with the main effect of climb training (F (1,36) = 41.96, P < 0.0001, eta = 0.538) and the effect of climb training on grip strength significantly increasing the grip strength of training groups as compared to sedentary groups. In addition, RES supplementation significantly increased the grip strength (F (1,36) = 25.2, P < 0.0001, eta = 0.412). Therefore, the Trained + RES group had significantly higher grip strength than the Sed + RES group, with a significant interaction effect (F (1,36) = 25.2, P = 0.048, eta = 0.150). A previous study found grip strength to correlate positively with anthropometric factors such as age, weight, and body mass index [25]. The similar analytic trends found in this study may further validate the results of grip strength adjusted to individual bodyweight, as seen in Figure 3B.

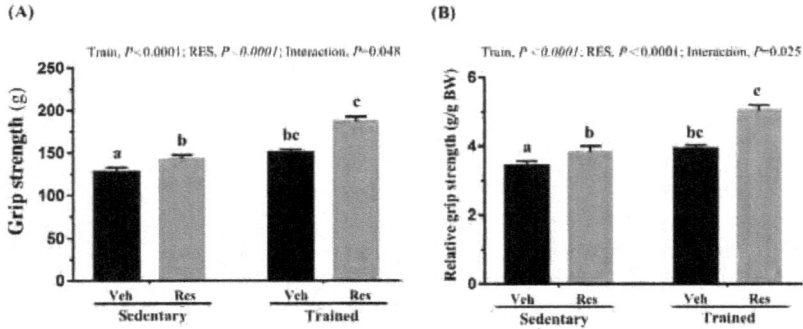

Figure 3. climb training (Trained) and/or resveratrol (RES) supplementation on absolute forelimb grip strength (**A**) and forelimb grip strength (%) relative to bodyweight (**B**). Data are mean ± SEM for $n = 10$ mice per group. Columns with different superscript letters (a, b, c) are significantly different at $p < 0.05$. The abbreviations Veh and RES represented the vehicle and resveratrol supplement, respectively.

3.2. The Effects of Climb Training and Resveratrol on Anaerobic Exercise Performance

Speed and anaerobic endurance performance were used to assess the indexes of anaerobic exercise performance. In terms of speed performance, as seen in Figure 4A, the climb training and RES supplementation significantly improved the time performance (climb training: $F (1,36) = 6.39$, $P = 0.016$, eta $= 0.151$; RES supplementation: $F (1,36) = 24.85$, $P < 0.0001$, eta $= 0.408$). However, the interaction effect did not show a significant difference ($F (1,36) = 3.61$, $P = 0.065$, eta $= 0.091$) even though the time performance of the Trained + RES group was significantly better than Sed + RES group ($P < 0.05$). In terms of anaerobic endurance capacity, the exhaustion times for repetitive climbing were also evaluated as shown in Figure 4B. The main effects of climb training and RES demonstrated significant differences (climb training: $F (1,36) = 6.19$, $P = 0.018$, eta $= 0.147$; RES supplementation: $F (1,36) = 15.1$, $P = 0.0004$, eta $= 0.296$). The Trained + RES group was significantly higher than the Sed + RES group, with a significant interaction effect ($F (1,36) = 17.21$, $P = 0.0002$, eta $= 0.323$).

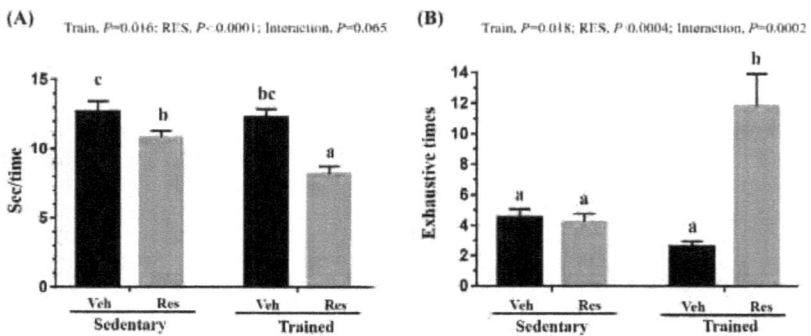

Figure 4. Effect of climb training (Trained) and/or resveratrol (RES) supplementation on anaerobic endurance performance, including time for each climbing (**A**) and exhaustion times for climbing (**B**). Data are mean ± SEM for $n = 10$ mice per group and the columns with different superscript letters (a, b, c) are significantly different at $P < 0.05$. The abbreviations Veh and RES represented the vehicle and resveratrol supplement, respectively.

3.3. The Effects of Climb Training and Resveratrol on Aerobic Exercise Performance

The treadmill test has been applied widely to assess cardiorespiratory ability (VO$_2$ max) and aerobic endurance capacity. In the exhaustive running test, shown in Figure 5, a significant difference was observed for the main effects of both training and RES (F (1,36) = 74.03, P < 0.0001, eta = 0.673 and F (1,36) = 21.73, P < 0.0001, eta = 0.376, respectively). The Sed + RES group and Trained + RES group were significantly higher than the Sed + Veh group and Trained + Veh group, respectively, although the training combined with RES treatment (Trained + RES group) did not show synergistic effects due to the lack of a significant interaction effect (F (1,36) = 1.78, P = 0.19, eta = 0.047).

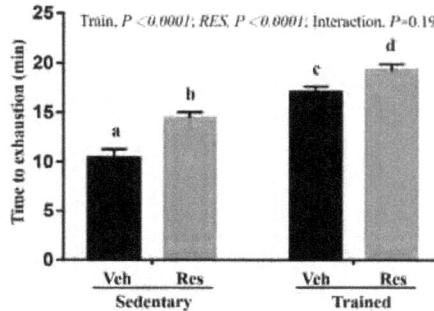

Figure 5. Effect of climb training (Trained) and/or resveratrol (RES) supplementation on aerobic endurance performance. Data are mean ± SEM for n = 10 mice per group and the columns with different superscript letters (a, b, c, d) are significantly different at P < 0.05. The abbreviations Veh and RES represented the vehicle and resveratrol supplement, respectively.

3.4. The Effects of Climb Training and Resveratrol on Fatigue-Associated Biochemistries

Table 1 shows the results of the assessment of the fatigue-associated indexes, including GLU, Lactate, BUN, CK and NH_3, that was conducted immediately after 15 min of acute exercise. No significant differences in GLU, BUN, or CK were observed among the 4 indicated groups discounting the main and interaction effects. In terms of lactate levels, the exercise training groups had significantly lower levels than the sedentary groups, with the main effect of exercise training (P = 0.0035) and RES supplement identified as the significant main effect (P < 0.0001). The interaction effect for training and supplementation was significant after the 4-week resistance training program. In addition, ammonia levels exhibited a significant difference in the supplement's main effect (P = 0.0075) but not in the main effect of training or interaction effect (P = 0.69 and 0.14, respectively).

Table 1. Effects of climb training (Trained) and/or resveratrol (RES) on fatigue-related biochemical assessments of serum after acute exercise.

					F Values for Two-Way ANOVA		
Parameter	Sed + Vehicle	Sed + RES	Train + Vehicle	Train + RES	Main Effect of RES	Main Effect of Climb	Interaction (RES × Climb)
GLU (mg/dL)	103 ± 5	116 ± 11	124 ± 9	123 ± 11	0.45	2.16	0.5
LACT (mmol/L)	4.9 ± 0.2 [b]	4.5 ± 0.2 [b]	4.7 ± 0.2 [b]	3.5 ± 0.2 [a]	19.84 *	9.79 *	4.77 *
BUN (mg/dL)	25.8 ± 0.8	23.9 ± 0.6	23.7 ± 1	23.9 ± 1	0.95	1.44	1.5
CK (U/L)	395 ± 65	349 ± 62	459 ± 73	364 ± 52	1.03	0.47	0.1
NH_3 (umol/L)	97 ± 46 [a,b]	90 ± 78 [a]	106 ± 28 [b]	85 ± 59 [a]	8.02 *	0.16	2.24

Values are the mean ± SEM for n = 10 mice in each group. Values in the same line with different superscripts letters (a, b) differ significantly; *: P < 0.05 by two-way analysis of variance (ANOVA). GLU: glucose; LACT: lactate; BUN: blood urine nitrogen; CK: creatine kinase; NH_3: ammonia.

3.5. The Effects of Climb Training and Resveratrol on Clinical Biochemistries

The serum was further analyzed at the end of the experiment for related clinical biochemistries, as seen in Table 2. No significant differences in main and interaction effects were identified on AST, TG, CK, LDH, BUN, Creatinine, ALB, TP, and GLU indexes and the indicated groups did not differ significantly. The ALT index showed significant differences in RES main effect (P = 0.008), with this effect significantly higher in the Sed + RES and Trained + RES groups than the Sed + Veh and Trained

+ Veh groups. However, the main effects and interaction effects of training were not significantly different. Besides, the UA index differed significantly not only in terms of the main effect of training but also in terms of the main effect of RES, with significantly higher effects in the Sed + RES and Trained + RES groups than the Sed + Veh and Trained + Veh groups but no significant differences in terms of the interaction effect ($P = 0.726$).

Table 2. Effects of climb training (Trained) and/or resveratrol (RES) on biochemical assessments of serum at the end of the experiment.

					F Values for Two-Way ANOVA		
Parameter	Sed + Vehicle	Sed + RES	Trained + Vehicle	Trained + RES	Main Effect of RES	Main Effect of Climb	Interaction (RES × Climb)
AST (U/L)	129 ± 12	149 ± 22	116 ± 8	174 ± 37	3	0.07	0.68
ALT (U/L)	44 ± 3 [a]	78 ± 12 [b]	50 ± 5 [a,b]	77 ± 17 [b]	7.9 *	0.06	0.1
TG (mg/dL)	114 ± 5	118 ± 9	124 ± 12	125 ± 9	0.06	0.81	0.02
CK (U/L)	400 ± 48	384 ± 83	360 ± 36	349 ± 61	0.05	0.4	0
LDH (U/L)	565 ± 46	672 ± 78	547 ± 28	634 ± 59	3.07	0.26	0.03
BUN (mg/dL)	24.5 ± 0.6	25.4 ± 1.1	25.8 ± 0.6	26.5 ± 1.3	0.64	1.5	0.01
CREA (mg/dL)	0.4 ± 0.01	0.4 ± 0.01	0.4 ± 0.01	0.4 ± 0.01	0	0	2
UA (mg/dL)	1.83 ± 0.14 [a]	2.91 ± 0.31 [b]	3.05 ± 0.39 [b,c]	3.90 ± 0.40 [c]	8.79 *	11.53 *	0.12
ALB (g/dL)	2.7 ± 0.1	2.7 ± 0.1	2.8 ± 0.1	2.8 ± 0.1	0.66	0.27	0.14
TP (g/dL)	5.4 ± 0.1	5.4 ± 0.1	5.5 ± 0.1	5.4 ± 0.1	0.67	0.05	0.12
GLU	148 ± 8	142 ± 10	157 ± 10	143 ± 6	1.34	0.28	0.25

Values are the mean ± SEM for $n = 10$ mice in each group. Values in the same line with different superscripts letters (a, b, c) differ significantly; *: $P < 0.05$ by two-way analysis of variance (ANOVA). Sed and Trained refer to the sedentary and climbing intervention, respectively. AST, aspartate aminotransferase; ALT, alanine aminotransferase; ALB, albumin; LDH, lactate dehydrogenase; TP, total protein; BUN, blood urea nitrogen; CREA, creatine; UA, uric acid; TG, triacylglycerol; GLU, glucose.

3.6. The Effects of Climb Training and Resveratrol on Tissue Glycogen Contents

Glycogen is primarily stored in the liver and muscle tissues for the purpose of energy homeostasis and demands. In terms of liver glycogen content, as seen in Figure 6A, the climb training regimen increased the liver glycogen content in the trained groups to a level significantly higher than that in the untrained groups ($F (1,36) = 19.05$, $P < 0.0001$, eta = 0.346). In terms of RES effects, the main effect of RES supplementation was not significant ($F (1,36) = 3.39$, $P = 0.074$, eta = 0.086). Furthermore, the synergistic effects of training and RES supplementation was not significant due to the lack of a significant interaction effect ($F (1,36) = 0.54$, $P = 0.47$). In terms of muscular glycogen content, shown in Figure 6B, while a significant main effect was not supported for RES supplementation ($F (1,36) = 0.58$, $P = 0.45$, eta = 0.016), it was supported for the training ($F (1,36) = 5.16$, $P = 0.029$, eta = 0.125). In addition, the synergistic effects of training and RES supplement were not significant due to the lack of a significant interaction effect ($F (1,36) = 0.4$, $P = 0.53$).

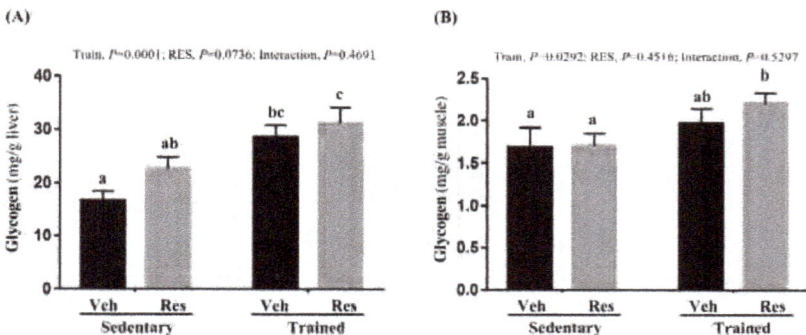

Figure 6. Effect of climb training (Trained) and/or resveratrol (RES) supplementation on hepatic (**A**) and muscle (**B**) glycogen level. Data are mean ± SEM for $n = 10$ mice per group. Bars with different superscript letters (a, b, c) are significantly different at $P < 0.05$. The abbreviations Veh and RES represented the vehicle and resveratrol supplement, respectively.

3.7. The Effects of Climb Training and Resveratrol on Growth and Body Composition

The growth curve over the duration of climb training did not significantly differ between the groups without main and interaction effects, as seen in Table 3. In terms of dietary data, the significant main and interaction effects of training were found in food and water consumption, with the Trained + Veh and Sed + RES groups significantly higher than the Sed + Veh group in this category ($P < 0.05$). Body composition variables, including liver, muscle, heart, lung, kidney, epididymal fat pad (EFP), and BAT, did not differ significantly between the groups without significant main and interaction effects. Remarkably, the thigh muscle (MT) showed a significant training main effect ($P = 0.035$), with the training groups earning significantly higher scores than the sedentary group. The percentage of organ and tissue weight, adjusted by individual weight, also exhibited the same analytic results (data not shown).

Table 3. General characteristics of the experimental groups.

Characteristic	Sed + Vehicle	Sed + RES	Trained + Vehicle	Trained + RES	Main Effect of RES	Main Effect of Climb	Interaction (RES × Climb)
					F Values for Two-Way ANOVA		
Initial BW (g)	31.0 ± 0.3	30.4 ± 0.3	30.3 ± 0.2	30.7 ± 0.4	—	—	—
Final BW (g)	38.5 ± 0.4	37.7 ± 0.6	38.4 ± 0.6	38.5 ± 0.6	0.16	0.21	0.31
Food intake (g/day)	7.28 ± 0.2 [a]	7.84 ± 0.2 [c]	7.6 ± 0.2 [b]	7.2 ± 0.2 [a]	0.46	5.6*	44.69 *
Water intake (mL/day)	9.5 ± 0.3 [a]	10.14 ± 0.2 [b]	10.73 ± 0.2 [c]	10.64 ± 0.2 [c]	7.9 *	77.81 *	14.27 *
Liver (g)	2.04 ± 0.17	2.04 ± 0.16	2.15 ± 0.12	2.10 ± 0.16	0.1	1.31	0.17
Muscle (g)	0.38 ± 0.05	0.36 ± 0.06	0.38 ± 0.05	0.39 ± 0.07	1.25	0.77	0.52
MT (g)	0.46 ± 0.02 [a]	0.48 ± 0.02 [a,b]	0.51 ± 0.02 [b,c]	0.53 ± 0.02 [c]	0.822	10.1 *	0.01
Heart (g)	0.17 ± 0.04	0.18 ± 0.04	0.18 ± 0.05	0.18 ± 0.04	0.56	0.2	0.2
Lung (g)	0.26 ± 0.07	0.23 ± 0.07	0.24 ± 0.05	0.23 ± 0.06	1.25	0.77	0.52
Kidney (g)	0.68 ± 0.06	0.67 ± 0.07	0.68 ± 0.07	0.68 ± 0.08	0.46	0.03	0.03
EFP (g)	0.39 ± 0.11	0.35 ± 0.14	0.39 ± 0.12	0.34 ± 0.12	0.98	0	0.01
BAT (g)	0.11 ± 0.04	0.10 ± 0.06	0.10 ± 0.04	0.16 ± 0.13	0.48	1	1.22

Values in the same line with different superscripts letters (a, b, c) differ significantly; *: $P < 0.05$ by two-way analysis of variance (ANOVA). Sed and Trained refer to the sedentary and climbing intervention, respectively. Muscle: gastrocnemius and soleus muscles; MT: muscle of thigh; EFP: epididymal fat pad; BAT: brown adipocyte tissue; RES: resveratrol.

3.8. The Effects of Climb Training and Resveratrol on Histological Observation

Figure 7 shows the results of the inspections of different tissues (liver, muscle, heart, kidney, and fat pad) for potential pathological changes with programmed training and resveratrol supplementation. The arrangement of sinusoid and hepatic cords in the liver showed no changes after the indicated treatments. In addition, Zenker's degeneration and hyperplasia were not observed in the skeletal muscles or cardiomyocytes, and the structure of the renal tubules and glomeruli did not differ between the treatment groups. The white adipose tissue (WAT) was composed of adipocytes, which are very large cells that have small, uniform nuclei and are usually located near the plasma membrane. Most of the cytoplasm in mice is occupied by a large lipid drop, which was found to be empty in most of the histological slides because fat was removed during the histological process. The cellular size of brown adipocytes (BAT) is usually smaller than that of white adipocytes. These morphologic differences may be because the cytoplasm is distributed with small, fatty droplets. Moreover, the nucleus is circular and located at the center of the cell.

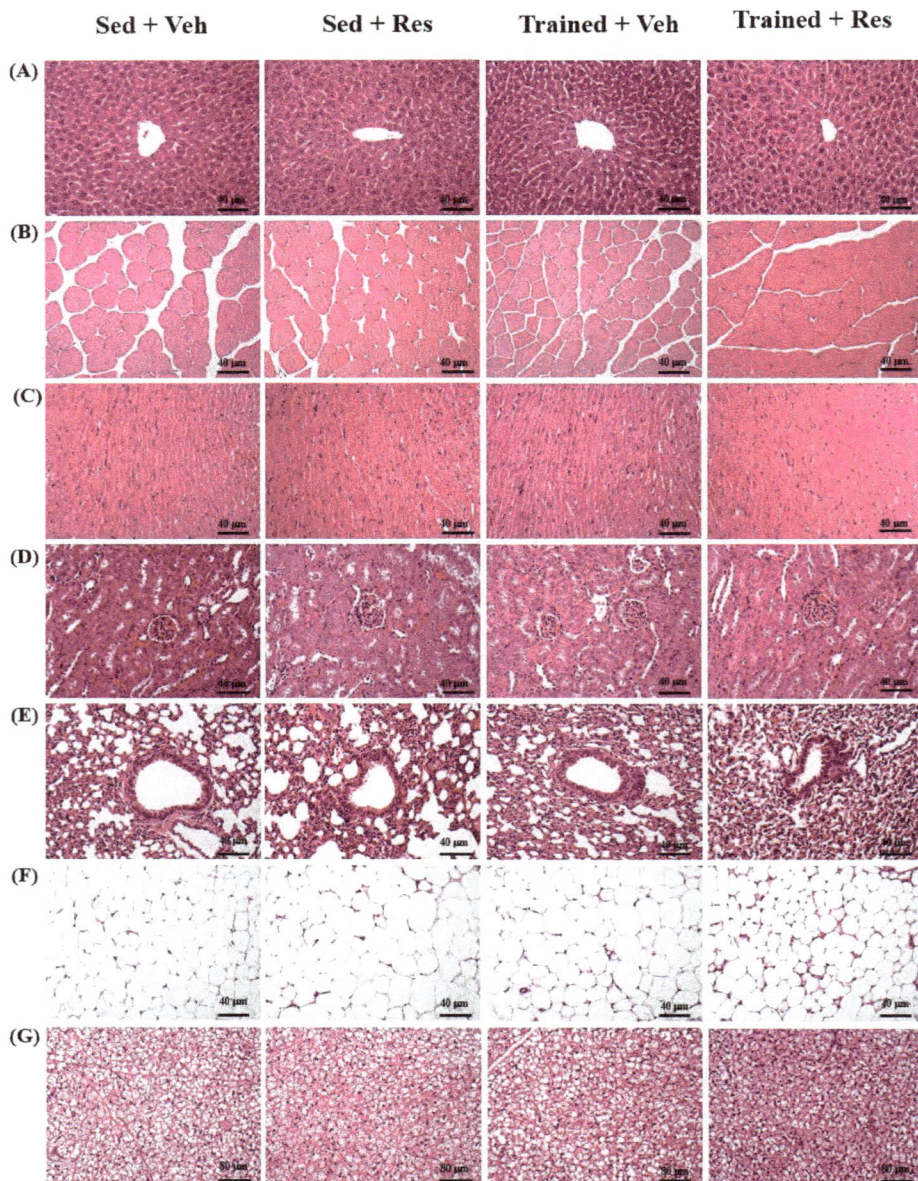

Figure 7. Effect of climb training (Trained) and/or resveratrol (RES) supplementation on the morphology of (**A**) liver; (**B**) skeletal muscle; (**C**) heart; (**D**) kidney; and (**E**) lung (**F**) white adipose tissue (WAT) (**G**) brown adipocytes (BAT) in mice. Specimens were photographed using light microscopy. (Hematoxylin and eosin stain, magnification: 200×; scale bar, 40 or 80 μm).

3.9. The Effects of Climb Training and Resveratrol on Muscle Types and Morphology

Figure 8A shows the results of further analysis of the type I and type II fiber proportions and cross section area (CSA) of the thigh muscle that was conducted to verify the effect of resistance exercise and

RES supplementation. Type I and type IIa were reddish in color, while type II was brownish in color. The proportions of muscular fiber in the different groups did not differ significantly after resistance training and/or RES treatment and the cross-section area of the indicated groups showed a significant training effect, as seen in Figure 8B,C. The CSA of the Trained + RES group was significantly higher than that of other groups.

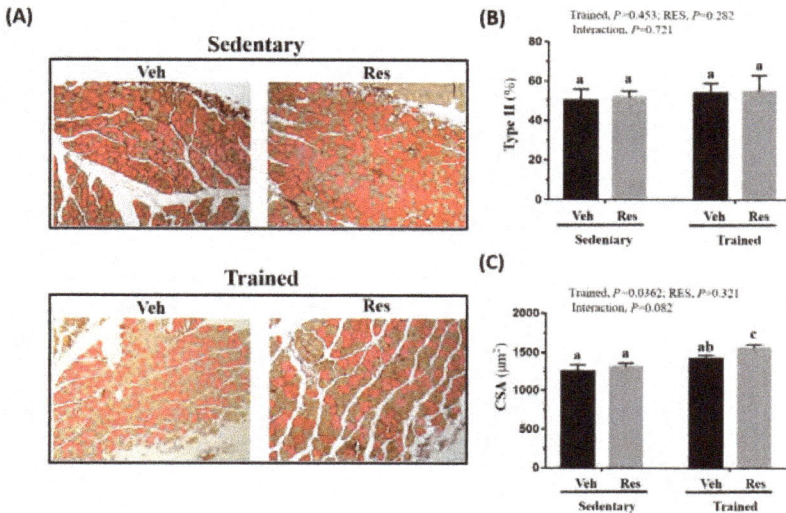

Figure 8. Effect of climb training (Trained) and/or resveratrol (RES) supplementation on the muscle of thigh with IHC staining (**A**), muscular type proportions (**B**), and cross section area (CSA) (**C**). Specimens were photographed under a light microscope. (Hematoxylin and eosin stain, magnification: 200×; scale bar, 40 μm). Bars with different superscript letters (a, b, c) are significantly different at $P < 0.05$. The abbreviations Veh and RES represented the vehicle and resveratrol supplement, respectively.

4. Discussion

In this study, RES and programmed resistance exercise elevated the aerobic endurance effectively over the 4-week intervention, possibly due to the modulation of lactate metabolite and glycogen content, which is a finding consistent with previous studies [17,26]. The resistance training was shown to improve strength and muscular hypertrophy, while the RES, in combination with the 4-week resistance training program, demonstrated a significantly synergistic increase not only in terms of anaerobic performance and endurance but also of the exercise-induced lactate production for better physiological adaption. The treatments of RES, programmed resistance training, and combination also elucidated the safety with growth curve, biochemistries, and histopathology.

Although aerobic capacity may be improved using traditional, low-intensity endurance training, or high-intensity resistance, circuit-based training also demonstrated a significantly positive effect on aerobic performance [27]. The data collected for this study, shown in Figure 5, demonstrated that a combination of RES supplementation and resistance training could significantly improve aerobic performance with respective main effects via a treadmill platform. This finding is consistent with previous studies regarding the effects of resistance exercise on cardiopulmonary fitness and the RES anti-fatigue effect [17], but no interaction effect was observed in the present result. In addition, the climb training with incremental load has been widely applied to animal studies as the resistance exercise model [28]. As shown in Figure 1B, the forelimb and pelvic limb are required to climb firmly and fight against the resistance generated by the screw washer. The elevation of grip strength was highly associated with both the resistance exercise [29] and the RES-improved ultrastructure of the myofibrils via the activating AMPK/sirt1 pathway [30]. However, this study found that RES in combination with resistance exercise demonstrated a significantly synergistic effect with the interaction effect in terms of both absolute and relative grip strength, as seen in Figure 3A,B.

Power (explosiveness) and speed endurance are important factors in the success of athletes in various sports. Resistance training has the potential to improve both strength and power as a result of hypertrophy and neural adaptations in beginner athletes, but not in advanced athletes [31]. Therefore, increasing strength increases power performance, while power training may assist in the development of endurance performance [32]. Thus, the time duration of each climb in the indicated groups permitted an assessment of muscular power capacity in a short time period due to rodent aquaphobia. In Figure 4A, RES and resistance also showed their respective main effects, while their combined effects demonstrated the significant interaction effect of the higher synergistic effect on power performance. The model of resistance exercise in this study models the concept of higher-intensity interval training for the improvement of cardiopulmonary and muscular endurance performance with similar aerobic and anaerobic adaptations [33]. Therefore, the aerobic performance, shown in Figure 5, and anaerobic endurance, shown in Figure 4B, may be explained as the main effect of training and possible interaction effect, respectively, in this study.

Different muscle groups may be involved in specific physical movements, as resistance exercise is known to induce muscle hypertrophy. The muscle groups that were involved in the exercise regimen in this study included the quadriceps, biceps femoris, gluteus maximus, and gastrocnemius muscles for functional movement, like climbing stairs or squats. The ladder-climbing animal model simulates the muscle hypertrophy in leg muscle groups caused by resistance exercise, especially with programmed weight loads. In previous studies, progressive resistance exercise was shown to induce muscle hypertrophy in the cross-section area [28] and tissue weight [34] in the rodent animal model. The results of this study found a significant difference in terms of the main effect of training, which means that resistance training contributed to hypertrophy in the muscle of thigh, as shown in Table 3. Moreover, analysis of the immunohistochemical staining and cross section area (CSA) on the muscle of thigh showed a significant increase in the CSA with the main effect of training but without an interaction effect, as shown in Figure 8. This result may directly explain the possible functional increase on grip strength and anaerobic performance.

The effects of the interventions were evaluated using the exercise-associated metabolites and energy content to infer physiological adaption. Lactate, which relates positively to exercise duration and intensity, releases hydrogen ions, which have potentially deleterious effects on metabolism and on the release of calcium during muscular contractions [35], eventually contributing to the sensation of fatigue. Previous reports have found that HIIT training improves insulin sensitivity and glycogen content [36]. In addition, resveratrol is known to improve insulin sensitivity and to mimic the effects of calorie restriction in terms of reducing blood glucose levels, insulin levels, and insulin like growth factor-1 (IGF-1) via the activation of the longevity gene SirT1 [37]. Furthermore, the resveratrol affects upregulated mitochondrial function and aerobic capacity through the activation of muscle SirT1 and PGC alpha [38]. Therefore, the aerobic capacity during the treadmill test may be elucidated by the possible effects of resveratrol and training. On the other hand, although the administrative dose of RES 25 mg/kg did not elevate the glycogen content, which was consistent with our previous report [17], the glycogen content of training combined with RES was significantly higher than in the other groups with the main effects of training in this study, as seen in Figure 6. The content and availability of glycogen have a critical effect on the anaerobic capacity of type II muscle fiber, as shown in the climbing test in Figure 4. However, while the proportions of muscular type were not significantly altered in the current intervention, the training combined with RES supplement was significantly higher than other indicated groups with the main effects of training as shown in Figure 8B,C.

This study presumed that the synergistic effects of resistance exercise combined with resveratrol supplement could not be observed in terms of aerobic performance, muscular fiber compositions, and muscular hypertrophy. Thus the two issues of resveratrol bioavailability and resistance exercise protocol should be examined further in order to understand their combinational benefits and mechanisms. The oral bioavailability of resveratrol in humans is quite limited, but may be increased significantly without any treatment-related adverse effects through the use of a liquid micellar formulation [39]. The dose in current animal studies could be further converted to human dose according to the conversion factor of 12.3-fold by body surface area difference, suggested by US Food and Drug Administration [40]. Before the clinical trial, we will test the resveratrol pharmacokinetics for bioavailability with different formulation. The preferred subject would be a non-athlete to avoid the training effects, and the programmed resistance training would be intervened with optimized resveratrol formulation supplement. In addition, the body composition, muscular strength, power, aerobic, and anaerobic capacities would be assessed for functional and physiological validation.

5. Conclusions

Exercise duration and loading intensity may be elevated further for better physiological adaptions. Therefore, there may be value in further studying the potential molecular mechanisms that underlie these combinational effects. In terms of practical applications, people have limited time for exercise. Therefore, effective and efficient methods of exercise are particularly appropriate for promoting public fitness and health. This study supports the hypothesis that resistance exercise in combination with resveratrol supplementation effectively induces muscular hypertrophy, physiological adaption, aerobic, and anaerobic performance.

Author Contributions: W.-C.H., and C.-C.H. designed the experiments. N.-W.K., M.-C.L., Y.-T.T. and C.-C.C. carried out the laboratory experiments. N.-W.K. and C.-C.H. contributed reagents, materials, and analysis platforms. N.-W.K. and Y.-T.T. analyzed the data. W.-C.H. and C.-C.H. interpreted the results, prepared the Figures, wrote the manuscript, and revised the manuscript. We also appreciate Jeff Miller for editing the manuscript.

Funding: This study was financially supported by the Ministry of Science and Technology in Taiwan (grant no. MOST 107-2410-H-227-007).

Acknowledgments: The authors are grateful to graduate students at the Sport Nutrition Laboratory, National Taiwan Sport University, for their technical assistance in conducting animal experiments.

Conflicts of Interest: The authors declare no conflict of interest.

References

1. Kulkarni, S.S.; Cantó, C. The molecular targets of resveratrol. *Biochim. Biophys. Acta* **2015**, *1852*, 1114–1123. [CrossRef] [PubMed]
2. Sales, J.M.; Resurreccion, A.V. Resveratrol in peanuts. *Crit. Rev. Food. Sci. Nutr.* **2014**, *54*, 734–770. [CrossRef] [PubMed]
3. Romero-Pérez, A.I.; Ibern-Gómez, M.; Lamuela-Raventós, R.M.; de La Torre-Boronat, M.C. Piceid, the major resveratrol derivative in grape juices. *J. Agric. Food Chem.* **1999**, *47*, 1533–1536. [CrossRef] [PubMed]
4. Biagi, M.; Bertelli, A.A. Wine, alcohol and pills: What future for the French paradox? *Life Sci.* **2015**, *131*, 19–22. [CrossRef] [PubMed]
5. Zheng, X.; Jia, B.; Song, X.; Kong, Q.Y.; Wu, M.L.; Qiu, Z.W.; Li, H.; Liu, J. Preventive Potential of Resveratrol in Carcinogen-Induced Rat Thyroid Tumorigenesis. *Nutrients* **2018**, *10*, 279. [CrossRef] [PubMed]
6. Marques, B.C.A.A.; Trindade, M.; Aquino, J.C.F.; Cunha, A.R.; Gismondi, R.O.; Neves, M.F.; Oigman, W. Beneficial effects of acute trans-resveratrol supplementation in treated hypertensive patients with endothelial dysfunction. *Clin. Exp. Hypertens.* **2018**, *40*, 218–223. [CrossRef] [PubMed]
7. Chen, S.; Zhao, Z.; Ke, L.; Li, Z.; Li, W.; Zhang, Z.; Zhou, Y.; Feng, X.; Zhu, W. Resveratrol improves glucose uptake in insulin-resistant adipocytes via Sirt1. *J. Nutr. Biochem.* **2018**, *55*, 209–218. [CrossRef] [PubMed]
8. Peñalver, P.; Belmonte-Reche, E.; Adán, N.; Caro, M.; Mateos-Martín, M.L.; Delgado, M.; González-Rey, E.; Morales, J.C. Alkylated resveratrol prodrugs and metabolites as potential therapeutics for neurodegenerative diseases. *Eur. J. Med. Chem.* **2018**, *146*, 123–138. [CrossRef] [PubMed]
9. Li, Y.R.; Li, S.; Lin, C.C. Effect of resveratrol and pterostilbene on aging and longevity. *Biofactors* **2018**, *44*, 69–82. [CrossRef] [PubMed]

10. Schoenfeld, B.J. The mechanisms of muscle hypertrophy and their application to resistance training. *J. Strength Cond. Res.* **2010**, *24*, 2857–2872. [CrossRef] [PubMed]

11. Flack, K.D.; Davy, K.P.; Hulver, M.W.; Winett, R.A.; Frisard, M.I.; Davy, B.M. Aging, resistance training, and diabetes prevention. *J. Aging Res.* **2010**, *2011*, 127315. [CrossRef] [PubMed]

12. Siparsky, P.N.; Kirkendall, D.T.; Garrett, W.E. Muscle Changes in Aging: Understanding Sarcopenia. *Sports Health* **2014**, *6*, 36–40. [CrossRef] [PubMed]

13. Barcelos, C.; Damas, F.; Nóbrega, S.R.; Ugrinowitsch, C.; Lixandrão, M.E.; Marcelino Eder Dos Santos, L.; Libardi, C.A. High-frequency resistance training does not promote greater muscular adaptations compared to low frequencies in young untrained men. *Eur. J. Sport Sci.* **2018**. [CrossRef] [PubMed]

14. Westcott, W.L. Resistance training is medicine: Effects of strength training on health. *Curr. Sports Med. Rep.* **2012**, *11*, 209–216. [CrossRef] [PubMed]

15. Buckner, S.L.; Jessee, M.B.; Dankel, S.J.; Mattocks, K.T.; Abe, T.; Loenneke, J.P. Resistance exercise and sports performance: The minority report. *Med. Hypotheses* **2018**, *113*, 1–5. [CrossRef] [PubMed]

16. Lloyd, R.S.; Faigenbaum, A.D.; Stone, M.H.; Oliver, J.L.; Jeffreys, I.; Moody, J.A.; Brewer, C.; Pierce, K.C.; McCambridge, T.M.; Howard, R.; et al. Position statement on youth resistance training: The 2014 International Consensus. *Br. J. Sports Med.* **2014**, *48*, 498–505. [CrossRef] [PubMed]

17. Wu, R.E.; Huang, W.C.; Liao, C.C.; Chang, Y.K.; Kan, N.W.; Huang, C.C. Resveratrol protects against physical fatigue and improves exercise performance in mice. *Molecules* **2013**, *18*, 4689–4702. [CrossRef] [PubMed]

18. Alway, S.E.; McCrory, J.L.; Kearcher, K.; Vickers, A.; Frear, B.; Gilleland, D.L.; Bonner, D.E.; Thomas, J.M.; Donley, D.A.; Lively, M.W.; et al. Resveratrol enhances exercise-Induced cellular and functional adaptations of skeletal muscle in older men and women. *J. Gerontol. A Biol. Sci. Med. Sci.* **2017**, *72*, 1595–1606. [CrossRef] [PubMed]

19. Gliemann, L.; Schmidt, J.F.; Olesen, J.; Biensø, R.S.; Peronard, S.L.; Grandjean, S.U.; Mortensen, S.P.; Nyberg, M.; Bangsbo, J.; Pilegaard, H.; et al. Resveratrol blunts the positive effects of exercise training on cardiovascular health in aged men. *J. Physiol.* **2013**, *591*, 5047–5059. [CrossRef] [PubMed]

20. Hornberger, T.A., Jr.; Farrar, R.P. Physiological hypertrophy of the FHL muscle following 8 weeks of progressive resistance exercise in the rat. *Can. J. Appl. Physiol.* **2004**, *29*, 16–31. [CrossRef] [PubMed]

21. Conover, C.A.; Bale, L.K.; Nair, K.S. Comparative gene expression and phenotype analyses of skeletal muscle from aged wild-type and PAPP-A-deficient Mice. *Exp. Gerontol.* **2016**, *80*, 36–42. [CrossRef] [PubMed]

22. Hsu, Y.J.; Huang, W.C.; Chiu, C.C.; Liu, Y.L.; Chiu, W.C.; Chiu, C.H.; Chiu, Y.S.; Huang, C.C. Capsaicin supplementation reduces physical fatigue and improves exercise performance in mice. *Nutrients* **2016**, *8*, 648. [CrossRef] [PubMed]

23. Huang, W.C.; Huang, C.C.; Chuang, H.L.; Chen, W.C.; Hsu, M.C. Cornu cervi pantotrichum supplementation improves physiological adaptions during intensive endurance training. *J. Vet. Med. Sci.* **2017**, *79*, 674–682. [CrossRef] [PubMed]

24. Hsiao, C.Y.; Chen, Y.M.; Hsu, Y.J.; Huang, C.C.; Sung, H.C.; Chen, S.S. Supplementation with Hualian No. 4 wild bitter gourd (Momordica charantia Linn. var. abbreviata ser.) extract increases anti-fatigue activities and enhances exercise performance in mice. *J. Vet. Med. Sci.* **2017**, *79*, 1110–1119. [CrossRef] [PubMed]

25. Musa, T.H.; Li, W.; Xiaoshan, L.; Guo, Y.; Wenjuan, Y.; Xuan, Y.; YuePu, P.; Pingmin, W. Association of normative values of grip strength with anthropometric variables among students, in Jiangsu Province. *Homo* **2018**, *69*, 70–76. [CrossRef] [PubMed]

26. Prestes, J.; Leite, R.D.; Pereira, G.B.; Shiguemoto, G.E.; Bernardes, C.F.; Asano, R.Y.; Sales, M.M.; Bartholomeu Neto, J.; Perez, S.E. Resistance training and glycogen content in ovariectomized rats. *Int. J. Sports Med.* **2012**, *33*, 550–554. [CrossRef] [PubMed]

27. Ramos-Campo, D.J.; Martínez-Guardado, I.; Olcina, G.; Marín-Pagán, C.; Martínez-Noguera, F.J.; Carlos-Vivas, J.; Alcaraz, P.E.; Rubio, J.Á. Effect of high-intensity resistance circuit-based training in hypoxia on aerobic performance and repeat sprint ability. *Scand. J. Med. Sci. Sports* **2018**. [CrossRef] [PubMed]

28. Hellyer, N.J.; Nokleby, J.J.; Thicke, B.M.; Zhan, W.Z.; Sieck, G.C.; Mantilla, C.B. Reduced ribosomal protein s6 phosphorylation after progressive resistance exercise in growing adolescent rats. *J. Strength Cond. Res.* **2012**, *26*, 16571666. [CrossRef] [PubMed]

29. Olvera-Soto, M.G.; Valdez-Ortiz, R.; López Alvarenga, J.C.; Espinosa-Cuevas Mde, L. Effect of resistance exercises on the indicators of muscle reserves and handgrip strength in adult patients on hemodialysis. *J. Ren. Nutr.* **2016**, *26*, 53–60. [CrossRef] [PubMed]

30. Liao, Z.Y.; Zhao, K.X.; Xiao, Q. Effect of resveratrol on forelimb grip strength and myofibril structure in aged rats. *Nan Fang Yi Ke Da Xue Xue Bao* **2017**, *37*, 1405–1409. [PubMed]

31. Wilson, G.J.; Newton, R.U.; Murphy, A.J.; Humphries, B.J. The optimal training load for the development of dynamic athletic performance. *Med. Sci. Sports Exerc.* **1993**, *25*, 1279–1286. [CrossRef] [PubMed]

32. Paavolainen, L.; Häkkinen, K.; Hämäläinen, I.; Nummela, A.; Rusko, H. Explosive-strength training improves 5-km running time by improving running economy and muscle power. *J. Appl. Physiol.* **1999**, *86*, 1527–1533. [CrossRef] [PubMed]

33. Buckley, S.; Knapp, K.; Lackie, A.; Lewry, C.; Horvey, K.; Benko, C.; Trinh, J.; Butcher, S. Multimodal high-intensity interval training increases muscle function and metabolic performance in females. *Appl. Physiol. Nutr. Metab.* **2015**, *40*, 1157–1162. [CrossRef] [PubMed]

34. Jung, S.; Ahn, N.; Kim, S.; Byun, J.; Joo, Y.; Kim, S.; Jung, Y.; Park, S.; Hwang, I.; Kim, K. The effect of ladder-climbing exercise on atrophy/hypertrophy-related myokine expression in middle-aged male Wistar rats. *J. Physiol. Sci.* **2015**, *65*, 515–521. [CrossRef] [PubMed]

35. Cairns, S.P. Lactic acid and exercise performance: Culprit or friend? *Sports Med.* **2006**, *36*, 279–291. [CrossRef] [PubMed]

36. Søgaard, D.; Lund, M.T.; Scheuer, C.M.; Dehlbaek, M.S.; Dideriksen, S.G.; Abildskov, C.V.; Christensen, K.K.; Dohlmann, T.L.; Larsen, S.; Vigelsø, A.H.; Dela, F.; et al. High-intensity interval training improves insulin sensitivity in older individuals. *Acta Physiol.* **2018**, *222*, e13009. [CrossRef] [PubMed]

37. Lekli, I.; Ray, D.; Das, D.K. Longevity nutrients resveratrol, wines and grapes. *Genes Nutr.* **2010**, *5*, 55–60. [CrossRef] [PubMed]

38. Momken, I.; Stevens, L.; Bergouignan, A.; Desplanches, D.; Rudwill, F.; Chery, I.; Zahariev, A.; Zahn, S.; Stein, T.P.; Sebedio, J.L.; et al. Resveratrol prevents the wasting disorders of mechanical unloading by acting as a physical exercise mimetic in the rat. *FASEB J.* **2011**, *25*, 3646–3660. [CrossRef] [PubMed]

39. Calvo-Castro, L.A.; Schiborr, C.; David, F.; Ehrt, H.; Voggel, J.; Sus, N.; Behnam, D.; Bosy-Westphal, A.; Frank, J. The Oral bioavailability of trans-resveratrol from a grapevine-shoot extract in healthy humans is significantly increased by micellar solubilization. *Mol. Nutr. Food Res.* **2018**, *62*, e1701057. [CrossRef] [PubMed]

40. Nair, A.B.; Jacob, S. A simple practice guide for dose conversion between animals and human. *J. Basic Clin. Pharm.* **2016**, *7*, 27–31. [CrossRef] [PubMed]

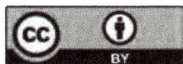

nutrients

MDPI

Article

Effect of Resveratrol, a Dietary-Derived Polyphenol, on the Oxidative Stress and Polyol Pathway in the Lens of Rats with Streptozotocin-Induced Diabetes

Lech Sedlak [1,2,*], Weronika Wojnar [3], Maria Zych [3], Dorota Wyględowska-Promieńska [1,2], Ewa Mrukwa-Kominek [1,2] and Ilona Kaczmarczyk-Sedlak [3]

[1] Department of Ophthalmology, University Clinical Center, Medical University of Silesia in Katowice, 40-514 Katowice, Poland; wpdorota@gmail.com (D.W.-P.); emrowka@poczta.onet.pl (E.M.-K.)
[2] Department of Ophthalmology, School of Medicine in Katowice, Medical University of Silesia in Katowice, 40-514 Katowice, Poland
[3] Department of Pharmacognosy and Phytochemistry, School of Pharmacy with the Division of Laboratory Medicine in Sosnowiec, Medical University of Silesia in Katowice, 41-200 Sosnowiec, Poland; wwojnar@sum.edu.pl (W.W.); mzych@sum.edu.pl (M.Z.); isedlak@sum.edu.pl (I.K.-S.)
* Correspondence: lech.sedlak@gmail.com; Tel.: +48-504-819-778

Received: 30 August 2018; Accepted: 27 September 2018; Published: 4 October 2018

Abstract: Resveratrol is found in grapes, apples, blueberries, mulberries, peanuts, pistachios, plums and red wine. Resveratrol has been shown to possess antioxidative activity and a variety of preventive effects in models of many diseases. The aim of the study was to investigate if this substance may counteract the oxidative stress and polyol pathway in the lens of diabetic rats. The study was conducted on the rats with streptozotocin-induced type 1 diabetes. After the administration of resveratrol (10 and 20 mg/kg *po* for 4 weeks), the oxidative stress markers in the lens were evaluated: activity of superoxide dismutase, catalase and glutathione peroxidase, as well as levels of total and soluble protein, level of glutathione, vitamin C, calcium, sulfhydryl group, advanced oxidation protein products, malonyldialdehyde, Total Oxidant Status and Total Antioxidant Reactivity. The obtained results indicate that the administration of resveratrol to the diabetic rats shows antioxidative properties. It is not a result of antiglycaemic activity but resveratrol probably directly affects the antioxidative system. Resveratrol did not affect the polyol pathway in the lens of diabetic rats. Our results may indirectly indicate benefits of consumption of foods as well as dietary supplements containing resveratrol in diminishing oxidative stress in lenses of individuals suffering from diabetes mellitus.

Keywords: diabetes; oxidative stress; polyol pathway; rats; resveratrol; streptozotocin; lens

1. Introduction

Resveratrol (3,4′,5-trihydroxy-stilbene) is a polyphenolic compound discovered in 1939. The first part of its name 'res' means that this compound is a derivative of resorcinol (benzene-1,3-diol) and the 'veratrol' part indicates the white hellebore—*Veratrum grandiflorum* (Maxim. ex Miq.) O.Loes.—the plant in which roots resveratrol was found for the first time. Resveratrol occurs in many plants such as apples, blueberries, mulberries, peanuts, pistachios, plums, raspberries and soy. The highest concentrations of this stilbene were found in the dried roots and rhizomes of Japanese knotweed—*Reynoutria japonica* Houtt. synonyms *Fallopia japonica* (Houtt.) Ronse Decr., *Polygonum cuspidatum* Siebold & Zucc.—which are used in a form of tea in Traditional Chinese Medicine. In Europe, its main sources are dark varieties of grapes (*Vitis vinifera* L.) and red wines, containing roughly 3- to 10-fold more resveratrol than white grape varieties or white wines. Resveratrol can be synthesized in larger amounts by plants in response to pathogens and abiotic stress [1].

It has been shown, in both experimental and clinical studies, that resveratrol reveals many beneficial effects. It may prevent cardiovascular diseases, neurological disorders, diabetes, obesity, non-alcoholic fatty liver disease, lung dysfunction in asthma, aging and cancer. Moreover, it also has a favourable effect on bone homeostasis and skeletal muscle atrophy [1,2]. There are also reports describing the potential role of resveratrol in prevention or treatment of some ocular impairments such as age-related macular degeneration, cataract, glaucoma, diabetic retinopathy, thyroid eye disease or retinopathy of prematurity. It may also inhibit the growth of uveal melanoma or retinoblastoma. The positive effect of this stilbene on the eye structures is connected mostly with its anti-oxidative, anti-apoptotic, anti-inflammatory, anti-angiogenic and vasodilatative activities [3–12].

The scientific literature indicates that there is a link between diabetes mellitus, oxidative stress and cataract formation. Long-term hyperglycaemia leads to overproduction of reactive oxygen species (ROS) in mitochondria and in results in the imbalance between ROS and endogenous defence mechanisms. Protein oxidation in the lens leads to an accumulation of insoluble aggregates and light scattering by lens opacity [13–15]. In diabetic patients, there is a higher risk of cataract development than in healthy people of the same age. What is more, cataract is more likely to develop earlier in diabetic patients than in healthy people [15]. There is also a higher complication rate in diabetic patients undergoing cataract surgery [16].

Resveratrol is proven to be a potent antioxidant. Its antiradical and antioxidative activity results from its structure. Antioxidative properties of polyphenols depend mainly on the redox properties of the hydroxyl groups in phenolic moieties and the potential for electron delocalization across their chemical structure. In resveratrol's structure, there are two phenolic rings: monophenol and diphenol, while an abstraction of a hydrogen atom from monophenolic hydroxyl group occurs rather easily. Moreover, resveratrol also has three hydroxyl groups, which play important role in radical scavenging, since it was reported, that antioxidant activity increases along with the number of –OH groups. These hydroxyl groups also help resveratrol to chelate metals, which is also an important feature in the prevention of ROS generation [17].

As hyperglycaemia may result in the development of cataract via oxidative stress, it seems to be reasonable to examine, whether dietary antioxidants may be helpful in the prevention or delaying of its onset. Therefore, the main goal of this study was to investigate if resveratrol administered orally at the doses of 10 and 20 mg/kg affects oxidative-stress related changes in the lens of diabetic rats.

2. Materials and Methods

2.1. Experiment Design, Animals and Diabetes Induction

The study was conducted with the approval of the Local Ethics Committee in Katowice, Poland (approval no. 36/2015).

Mature (3-month-old) Wistar male rats were provided by the Centre of Experimental Medicine at the Medical University of Silesia. The rats were divided into 4 experimental groups (n = 8–9): C—control, healthy rats, D—control diabetic rats, D+R10—diabetic rats treated orally with resveratrol at a dose of 10 mg/kg and D+R20—diabetic rats treated orally with resveratrol at a dose of 20 mg/kg. In the D, D+R10 and D+R20 groups of rats, diabetes was induced by a single intraperitoneal injection of streptozotocin (60 mg/kg) [18,19]. Streptozotocin was prepared as a solution in 0.1 M citric buffer, pH = 4.5. The C group received a single injection only with citric buffer. 14 days after streptozotocin injection, blood glucose level was measured with the MicroDot glucometer. The rats in which blood glucose level exceeded 200 mg/dL were classified to the further stage of the experiment. Resveratrol suspension in water was administered orally for 4 weeks to the D+R10 and D+R20 groups via intragastric tube, once a day. The rats in the C and D groups received only water. To ensure the proper dose of resveratrol, the rats were weighted at the whole time of the experiment. Moreover, body mass was recorded at the day of STZ injection (initial body mass), after 2 weeks from STZ injection (start body mass) and after 4 weeks of resveratrol and water administration (final body mass). The difference between final and start body mass represents body mass gain.

After 4 weeks of resveratrol administration, the rats were euthanized by injection of ketamine + xylazine mixture and cardiac exsanguination. The collected blood was centrifuged in order to obtain the serum. In the serum, the glucose and fructosamine levels were assessed. The lenses were extracted from the eyeball, weighted, then homogenized in the PBS buffer (10% *v/w*). In the total homogenate, the total protein level and malondialdehyde level was assayed. Remaining homogenate was centrifuged (4 °C, 15 min, 10,000× *g*), the supernatant was collected, divided into parts and frozen until use.

2.2. Glucose and Fructosamine Concentration in the Serum

The assessment of serum glucose and fructosamine concentrations was carried out using the commercially available kits (Glucose kit no. 11504, Fructosamine kit no. 11043; BioSystems S.A., Barcelona, Spain).

2.3. Enzymes and Sugars Related to Polyol Pathway in the Lens

Aldose reductase (AR) activity was evaluated according to the procedure described by Patel et al.: phosphate buffer (pH 6.2) and NADPH solution were added to the lens homogenates. The reaction was initiated by addition of D,L-glyceraldehyde. The plate was read for 5 min at 340 nm [20]. Sorbitol dehydrogenase activity was analysed using QuantiChrom™ Sorbitol Dehydrogenase Assay Kit (kit no. DSDH-100; BioAssay Systems, Hayward, CA, USA). Glucose and fructose concentrations were assessed using BioSystems kits (Glucose kit no. 11504, Fructose kit no. 23794) and sorbitol concentration was measured with EnzyChrom™ Sorbitol Assay Kit (kit no. ESBT-100; BioAssay Systems).

2.4. Total and Soluble Protein in the Lens

Estimation of total and soluble protein content was carried out as described in Lowry [21]: the mixture of 2% Na_2CO_3 solution in 0.1 M NaOH, 1% $CuSO_4$ and 2% potassium-sodium tartrate was added to the aliquot of the homogenate. After 10 min, the Folin-Ciocalteu reagent was added and after 30 min of incubation, 200 μL of the mixture was transferred into the 96-well plate, then read at 750 nm. The standard curve was prepared with bovine serum albumin.

2.5. Advanced Glycation End Products and Total Sulfhydryl Groups in the Lens

Evaluation of advanced glycation end products (AGEs) content was conducted with OxiSelect™ Competitive ELISA Kit (Cell Biolabs, Inc., San Diego, CA, USA). Total sulfhydryl groups (-SH groups) content was estimated basing the protocol described by Ellmann: a phosphate buffer (pH 8.0) and DTNB reagent were added to the samples and after colour development, the reaction was read at 412 nm. Obtained results were calculated with the use of extinction coefficient = 13,600/M/cm [22].

2.6. Enzymatic Oxidative Stress Parameters in the Lens

Superoxide dismutase (SOD), catalase (CAT) and glutathione peroxidase (GPx) activity was assayed using Cayman kits (SOD kit no. 706002, CAT kit no. 707002. GPx kit no. 703102; Cayman Chemicals, Ann Arbor, MI, USA).

2.7. Non-Enzymatic Oxidative Stress Parameters Content in the Lens

Reduced glutathione (GSH) content was measured according to the method described by Sedlak and Lindsay: the homogenates 10% trichloroacetic acid was added to the homogenates in order to deprotein the samples. After centrifuging, the obtained supernatants were collected and transferred to the 96-well plate, then the phosphate buffer (pH 8.0) and 0.01 M DTNB were added. GSH standard was used as a reference. The reaction was measured at 412 nm [23]. Vitamin C level was assessed basing the Jagota and Dani method, in which trichloroacetic acid is used to deprotein the samples and acidify the reaction environment. In low pH, Folin-Ciocalteu reagent reacts specifically with vitamin C [24]. Advanced oxidation protein products (AOPP) estimation was conducted according to the protocol described by Witko-Sarsat et al. 1.16 M solution of potassium iodide and glacial acetic acid were added to the samples. The samples were read at 340 nm with chloramine-T used as a reference [25]. As a marker for lipid peroxidation malondialdehyde (MDA) was examined as described in Ohkawa et al. To the probes following reagents were added: 8.1% SDS, 20% acetic acid and 0.8% TBA. After thorough mixing, the mixture was heated for 60 min in boiling water. Afterwards, the probes were cooled and the mixture of pyridine with n-butanol was added. Probes were mixed and centrifuged at $4000\times g$ for 5 min. Obtained supernatants were transferred to the 96-well plate and measured at 532 nm with 1,1,3,3-tetraethoxypropane used as a reference [26]. Calcium level was estimated with the Pointe Sci. kit (kit no. C7503, Pointe Scientific, Canton, MI, USA).

2.8. Total Oxidant Status and Total Antioxidant Response in the Lens

Total Oxidant Status (TOS) was assayed as described by Erel: to the probes the reagent 1 (consisted of mixture of 150 μM xylenol orange, mM NaCl 140 and 1.35 M glycerol in 25 mM H_2SO_4) and reagent 2 (5 mM ferrous ion and 10 mM o-dianisidine in 25 mM H_2SO_4) were added. The first absorbance (at 560 nm and 800 nm as reference) was taken before the mixing of reagents 1 and 2 and the last absorbance was taken after 4 min of mixing probes with reagent 2. The standard curve was prepared with H_2O_2 [27]. Total Antioxidant Response (TAR) estimation was conducted following the Erel protocol: the probes were mixed with reagent 1 (10 mM o-dianisidine, 45 μM ferrous ion in the 75 mM Clark and Lubs solution, pH 1.8) and with reagent 2 (7.5 mM H_2O_2 in the Clark and Lubs solution). Similarly like in TOS method, the first absorbance (at 444 nm) was taken before the mixing of reagents 1 and 2 and the last absorbance was taken after 4 min of mixing probes with reagent 2. The standard curve was prepared with Trolox [28]. Results obtained from TOS and TAR were used to calculate the TAR/TOS ratio.

2.9. Results Analysis

All measurements were conducted in microplate reader Tecan Infinite M200 PRO with Magellan 7.2 Software. Obtained results were subjected to statistical analysis with one-way ANOVA followed with Tukey post-hoc test in Statistica 10 Software (StatSoft, Tulsa, OK, USA). All results are presented as arithmetical mean $\pm$ SEM. Results were considered statistically significant if *p*-value < 0.05.

3. Results

3.1. Effect of Resveratrol on the Body Mass and Lens Mass in Diabetic Rats

In the non-diabetic animals (C group), the initial body mass was 281.2 ± 3.8 g. After 2 weeks of the experiment, the body mass (start body mass) was 312.8 ± 5.9 g. After the following 4 weeks, the final body mass in C rats was 344.9 ± 5.5 g. In the control diabetic rats (D group), 2 weeks after the administration of streptozotocin (STZ), the body mass (start body mass) was lower ($p < 0.001$) in comparison with the result obtained in C rats. The final body mass (after a further 4 weeks) was lower ($p < 0.001$) when compared to the C rats. In the diabetic rats receiving resveratrol at a dose of 10 mg/kg (D+R10) and 20 mg/kg (D+R20), the final body mass was similar to that observed in the D rats (Table 1).

The mass of the lens in the D, D+R10 and D+R20 groups was significantly lower ($p < 0.001$) as compared to the C group. No significant changes were noted in D+R10 or D+R20 groups when compared to the D group (Table 1).

Table 1. Effect of resveratrol on the body mass, lens mass, blood glucose concentration and blood fructosamine concentration in diabetic rats.

Parameter/Group	C	D	D+R10	D+R20
Initial body mass (g)	281.2 ± 3.8	283.2 ± 6.2	282.0 ± 3.7	276.6 ± 5.5
Start body mass (g)	312.8 ± 5.9	250.2 ± 8.7 ***	239.4 ± 4.9 ***	242.8 ± 6.6 ***
Final body mass (g)	344.9 ± 5.5	228.2 ± 10.9 ***	212.2 ± 5.7 ***	228.1 ± 7.4 ***
Body mass gain (g)	32.1 ± 2.8	−22.0 ± 5.1 ***	−27.2 ± 4.9 ***	−14.7 ± 3.5 ***
Lens mass (mg)	47.2 ± 0.5	42.9 ± 1.7 ***	42.8 ± 0.4 ***	43.7 ± 0.5 ***
Glucose in the blood (mg/dL)	141.4 ± 11.0	641.9 ± 28.6 ***	613.9 ± 55.5 ***	641.7 ± 51.6 ***
Fructosamine in the blood (μmol/L albumin)	275.1 ± 8.1	498.4 ± 21.3 ***	489.7 ± 19.4 ***	471.5 ± 54.7 **

C—control, non-diabetic rats; D—diabetic rats; D+R10—diabetic rats receiving resveratrol (10 mg/kg *po* for 4 weeks); D+R20—diabetic rats receiving resveratrol (20 mg/kg *po* for 4 weeks). Results are presented as means ± SEM ($n = 8$–9). ** $p < 0.01$, *** $p < 0.001$—statistically significantly different from the C group.

3.2. Effect of Resveratrol on the Blood Glucose Concentration and Blood Fructosamine Concentration

Before STZ injection, the blood glucose concentration in all groups of rats was between 103 and 141 mg/dL (below 200 mg/dL). 2 weeks after STZ injection, the blood glucose concentration in the D, D+R10 and D+R20 groups exceeded the 200 mg/dL concentration and even reached values above 600 mg/dL. After 4 weeks of resveratrol administration, there were no significant changes with regard to this parameter in the D+R10 and D+R20 groups (Table 1).

In comparison with the C rats, in the D rats an increase of the fructosamine concentration in blood ($p < 0.001$) was observed. No statistically significant changes between D+R10, D+R20 and D groups were noted (Table 1).

3.3. Effect of Resveratrol on Polyol Pathway in the Lens of the Diabetic Rats

In the D rats, the lens glucose concentration was higher ($p < 0.001$), in comparison with the C rats. In the diabetic rats receiving resveratrol, the lens glucose concentration was similar to that observed in the D rats (Table 2).

Table 2. Effect of resveratrol on polyol pathway and the advanced glycation end products (AGEs) content and sulfhydryl groups (-SH groups) content in lens in diabetic rats.

Parameter/Group	C	D	D+R10	D+R20
Glucose in the lens (mg/g lens)	0.16 ± 0.03	0.83 ± 0.07 ***	1.02 ± 1.00 ***	0.80 ± 0.07 ***
Sorbitol (μmol/g lens)	1.26 ± 0.05	30.10 ± 0.47 ***	29.42 ± 0.70 ***	30.73 ± 0.66 ***
Fructose in the lens (μmol/g lens)	0.08 ± 0.01	0.13 ± 0.01 ***	0.14 ± 0.01 ***	0.13 ± 0.01 ***
Aldose reductase (nmol/min/mg protein)	0.085 ± 0.003	0.107 ± 0.008 *	0.102 ± 0.003 **	0.109 ± 0.005 *
Sorbitol dehydrogenase (μU/mg protein)	1.94 ± 0.18	3.01 ± 0.34 *	2.33 ± 0.14	2.67 ± 0.15 *
AGEs (μg/g lens)	5.80 ± 0.12	10.17 ± 0.29 ***	10.30 ± 0.12 ***	9.94 ± 0.50 ***
-SH groups (nmol/g lens)	3.63 ± 0.13	3.09 ± 0.15	3.38 ± 0.20	3.91 ± 0.34

C—control, non-diabetic rats; D—diabetic rats; D+R10—diabetic rats receiving resveratrol (10 mg/kg *po* for 4 weeks); D+R20—diabetic rats receiving resveratrol (20 mg/kg *po* for 4 weeks). Results are presented as means ± SEM ($n = 8$–9). * $p < 0.05$, ** $p < 0.01$, *** $p < 0.001$—statistically significantly different from the C group.

The sorbitol and the fructose concentration in the lens was higher ($p < 0.001$ and $p < 0.001$, respectively) in the lens of the D rats, as compared to the C rats. No significant changes were observed in the sorbitol and fructose concentration after administration of resveratrol in diabetic rats (D+R10, D+R20 groups) when compared to the D rats (Table 2).

There was an increase of the aldose reductase activity and the sorbitol dehydrogenase activity in the lens of the D rats ($p < 0.05$) in comparison with the C rats. In the D+R10 and D+R20 groups, the activity of these enzymes was similar to those observed in the D rats (Table 2).

3.4. Effect of Resveratrol on the Advanced Glycation End Products (AGEs) Content and Sulfhydryl Group (-SH Groups) Content in the Lens of the Diabetic Rats

In comparison with the C rats, in the D rats an increase of the AGEs content in the lens was observed ($p < 0.001$). No significant changes were observed in the AGEs content after administration of resveratrol in diabetic rats (D+R10, D+R20 groups) when compared to the D rats (Table 2).

The -SH groups content in the lens of the D rats was lower, as compared to the C rats (not statistically significant). In the diabetic rats which received resveratrol (D+R10, D+R20 groups), the -SH groups content was similar to that observed in the C rats. When compared to the D group, in the D+R10 and D+R20 groups, the -SH groups content was elevated. The changes were not statistically significant (Table 2).

3.5. The Effect of Resveratrol on the Total and Soluble Protein Content in the Lens of the Diabetic Rats

No significant changes were observed in the total protein content after diabetes induction in rats (D group) as compared to the C rats. In the diabetic rats which received resveratrol (D+R10 and D+R20 groups), the total protein content was similar to that observed in the D and C rats (Table 3).

Table 3. Effect of resveratrol on the total and soluble protein content in the lens in diabetic rats.

Parameter/Group	C	D	D+R10	D+R20
Total protein (mg/g lens)	563.2 ± 33.2	536.4 ± 43.6	511.5 ± 13.4	559.8 ± 26.9
Soluble protein (mg/g lens)	443.8 ± 8.4	408.5 ± 13.9 *	453.5 ± 8.6 ^	428.0 ± 12.0

C—control, non-diabetic rats; D—diabetic rats; D+R10—diabetic rats receiving resveratrol (10 mg/kg *po* for 4 weeks); D+R20—diabetic rats receiving resveratrol (20 mg/kg *po* for 4 weeks). Results are presented as means $\pm$ SEM ($n = 8$–9). * $p < 0.05$ – statistically significantly different from the C group. ^ $p < 0.05$ – statistically significantly different from the D group.

In the D group, the soluble protein content in the lens was lower ($p < 0.05$) in comparison with the C rats. The administration of resveratrol to the diabetic rats resulted in an increase of the soluble protein content in the D+R10 group ($p < 0.05$) and in the D+R20 group (not statistically significant) when compared to the D rats, while no changes in this parameter were recorded in comparison with the C group (Table 3).

3.6. Effect of Resveratrol on the Enzymatic Oxidative Stress Parameters in the Lens of the Diabetic Rats

The SOD activity in the lens of the D rats was higher ($p < 0.001$) in comparison with the C rats. When compared to the C group, an activity of the SOD was elevated in the D+R10 group and D+R20 group ($p < 0.05$) but administration of resveratrol at both the doses led to a decrease ($p < 0.01$ and $p < 0.05$, respectively) in this parameter as compared to the D group (Figure 1).

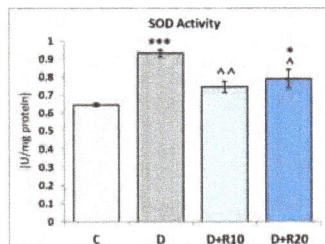

Figure 1. Effect of resveratrol administration on the superoxide dismutase (SOD) activity in the lens of the diabetic rats. C—control, non-diabetic rats; D—diabetic rats; D+R10—diabetic rats receiving resveratrol (10 mg/kg *po* for 4 weeks); D+R20—diabetic rats receiving resveratrol (20 mg/kg *po* for 4 weeks). Results are presented as means $\pm$ SEM ($n = 8$–9). * $p < 0.05$, *** $p < 0.001$—statistically significantly different from the C group. ^ $p < 0.05$, ^^ $p < 0.01$—statistically significantly different from the D group.

In comparison with the C rats, in the D rats an increase of the CAT activity in the lens was observed ($p < 0.001$). In the D+R10 and D+R20 groups, there was a decrease of the CAT activity when compared to the D rats (not statistically significant) and an increase in this parameter when compared to the C rats ($p < 0.05$ and $p < 0.01$, respectively) (Figure 2).

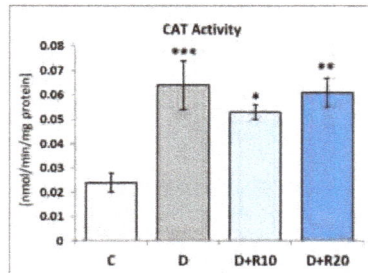

Figure 2. Effect of resveratrol administration on the catalase (CAT) activity in the lens of the diabetic rats. C—control, non-diabetic rats; D—diabetic rats; D+R10—diabetic rats receiving resveratrol (10 mg/kg *po* for 4 weeks); D+R20—diabetic rats receiving resveratrol (20 mg/kg *po* for 4 weeks). Results are presented as means $\pm$ SEM ($n = 8$–9). * $p < 0.05$, ** $p < 0.01$, *** $p < 0.001$—statistically significantly different from the C group.

The activity of GPx in the lens was insignificantly higher in the D rats than in the C rats. When compared to the D group, in the D+R10 and D+R20 groups, activity of the GPx was decreased ($p < 0.05$ in D+R10). No statistically significant changes between D+R10, D+R20 and C groups were noted (Figure 3).

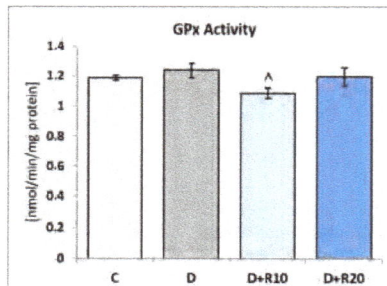

Figure 3. Effect of resveratrol administration on the glutathione peroxidase (GPx) activity in the lens of the diabetic rats. C—control, non-diabetic rats; D—diabetic rats; D+R10—diabetic rats receiving resveratrol (10 mg/kg *po* for 4 weeks); D+R20—diabetic rats receiving resveratrol (20 mg/kg *po* for 4 weeks). Results are presented as means $\pm$ SEM ($n = 8$–9). ^ $p < 0.05$ – statistically significantly different from the D group.

3.7. Effect of Resveratrol on the Non-Enzymatic Oxidative Stress Parameters Content in the Lens of the Diabetic Rats

In the lens of the D rats the content of GSH and vitamin C was lower ($p < 0.001$ and $p < 0.05$, respectively) in comparison with the C rats. Administration of resveratrol to the diabetic rats did not affect these parameters when compared to the D rats (Table 4).

In the lens of the D rats, the content of calcium was higher ($p < 0.05$) in comparison with the C rats. Administration of resveratrol at both doses did not affect the content of calcium when compared to the D rats. In comparison with the C group, in the D+R10 and D+R20 groups, this parameter was higher ($p < 0.01$ and not statistically significant, respectively) (Table 4).

Table 4. Effect of resveratrol on the glutathione (GSH), vitamin C and calcium content in the lens in diabetic rats.

Parameter/Group	C	D	D+R10	D+R20
GSH (μmol/g lens)	4.10 ± 0.61	0.78 ± 0.13 ***	0.75 ± 0.11 ***	0.74 ± 0.10 ***
Vitamin C (μg/g lens)	7.69 ± 0.05	7.17 ± 0.02 *	7.20 ± 0.02 *	7.21 ± 0.06 *
Calcium (μg/g lens)	42.6 ± 2.1	53.8 ± 3.1 *	60.3 ± 2.5 **	50.4 ± 4.9

C—control, non-diabetic rats; D—diabetic rats; D+R10—diabetic rats receiving resveratrol (10 mg/kg *po* for 4 weeks); D+R20—diabetic rats receiving resveratrol (20 mg/kg *po* for 4 weeks). Results are presented as means ± SEM (n = 8–9). * $p < 0.05$, ** $p < 0.01$, *** $p < 0.001$ – statistically significantly different from the C group.

In the D rats the AOPP content in the lens was higher ($p < 0.05$) as compared to the C rats. In comparison with the D rats, in the D+R10 and D+R20 groups, this parameter was lower ($p < 0.05$ and $p < 0.001$, respectively) and lower in comparison with the C group too (not statistically significant) (Figure 4).

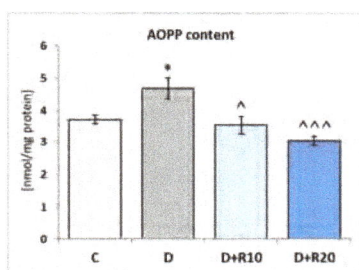

Figure 4. Effect of resveratrol administration on the advanced oxidation protein products (AOPP) content in the lens of the diabetic rats. C—control, non-diabetic rats; D—diabetic rats; D+R10—diabetic rats receiving resveratrol (10 mg/kg *po* for 4 weeks); DR20—diabetic rats receiving resveratrol (20 mg/kg *po* for 4 weeks). Results are presented as means ± SEM (n = 8–9). * $p < 0.05$—statistically significantly different from the C group. ^ $p < 0.05$, ^^^ $p < 0.001$—statistically significantly different from the D group.

The MDA content was higher ($p < 0.001$) in the lens of the D rats than in the C rats. Administration of resveratrol at both doses resulted in a decrease of the MDA content ($p < 0.05$) when confronted with the D group. In comparison with the C rats, in the D+R10 and D+R20 groups, this parameter was higher (not statistically significant) (Figure 5).

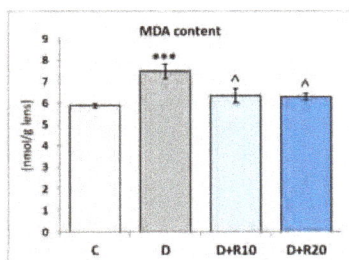

Figure 5. Effect of resveratrol administration on the malondialdehyde (MDA) content in the lens of the diabetic rats. C—control, non-diabetic rats; D—diabetic rats; D+R10—diabetic rats receiving resveratrol (10 mg/kg *po* for 4 weeks); D+R20—diabetic rats receiving resveratrol (20 mg/kg *po* for 4 weeks). Results are presented as means ± SEM (n = 8–9). *** $p < 0.001$—statistically significantly different from the C group. ^ $p < 0.05$—statistically significantly different from the D group.

3.8. Effect of Resveratrol on the Total Antioxidant Reactivity (TAR) Total Antioxidant Reactivity (TAR) and Total Oxidant Status (TOS) in the Lens of the Diabetic Rats

In the D rats the TAR in the lens was lower as compared to the C rats (not statistically significant). In comparison with the D rats, in the D+R10 and D+R20 groups, this parameter was higher and higher in comparison with the C group too (not statistically significant) (Figure 6).

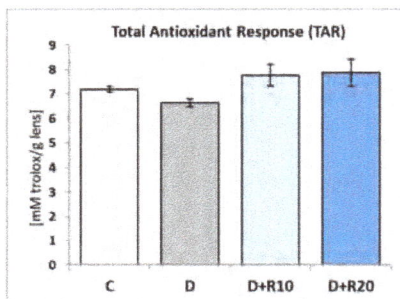

Figure 6. Effect of resveratrol administration on the Total Antioxidant Response (TAR) in the lens of the diabetic rats. C—control, non-diabetic rats; D—diabetic rats; D+R10—diabetic rats receiving resveratrol (10 mg/kg *po* for 4 weeks); D+R20—diabetic rats receiving resveratrol (20 mg/kg *po* for 4 weeks). Results are presented as means $\pm$ SEM (n = 8–9).

The TOS in the lens of the D rats was not statistically significantly higher, as compared to the C rats. When compared to the C group, in the D+R10 group and D+R20 group ($p < 0.01$), TOS was reduced and administration of resveratrol at both doses led to the decrease ($p < 0.05$ and $p < 0.001$, respectively) in this parameter, when compared to the D group (Figure 7).

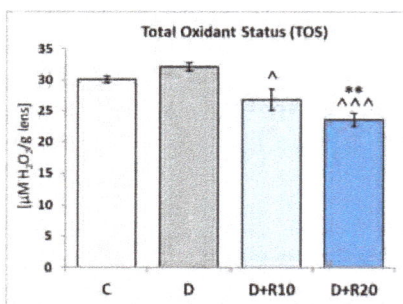

Figure 7. Effect of resveratrol administration on the Total Oxidant Status (TOS) in the lens of the diabetic rats. C—control, non-diabetic rats; D—diabetic rats; D+R10—diabetic rats receiving resveratrol (10 mg/kg *po* for 4 weeks); D+R20—diabetic rats receiving resveratrol (20 mg/kg *po* for 4 weeks). Results are presented as means $\pm$ SEM (n = 8–9). ** $p < 0.01$—statistically significantly different from the C group. ^ $p < 0.05$, ^^^ $p < 0.001$—statistically significantly different from the D group.

The TAR/TOS ratio in the lens was not statistically significantly lower in the D rats than in the C rats. When compared to the C group, in the D+R10 and D+R20 groups TAR/TOS ratio was elevated (not statistically significantly and $p < 0.05$, respectively). Administration of resveratrol at both doses resulted in an increase of the TAR/TOS ratio ($p < 0.01$ and $p < 0.001$, respectively), when confronted with the D group (Figure 8).

No statistically significant changes between the D+R10 and D+R20 group in the all parameters were reported.

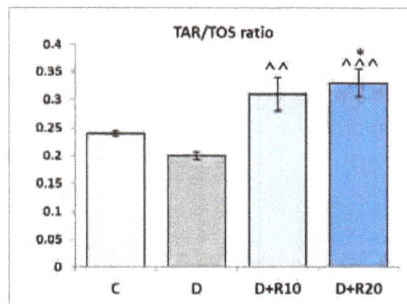

Figure 8. Effect of resveratrol administration on the TAR/TOS ratio in the lens of the diabetic rats. C—control, non-diabetic rats; D—diabetic rats; D+R10—diabetic rats receiving resveratrol (10 mg/kg *po* for 4 weeks); D+R20—diabetic rats receiving resveratrol (20 mg/kg *po* for 4 weeks). Results are presented as means ± SEM ($n = 8$–9). * $p < 0.05$—statistically significantly different from the C group. ˄˄ $p < 0.01$, ˄˄˄ $p < 0.001$—statistically significantly different from the D group.

4. Discussion

Diabetes mellitus (DM) is a disease characterized by chronic hyperglycaemia and disturbances of carbohydrate, fat and protein metabolism resulting from an absolute or relative deficiency of insulin. Increased oxidative stress is thought to play an important role in the pathogenesis of diabetic complications, as supported by increased levels of oxidized DNA, proteins and lipids. The induction of oxidative stress in DM can result from multiple mechanisms both non-enzymatic and enzymatic mechanisms.

In our study, the standard model of type 1 diabetes induced by streptozotocin was used [18,19]. We have noted, that an induction of type 1 diabetes in rats resulted in an increased blood glucose concentrations, blood fructosamine concentrations, lens glucose concentration and a decrease in the body mass of rats. This result overlaps with other studies conducted in diabetic rats [29–31].

It is known, that high glucose levels can stimulate oxidative stress by auto-oxidation of glucose and via non-enzymatic process of advanced glycation end products (AGEs) formation. We observed an increase of AGEs in the lens of rats with STZ-induced type 1 diabetes. An elevated lens AGEs level in diabetic rats was also described elsewhere [29,32]. Scientific evidences indicate that accumulation of AGEs in lens leads to accelerated cataractogenesis in hyperglycaemic experimental animals as well as in humans [33,34].

Another important mechanism whereby high glucose levels can induce oxidative stress is the polyol pathway. In our study, activation of the polyol pathway results in an increase of the sorbitol and fructose content in the lens of diabetic. This fact may be linked to an elevated glucose concentration in this tissue. Excessive accumulation of sorbitol increases osmotic stress, along with cross-linking with proteins of the lens by non-enzymatic glycosylation, promoting the formation of high molecular weight insoluble proteins which are responsible for the loss of transparency of the lens [35,36]. We have also noted an increased activity of polyol pathway enzymes—sorbitol dehydrogenase and aldose reductase.

We assume that lower body mass of rats with diabetes is associated with lower lens mass. These results also overlap with previous reports [30,31,37]. In the present study, the reason of the decrease in the lens mass was not a protein impoverishment because the total content of protein in the lens of the diabetic rats was the same as that in the non-diabetic rats. However, induction of diabetes in rats caused a decrease of content of soluble protein in the lens. This observation is confirmed by other studies [30,31]. Crystallins, soluble proteins of the lens, are important for the maintenance of lens transparency and the prevention of cataracts.

In the course of diabetes, the formation of protein aggregates in lens results from a decrease of sulfhydryl groups content in protein [38]. Similarly, in our study, we report a decrease of sulfhydryl groups content in the lens of rats with diabetes.

It has been well established that an increase of AOPP content is related to numerous different pathological states, underlined directly by oxidative stress, including diabetes [34]. AOPP content has increased in the lens in our study.

There are several reports in the literature demonstrating the elevated content of malondialdehyde (final products of polyunsaturated fatty acids peroxidation) in the lens [31] and other tissues [39–46] in STZ-induced diabetes in rats. The results of the present study are also in line with the previous reports.

Endogenous antioxidative mechanisms include both enzymatic and non-enzymatic processes. Two antioxidants (GSH and vitamin C) are fundamentally important for scavenging and correcting any damage due to ROS in the lens [47]. We observed, that GSH content and vitamin C content were reduced in the lens of diabetic rats. This result overlaps with other studies conducted on the lens of diabetic rats [29–31].

Some of the principal components of the oxidative defence system include SOD, CAT and GPx. Numerous previous studies indicate that changes in the activity of these enzymes are one of the major causes of diabetic cataractogenesis due to the imbalance between free radicals and antioxidants [35]. In the present study, oxidative stress in the lens of diabetic rats intensified antioxidant response by an increase of activity of SOD, CAT and GPx. These findings are in agreement with previous studies in diabetic animal [30,31,35,37].

Proper lens calcium concentration provides transparency of this tissue and its increase is associated with both human and animal lens opacification [29,48]. Likewise, in our study, we noted an elevated calcium concentration in the lens of diabetic rats.

In this study, the presence of oxidative stress in the diabetic lens was evidenced by the increased TOS and a decrease in TAR together with a reduction in TAR/TOS ratio. Many researchers have confirmed the changes of parameters of oxidative stress in the lens in the animal model of diabetes, thus indicating the contribution of ROS in the pathogenesis of lens opacity [35,49,50].

Resveratrol, as a dietary stilbene, is present in many plant-derived products (products made from grapes, soybeans, apples, blueberries, mulberries, peanuts, pistachios, plums, raspberries) and dietary supplement. In the present study, we examined, for the first time, the effect of orally administered resveratrol at the doses of 10 and 20 mg/kg on parameters of oxidative stress in vivo in the lens of the rats with STZ-induced type 1 diabetes. No changes in action after using both doses of resveratrol were observed. Doses of resveratrol were chosen based on the literature [38,42,44,45,51–54].

Administration of resveratrol did not influence the body mass and blood glucose and fructosamine concentrations of the diabetic rats. Likewise, the use of resveratrol did not change an increased glucose and fructose concentration in the lens of diabetic rats. Sorbitol content, as well as the activity of sorbitol dehydrogenase and aldose reductase associated with polyol pathway in lens, were not altered by resveratrol.

Since no effect on body mass, blood glucose concentration, blood fructosamine concentration, glucose and fructose concentration in the lens, which was observed after resveratrol administration, it can be presumed, that this stilbene shows no strict antidiabetic effect in this experimental model. Varsha et al., Ates et al., Schmatz et al., Yu et al., Bagatini et al., Faid et al. have documented that resveratrol administered to rats with streptozotocin-induced type 1 diabetes does not cause changes in blood glucose concentrations and does not affect the body mass [29,39,42,43,51,55]. Other studies have demonstrated that resveratrol decreases blood glucose in animals with hyperglycaemia [40,44,45,54]. Similarly, ambiguous results are obtained in humans [2,56,57].

However, despite the lack of effect of resveratrol on hyperglycaemia in our studies, we have observed that this compound shows other beneficial effects in the lens of diabetic rats. Soluble protein content and the sulfhydryl groups content were increased in the lens. To the best of our knowledge, there is only one study of influence on sulfhydryl groups content after administration of resveratrol.

Asadi et al. reported an increase of sulfhydryl groups content in the serum after the use of resveratrol at the dose of 10 mg/kg for 30 days in rats with diabetes [38].

Furthermore, administration of resveratrol resulted in favourable changes in oxidative stress parameters in the lens of the streptozotocin-induced diabetic rats. The studied substance also normalizes an increased activity of basic enzymes taking part in oxidative stress id est SOD, CAT and GPx. In diabetic rats, resveratrol used in doses from 5 to 20 mg/kg demonstrated beneficial effect on SOD and CAT activity in blood [38], aorta [54], kidney [42,45], brain [44,46], corpus cavernosus penis [43] and liver [42,54].

These findings are also confirmed by other oxidative stress-related parameters which were assessed in the lens—AOPP and MDA content. Both parameters increased by diabetes induction and decreased after administration of resveratrol. Doganay et al. triggered oxidative stress and cataract in rat pups by injection of sodium selenite subcutaneously. Afterwards, the animals have been receiving resveratrol for 21 days (40 mg/kg intraperitoneal). The researchers observed that resveratrol suppressed lens opacification in rats. This protective effect was supported by lower MDA content in lens [6]. In sugar-induced lens opacity ex vivo model, resveratrol showed a significant protective effect preventing a decrease in transparency and formation of polyols in cattle lens [32]. Numerous scientific reports indicate that MDA level decreases under the influence of resveratrol in different tissues of diabetic rats: brain [39,41,44,46], liver [42,52,54], kidneys [40,42,45,53], corpus cavernosus penis [43].

Resveratrol does not influence GSH content in diabetic rats in our study. This is in line with observations made by Sadi and Konat [41], who did not find an effect of resveratrol on GSH content in the brain of diabetic rats.

In our study, we confirmed an indirect evidence for the antioxidant effect of resveratrol in the diabetic lens by noting a significant decrease of TOS, as well as an increase of TAR and TOS/TAR ratio. Administration of resveratrol to diabetic rats decreased TOS in the brain [41], blood [38], liver [52] and increased TAR in the brain [52]. Among the different beneficial effects of resveratrol found in diabetes, the ability of this compound to reduce oxidative stress seems to be best documented.

It can be concluded from our study that resveratrol shows antioxidative properties also in the lens of diabetic rats. It is not a result of antiglycaemic activity but resveratrol probably directly affects the antioxidative system. This conclusion might be confirmed by a fact of increasing defence antioxidant system by resveratrol in different tissues of healthy animals. Venturini et al. demonstrated that treatment with resveratrol administered to healthy rats at the dose of 20 mg for 21 days increases antioxidant capacities in the brain of healthy rats (an increase of SOD activity in striatum and CAT activity in the hippocampus, a decrease of MDA level in the striatum and frontal cortex) [46]. Faid et al. also reported a raised antioxidant potential in testes of healthy animals as an effect of the increased activity of SOD, CAT, GPx [55]. In another study, administration of resveratrol resulted in an increase in antioxidant defence system, namely SOD and CAT activity and a decrease of MDA level in the liver of normal rats [58].

Our results may indirectly indicate benefits of consumption of foods as well as dietary supplements containing resveratrol in diminishing oxidative stress in lenses of individuals suffering from diabetes mellitus. It requires further research.

Author Contributions: Conceptualization, I.K.-S.; Formal analysis, L.S.; Investigation, W.W. and M.Z.; Methodology, W.W. and M.Z.; Supervision, I.K.-S.; Visualization, D.W.-P.; Writing—original draft, L.S.; Writing—review & editing, D.W.-P. and E.M.-K.

Funding: This study was supported by grant no. KNW-1-088/N/7/0.

Conflicts of Interest: The authors declare no conflict of interest.

References

1. Weiskirchen, S.; Weiskirchen, R. Resveratrol: How Much Wine Do You Have to Drink to Stay Healthy? *Adv. Nutr.* **2016**, *7*, 706–718. [CrossRef] [PubMed]

Nutrients **2018**, *10*, 1423

2.   Berman, A.Y.; Motechin, R.A.; Wiesenfeld, M.Y.; Holz, M.K. The therapeutic potential of resveratrol: A review of clinical trials. *NPJ Precis. Oncol.* **2017**, *1*. [CrossRef] [PubMed]
3.   Abu-Amero, K.K.; Kondkar, A.A.; Chalam, K.V. Resveratrol and Ophthalmic Diseases. *Nutrients* **2016**, *8*, 200. [CrossRef] [PubMed]
4.   Pintea, A.; Rugină, D.; Pop, R.; Bunea, A.; Socaciu, C.; Diehl, H.A. Antioxidant effect of trans-resveratrol in cultured human retinal pigment epithelial cells. *J. Ocul. Pharmacol. Ther.* **2011**, *27*, 315–321. [CrossRef] [PubMed]
5.   Villalba, J.M.; Alcaín, F.J. Sirtuin activators and inhibitors. *Biofactors* **2012**, *38*, 349–359. [CrossRef] [PubMed]
6.   Doganay, S.; Borazan, M.; Iraz, M.; Cigremis, Y. The effect of resveratrol in experimental cataract model formed by sodium selenite. *Curr. Eye Res.* **2006**, *31*, 147–153. [CrossRef] [PubMed]
7.   Luna, C.; Li, G.; Liton, P.B.; Qiu, J.; Epstein, D.L.; Challa, P.; Gonzalez, P. Resveratrol prevents the expression of glaucoma markers induced by chronic oxidative stress in trabecular meshwork cells. *Food Chem. Toxicol.* **2009**, *47*, 198–204. [CrossRef] [PubMed]
8.   Li, C.; Wang, L.; Huang, K.; Zheng, L. Endoplasmic reticulum stress in retinal vascular degeneration: Protective role of resveratrol. *Investig. Ophthalmol. Vis. Sci.* **2012**, *53*, 3241–3249. [CrossRef] [PubMed]
9.   Losso, J.N.; Truax, R.E.; Richard, G. trans-Resveratrol inhibits hyperglycaemia-induced inflammation and connexin downregulation in retinal pigment epithelial cells. *J. Agric. Food Chem.* **2010**, *58*, 8246–8252. [CrossRef] [PubMed]
10. Van Ginkel, P.R.; Darjatmoko, S.R.; Sareen, D.; Subramanian, L.; Bhattacharya, S.; Lindstrom, M.J.; Albert, D.M.; Polans, A.S. Resveratrol inhibits uveal melanoma tumor growth via early mitochondrial dysfunction. *Investig. Ophthalmol. Vis. Sci.* **2008**, *49*, 1299–1306. [CrossRef] [PubMed]
11. Sareen, D.; van Ginkel, P.R.; Takach, J.C.; Mohiuddin, A.; Darjatmoko, S.R.; Albert, D.M.; Polans, A.S. Mitochondria as the primary target of resveratrol-induced apoptosis in human retinoblastoma cells. *Investig. Ophthalmol. Vis. Sci.* **2006**, *47*, 3708–3716. [CrossRef] [PubMed]
12. Kim, W.T.; Suh, E.S. Retinal protective effects of resveratrol via modulation of nitric oxide synthase on oxygen-induced retinopathy. *Korean J. Ophthalmol.* **2010**, *24*, 108–118. [CrossRef] [PubMed]
13. Moussa, S.A. Oxidative stress in diabetes mellitus. *Romanian J. Biophys.* **2008**, *18*, 225–236.
14. Rolo, A.P.; Palmeira, C.M. Diabetes and mitochondrial function: Role of hyperglycaemia and oxidative stress. *Toxicol. Appl. Pharmacol.* **2006**, *212*, 167–178. [CrossRef] [PubMed]
15. Sayin, N.; Kara, N.; Pekel, G. Ocular complications of diabetes mellitus. *World J. Diabetes* **2015**, *6*, 92–108. [CrossRef] [PubMed]
16. Pollreisz, A.; Schmidt-Erfurth, U. Diabetic cataract - pathogenesis, epidemiology and treatment. *J. Ophthalmol.* **2010**. [CrossRef] [PubMed]
17. Gülçin, İ. Antioxidant properties of resveratrol: A structure–activity insight. *Innov. Food Sci. Emerg. Technol.* **2010**, *11*, 210–218. [CrossRef]
18. Szkudelski, T. The mechanism of alloxan and streptozotocin action in B cells of the rat pancreas. *Physiol. Res.* **2001**, *50*, 536–546.
19. Yümün, G.; Kahaman, C.; Kahaman, N.; Yalçınkaya, U.; Akçılar, A.; Akgül, E.; Vural, A.H. Effects of hyperbaric oxygen therapy combined with platelet-rich plasma on diabetic wounds: An experimental rat model. *Arch. Med. Sci.* **2016**, *12*, 1370–1376. [CrossRef] [PubMed]
20. Patel, D.; Kumar, R.; Kumar, M.; Sairam, K.; Hemalatha, S. Evaluation of in vitro aldose reductase inhibitory potential of different fraction of Hybanthus enneaspermus Linn F. Muell. *Asian Pac. J. Trop. Biomed.* **2012**, *2*, 134–139. [CrossRef]
21. Lowry, O.H.; Rosebrough, N.J.; Farr, A.L.; Randall, R.J. Protein measurement with the Folin phenol reagent. *J. Biol. Chem.* **1951**, *193*, 265–275. [PubMed]
22. Ellman, G.L. Tissue sulfhydryl groups. *Arch. Biochem. Biophys.* **1959**, *82*, 70–77. [CrossRef]
23. Sedlak, J.; Lindsay, R.H. Estimation of total, protein-bound and nonprotein sulfhydryl groups in tissue with Ellman's reagent. *Anal. Biochem.* **1968**, *25*, 192–205. [CrossRef]
24. Jagota, S.K.; Dani, H.M. A new colorimetric technique for the estimation of vitamin C using Folin phenol reagent. *Anal. Biochem.* **1982**, *127*, 178–182. [CrossRef]
25. Witko-Sarsat, V.; Friedlander, M.; Capeillère-Blandin, C.; Nguyen-Khoa, T.; Nguyen, A.T.; Zingraff, J.; Jungers, P.; Descamps-Latscha, B. Advanced oxidation protein products as a novel marker of oxidative stress in uremia. *Kidney Int.* **1996**, *49*, 1304–1313. [CrossRef] [PubMed]

26. Ohkawa, H.; Ohishi, N.; Yagi, K. Assay for lipid peroxides in animal tissues by thiobarbituric acid reaction. *Anal. Biochem.* **1979**, *95*, 351–358. [CrossRef]

27. Erel, O. A new automated colorimetric method for measuring total oxidant status. *Clin. Biochem.* **2005**, *38*, 1103–1111. [CrossRef] [PubMed]

28. Erel, O. A novel automated method to measure total antioxidant response against potent free radical reactions. *Clin. Biochem.* **2004**, *37*, 112–119. [CrossRef] [PubMed]

29. Varsha, M.K.S.; Raman, T.; Manikandan, R. Inhibition of diabetic-cataract by vitamin K1 involves modulation of hyperglycaemia-induced alterations to lens calcium homeostasis. *Exp. Eye Res.* **2014**, *128*, 73–82. [CrossRef] [PubMed]

30. Kaczmarczyk-Sedlak, I.; Folwarczna, J.; Sedlak, L.; Zych, M.; Wojnar, W.; Szumińska, I.; Wyględowska-Promieńska, D.; Mrukwa-Kominek, E. Effect of caffeine on the biomarkers of oxidative stress in lenses of rats with streptozotocin-induced diabetes. *Arch. Med. Sci.* **2018**, in press.

31. Wojnar, W.; Kaczmarczyk-Sedlak, I.; Zych, M. Diosmin ameliorates the effects of oxidative stress in lenses of streptozotocin-induced type 1 diabetic rats. *Pharmacol. Rep.* **2017**, *69*, 995–1000. [CrossRef] [PubMed]

32. Ciddi, V.; Dodda, D. Therapeutic potential of resveratrol in diabetic complications: In vitro and in vivo studies. *Pharmacol. Rep.* **2014**, *66*, 799–803. [CrossRef] [PubMed]

33. Reddy, P.Y.; Giridharan, N.V.; Reddy, G.B. Activation of sorbitol pathway in metabolic syndrome and increased susceptibility to cataract in Wistar-Obese rats. *Mol. Vis.* **2012**, *18*, 495–503. [PubMed]

34. Kalousová, M.; Skrha, J.; Zima, T. Advanced glycation end-products and advanced oxidation protein products in patients with diabetes mellitus. *Physiol. Res.* **2002**, *51*, 597–604. [PubMed]

35. Suryanarayana, P.; Saraswat, M.; Mrudula, T.; Krishna, P.T.; Krishnaswamy, K.; Reddy, G.B. Curcumin and turmeric delay streptozotocin-induced diabetic cataract in rats. *Investig. Ophthalmol. Vis. Sci.* **2005**, *46*, 2092–2099. [CrossRef] [PubMed]

36. Lorenzi, M. The polyol pathway as a mechanism for diabetic retinopathy: Attractive, elusive and resilient. *Exp. Diabetes Res.* **2007**. [CrossRef] [PubMed]

37. Patil, M.A.; Suryanarayana, P.; Putcha, U.K.; Srinivas, M.; Reddy, G.B. Evaluation of neonatal streptozotocin induced diabetic rat model for the development of cataract. *Oxid. Med. Cell Longev.* **2014**. [CrossRef] [PubMed]

38. Asadi, S.; Moradi, M.N.; Khyripour, N.; Goodarzi, M.T.; Mahmoodi, M. Resveratrol attenuates copper and zinc homeostasis and ameliorates oxidative stress in type 2 diabetic rats. *Biol. Trace Elem. Res.* **2017**, *177*, 132–138. [CrossRef] [PubMed]

39. Ates, O.; Cayli, S.R.; Yucel, N.; Altinoz, E.; Kocak, A.; Durak, M.A.; Turkoz, Y.; Yologlu, S. Central nervous system protection by resveratrol in streptozotocin-induced diabetic rats. *J. Clin. Neurosci.* **2007**, *14*, 256–260. [CrossRef] [PubMed]

40. Elbe, H.; Vardi, N.; Esrefoglu, M.; Ates, B.; Yologlu, S.; Taskapan, C. Amelioration of streptozotocin-induced diabetic nephropathy by melatonin, quercetin and resveratrol in rats. *Hum. Exp. Toxicol.* **2015**, *34*, 100–113. [CrossRef] [PubMed]

41. Sadi, G.; Konat, D. Resveratrol regulates oxidative biomarkers and antioxidant enzymes in the brain of streptozotocin-induced diabetic rats. *Pharm. Biol.* **2016**, *54*, 1156–1163. [CrossRef] [PubMed]

42. Schmatz, R.; Perreira, L.B.; Stefanello, N.; Mazzanti, C.; Spanevello, R.; Gutierres, J.; Bagatini, M.; Martins, C.C.; Abdalla, F.H.; Daci da Silva Serres, J. Effects of resveratrol on biomarkers of oxidative stress and on the activity of delta aminolevulinic acid dehydratase in liver and kidney of streptozotocin-induced diabetic rats. *Biochimie* **2012**, *94*, 374–383. [CrossRef] [PubMed]

43. Yu, W.; Wan, Z.; Qiu, X.F.; Chen, Y.; Dai, Y.T. Resveratrol, an activator of SIRT1, restores erectile function in streptozotocin-induced diabetic rats. *Asian J. Androl.* **2013**, *15*, 646–651. [CrossRef] [PubMed]

44. Tian, X.; Liu, Y.; Ren, G.; Yin, L.; Liang, X.; Geng, T.; Dang, H.; An, R. Resveratrol limits diabetes-associated cognitive decline in rats by preventing oxidative stress and inflammation and modulating hippocampal structural synaptic plasticity. *Brain Res.* **2016**, *1650*, 1–9. [CrossRef] [PubMed]

45. Sharma, S.; Anjaneyulu, M.; Kulkarni, S.K.; Chopra, K. Resveratrol, a polyphenolic phytoalexin, attenuates diabetic nephropathy in rats. *Pharmacology* **2006**, *76*, 69–75. [CrossRef] [PubMed]

46. Venturini, C.D.; Merlo, S.; Souto, A.A.; Fernandes Mda, C.; Gomez, R.; Rhoden, C.R. Resveratrol and red wine function as antioxidants in the nervous system without cellular proliferative effects during experimental diabetes. *Oxid. Med. Cell Longev.* **2010**, *3*, 434–441. [CrossRef] [PubMed]

47. Abdelkader, H.; Alany, R.G.; Pierscionek, B. Age-related cataract and drug therapy: Opportunities and challenges for topical antioxidant delivery to the lens. *J. Pharm. Pharmacol.* **2015**, *67*, 537–550. [CrossRef] [PubMed]

48. Shearer, T.R.; David, L.L. Role of calcium in selenium cataract. *Curr. Eye Res.* **1982**, *2*, 777–784. [CrossRef] [PubMed]

49. Gong, X.; Zhang, Q.; Tan, S. Inhibitory effect of r-hirudin variant III on streptozotocin-induced diabetic cataracts in rats. *Sci. World J.* **2013**, *630651*, 1–8. [CrossRef] [PubMed]

50. Saraswat, M.; Suryanarayana, P.; Reddy, P.Y.; Patil, M.A.; Balakrishna, N.; Reddy, G.B. Antiglycating potential of Zingiber officinalis and delay of diabetic cataract in rats. *Mol. Vis.* **2010**, *16*, 1525–1537. [PubMed]

51. Bagatini, P.B.; Xavier, L.L.; Bertoldi, K.; Moysés, F.; Lovatel, G.; Neves, L.T.; Barbosa, S.; Saur, L.; de Senna, P.N.; Souto, A.A. An evaluation of aversive memory and hippocampal oxidative status in streptozotocin-induced diabetic rats treated with resveratrol. *Neurosci. Lett.* **2017**, *636*, 184–189. [CrossRef] [PubMed]

52. Khazaei, M.; Karimi, J.; Sheikh, N.; Goodarzi, M.T.; Saidijam, M.; Khodadadi, I.; Moridi, H. Effects of resveratrol on receptor for advanced glycation end products (RAGE) expression and oxidative stress in the liver of rats with type 2 diabetes. *Phytother. Res.* **2016**, *30*, 66–71. [CrossRef] [PubMed]

53. Moridi, H.; Karimi, J.; Sheikh, N.; Goodarzi, M.T.; Saidijam, M.; Yadegarazari, R.; Khazaei, M.; Khodadadi, I.; Tavilani, H.; Piri, H. Resveratrol-dependent down-regulation of receptor for advanced glycation end-products and oxidative stress in kidney of rats with diabetes. *Int. J. Endocrinol. Metab.* **2015**, *13*, E23542. [CrossRef] [PubMed]

54. Roghani, M.; Baluchnejadmojarad, T. Mechanisms underlying vascular effect of chronic resveratrol in streptozotocin-diabetic rats. *Phytother. Res.* **2010**, *24*, S148–S154. [CrossRef] [PubMed]

55. Faid, I.; Al-Hussaini, H.; Kilarkaje, N. Resveratrol alleviates diabetes-induced testicular dysfunction by inhibiting oxidative stress and c-Jun N-terminal kinase signaling in rats. *Toxicol. Appl. Pharmacol.* **2015**, *289*, 482–494. [CrossRef] [PubMed]

56. Öztürk, E.; Arslan, A.K.K.; Yerer, M.B.; Bishayee, A. Resveratrol and diabetes: A critical review of clinical studies. *Biomed. Pharmacother.* **2017**, *95*, 230–234. [CrossRef] [PubMed]

57. Erdogan, C.S.; Vang, O. Challenges in analyzing the biological effects of resveratrol. *Nutrients* **2016**, *8*, 353. [CrossRef] [PubMed]

58. Hamadi, N.; Mansour, A.; Hassan, M.H.; Khalifi-Touhami, F.; Badary, O. Ameliorative effects of resveratrol on liver injury in streptozotocin-induced diabetic rats. *J. Biochem. Mol. Toxicol.* **2012**, *26*, 384–392. [CrossRef] [PubMed]

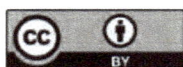

nutrients

MDPI

Article

Do the Effects of Resveratrol on Thermogenic and Oxidative Capacities in IBAT and Skeletal Muscle Depend on Feeding Conditions?

Iñaki Milton-Laskibar [1,2], Leixuri Aguirre [1,2,*], Usune Etxeberria [3,4], Fermin I. Milagro [2,5], J. Alfredo Martínez [2,5,6] and Maria P. Portillo [1,2]

[1]   Nutrition and Obesity Group, Department of Nutrition and Food Science, Lucio Lascaray Research Institute, University of the Basque Country (UPV/EHU), 01006 Vitoria, Spain; inaki.milton@ehu.eus (I.M.-L.); mariapuy.portillo@ehu.eus (M.P.P.)
[2]   CIBERobn Physiopathology of Obesity and Nutrition, Institute of Health Carlos III, 28029 Madrid, Spain; fmilagro@unav.es (F.I.M.); jalfmtz@unav.es (J.A.M.)
[3]   BCC Innovation, Technological Center of Gastronomy, 20009 Donostia, Spain; uetxeberria@bculinary.com
[4]   Basque Culinary Center, Mondragon Unibertsitatea, 20009 San Sebastián, Spain
[5]   Department of Nutrition, Food Sciences and Physiology, Centre for Nutrition Research, University of Navarra, 31008 Pamplona, Spain
[6]   IMDEA Food, 28049 Madrid, Spain
*   Correspondence: leixuri.aguirre@ehu.eus; Tel.: +34-945014298; Fax: +34-945013014

Received: 14 September 2018; Accepted: 29 September 2018; Published: 6 October 2018

Abstract: The aim of this study was to compare the effects of mild energy restriction and resveratrol on thermogenic and oxidative capacity in interscapular brown adipose tissue (IBAT) and in skeletal muscle. Rats were fed a high-fat high-sucrose diet for six weeks, and divided into four experimental groups fed a standard diet: a control group, a resveratrol-treated group, an energy-restricted group and an energy-restricted group treated with resveratrol. Weights of IBAT, gastrocnemius muscle and fat depots were measured. Activities of carnitine palmitoyltransferase (CPT) and citrate synthase (CS), protein levels of sirtuin (SIRT1 and 3), uncoupling proteins (UCP1 and 3), glucose transporter (GLUT4), mitochondrial transcription factor (TFAM), nuclear respiratory factor (NRF1), peroxisome proliferator-activated receptor (PPARα) and AMP activated protein kinase (AMPK) and peroxisome proliferator-activated receptor gamma coactivator (PGC1α) activation were measured. No changes in IBAT and gastrocnemius weights were found. Energy-restriction, but not resveratrol, decreased the weights of adipose depots. In IBAT, resveratrol enhanced thermogenesis activating the SIRT1/PGC1α/PPARα axis. Resveratrol also induced fatty acid oxidation and glucose uptake. These effects were similar when resveratrol was combined with energy restriction. In the case of gastrocnemius muscle, the effects were not as clear as in the case of IBAT. In this tissue, resveratrol increased oxidative capacity. The combination of resveratrol and energy restriction seemingly did not improve the effects induced by the polyphenol alone.

Keywords: resveratrol; energy restriction; thermogenesis; high-fat high-sucrose diet; rat

1. Introduction

The phenomenon of adaptive thermogenesis, also known as non-shivering or facultative thermogenesis, is a phenomenon characterized by heat production in response to environmental temperature or diet [1]. It is mediated by the action of uncoupling proteins (UCPs), a type of protein embedded in the inner mitochondrial membrane which uncouples the oxidative phosphorylation. As a result, the proton gradient is dissipated and used to produce heat instead of synthetizing adenosine triphosphate (ATP) [2]. In this regard, brown adipose tissue (BAT) has been identified as the main thermogenic tissue, due to its high content in mitochondria [3,4]. This tissue was thought to exist only in small mammals and newborns, but the recent discovery of BAT in adult humans has reactivated the interest of the scientific community in this tissue as a possible means of body weight management [5–7].

To produce heat, the lipids stored in BAT are firstly used as substrates [8] and then, in order to maintain this thermogenic activity, triglycerides from circulation are used [9]. Moreover, circulating glucose is also used by BAT as a substrate for thermogenesis [9]. As a result, both plasma triglyceride levels as well as plasma glucose levels are decreased by BAT thermogenic activity [9]. All these observations highlighted BAT as an interesting target-tissue for obesity and metabolic syndrome management.

Along with BAT, the other main thermogenic tissue in human body is skeletal muscle, which is the largest organ of the human body and determines the basal metabolic rate [10,11]. UCP3 is the characteristic uncoupling protein present in this tissue [12]. Although UCP3 was at first thought to participate in thermogenesis and energy expenditure (as does its more abundant ortholog UCP1, present in BAT), it has been proposed that its function is more related to glucose and fatty acid metabolism [13,14].

As previously mentioned, diet is one of the main modulators of thermogenesis, mediating this process in two different ways. It has been reported that macronutrient composition of the diet can influence thermogenic activity in animal models not only in BAT, but also in skeletal muscle [15]. Moreover, a reduction in energy intake has also been related to thermogenesis regulation. In this regard, while excess food intake (hyperphagia) has been related to increased thermogenesis (diet-induced thermogenesis), reductions in UCP1 mRNA in BAT have been identified in conditions of food scarcity [16].

In recent years interest in natural compounds with positive health effects has increased within scientific community. One of these bioactive compounds, resveratrol (3,5,4′-trihydroxy-*trans*-stilbene), a phenolic compound belonging to the stilbene group, has attracted a great deal of attention [17–19]. As reported by several authors, resveratrol is able to mimic the effects induced by dietary energy restriction without reducing caloric intake [20,21]. In addition, many studies have described resveratrol as a potential inducer of thermogenesis in rodent models fed obesogenic [22] or standard [23] diets.

In this context, the present study aimed to compare the effects of mild energy restriction and resveratrol on thermogenic capacity of BAT and skeletal muscle, in terms of efficiency and mechanisms of action. Moreover, the capacity of resveratrol to induce thermogenesis under energy restriction feeding conditions was also studied.

2. Material and Methods

2.1. Animals, Diets and Experimental Design

The experiment was conducted using 36 six-week-old male Wistar rats (Harlan Ibérica, Barcelona, Spain), and conducted in accordance with the University of the Basque Country's Guide for the Care and Use of Laboratory Animals (Reference protocol approval M20_2016_039). The rats, individually housed in polycarbonate metabolic cages (Tecniplast Gazzada, Buguggiate, Italy), were placed in a controlled air-conditioned room (22 ± 2 °C) with a 12-h light-dark cycle. After a 6-day adaptation period, animals were fed a high-fat high-sucrose (HFHS) diet (OpenSource Diets, Lynge, Denmark; Ref. D12451) for 6 weeks (45% of energy as fat, 13% of energy as sucrose and 4.7 kcal/g of energy) (Table S1 A). After this period, the animals were fed over 6 additional weeks with a standard semi-purified diet (OpenSource Diets, Lynge, Denmark; Ref. D10012G) which provided 3.9 kcal/g, 16% as fat, 64% as carbohydrates and 20% as protein (Table S1 B), and randomly distributed into four experimental groups ($n = 9$): the control group (C), the resveratrol group (RSV), the restricted group (R) and the combined group (RR) (Figure S1). The RSV group was treated with a dose of 30 mg/kg body weight/day of resveratrol, the R group was submitted to a mild energy restriction of 15% of total daily energy intake and the combined group was submitted to a mild energy restriction (15%) and treated with resveratrol (30 mg/kg body weight/day). In the case of C and RSV groups, the animals had free access to food and water (ad libitum). The selected resveratrol dose was based on the previous experience of our group [24]. In order to calculate the exact diet amount provided to the animals in the restricted groups, the spontaneous food intake of the C group rats was taken into account.

Once the whole experimental period (12 weeks) was completed, animals from the four experimental groups were sacrificed after an overnight fasting (12 h) under anesthesia (chloral hydrate) by cardiac exsanguination. Interscapular BAT (IBAT), gastrocnemius muscles and white adipose tissue depots from different anatomical locations (subcutaneous, mesenteric, perirenal and epididymal) were dissected, weighed, and immediately frozen in liquid nitrogen. All the samples were stored at −80 °C until analysis.

2.2. Enzyme Activities

The activity of carnitine palmitoyltransferase-1a and b (CPT-1a and CPT-1b) was measured spectrophotometrically in the mitochondrial fraction of IBAT and gastrocnemius muscle, respectively. Briefly, tissue samples (200 mg) were homogenized in 3 volumes (*wt/vol*) of buffer containing 10 mmol/L Tris-HCl, 1 mmol/L EDTA and 0.25 mol/L sucrose (pH 7.4), and then centrifuged (700× *g* for 10 min at 4 °C). After this first centrifugation, the supernatants were collected and centrifuged again (12,000× *g* for 15 min at 4 °C). The pellets were resuspended in resuspension buffer (220 mmol/L mannitol, 70 mmol/L sucrose, 1 mmol/L ethylenediaminetetraacetic acid (EDTA) and 2 mmol/L 4-(2-Hydroxyethyl)piperazine-1-ethanesulfonic acid (HEPES), pH 7.4), and the protein content determined according to the Bradford method [25]. The activity of CPT-1a and CPT-1b was measured by using the Bieber et al. method [26,27]. The activity of the enzyme was represented as nanomoles CoA formed per minute, per milligram of protein.

In the case of citrate synthase (CS), activity was also assessed spectrophotometrically, following the Srere method [27] by measuring the appearance of free CoA. Briefly, frozen IBAT and gastrocnemius muscle samples (50 and 100 mg respectively) were homogenized in 25 vol (*wt/vol*) of 0.1 M Tris-HCl buffer (pH 8.0). Homogenates were incubated for 2 min at 30 °C with 0.1 M Tris-HCl buffer containing 0.1 mM 5,5′-dithio-bis-[2-nitrobenzoic acid] (DTNB), 0.25 Triton X-100, 0.5 mM oxalacetate and 0.31 mM acetyl CoA, and readings were taken at 412 nm. CS activity was expressed as nmol CoA formed per minute, per milligram of protein. The protein content of the samples was determined by the Bradford method [25], using bovine serum albumine as standard.

2.3. Western Blot

For sirtuin 1 and 3 (SIRT1 and SIRT3), AMP activated protein kinase (AMPK), glucose transporter 4 (GLUT4), mitochondrial transcription factor A (TFAM), uncoupling proteins 1 and 3 (UCP1 and UCP3) and Tubulin, IBAT and gastrocnemius muscle samples (100 mg) were homogenized in 1000 μL of cellular phosphate buffer saline (PBS) (pH 7.4), containing protease inhibitors (100 mM phenylmethylsulfonyl fluoride and 100 mM iodoacetamide). Homogenates were centrifuged at 800× *g* for 10 min at 4 °C. Protein concentration in homogenates was measured by Bradford method (Bradford et al., 1976) using bovine serum albumin as standard. In the case of peroxisome proliferator-activated receptor gamma coactivator 1-alpha (PGC1α), nuclear respiratory factor 1 (NRF1), peroxisome proliferator-activated receptor alpha and beta/delta (PPARα and PPARβ/δ) and histone H3 (Histone H3), nuclear protein extraction were carried out with 100 mg of IBAT and gastrocnemius muscle, as previously described [28].

Immunoblot analyses were carried out using 50 μg and 40 μg of IBAT and gastrocnemius muscle total protein extracts (respectively), and 35 μg and 60 μg of IBAT and gastrocnemius muscle nuclear protein extracts (respectively), separated by electrophoresis in precast 4–15% sodium dodecyl sulfate (SDS)-polyacrylamide gradient gels (Bio-Rad, Hercules, CA, USA) and transferred to PVDF membranes (Bio-Rad, Hercules, CA, USA). The membranes were then blocked with 5% caseine PBS-Tween buffer for 2 h at room temperature. Subsequently, they were blotted with the appropriate antibodies overnight at 4 °C. Protein levels were detected via specific antibodies (Table S2) for SIRT3 (1:500), UCP1 (1:500),

UCP3 (1:500), TFAM (1:500), GLUT4 (1:5000), PPARβ/δ (1:500) (Santa Cruz Biotech, Dallas, TX, USA), AMPK (1:1000), Tubulin (1:5000), Histone H3 (1:1000) (Cell Signaling Technology, Danvers, MA, USA) and SIRT1 (1:1000), PGC1α (1:1000), NRF1 (1:1000), PPARα (1:1000) (Abcam, Cambridge, UK). Afterward, polyclonal anti-mouse for SIRT3 (1:5000) (Santa Cruz Biotech, Dallas, TX, USA), anti-goat for UCP1, UCP3, TFAM and GLUT4 (1:5000) (Santa Cruz Biotech, Dallas, TX, USA) and anti-rabbit for SIRT1, AMPK, Tubulin, Histone H3, PGC1α, NRF1, PPARα and PPAR β/δ (1:5000) (Santa Cruz Biotech, Dallas, TX, USA) were incubated for 2 h at room temperature, and the levels of the aforementioned proteins were measured (Table S2). After antibody stripping, the membranes were blocked and then incubated with phosphorylated AMPK (threonine 172, 1:1000), and acetylated lysine (1:1000) (Cell Signaling Technology, Danvers, MA, USA) antibodies (Table S2). The bound antibodies were visualized by an electrochemiluminescence (ECL) system (Thermo Fisher Scientific Inc., Rockford, IL, USA) and quantified by a ChemiDoc MP Imaging System (Bio-Rad, Hercules, CA, USA). Specific bands were identified by using a standard loading buffer (Precision Plus protein standards dual color; Ref. 161-0374 Bio-Rad).

2.4. Statistical Analysis

Results are presented as mean ± standard error of the mean (SEM). Statistical analysis was performed using SPSS 21.0 (SPSS, Chicago, IL, USA). All the variables were normally-distributed according to the Shapiro-Wilks test. Data were analyzed by one-way analysis of variance (ANOVA) followed by the Newman–Keuls post hoc test. Significance was assessed at the $p < 0.05$ level.

3. Results

3.1. Body Weight, Food Intake, Adipose Tissue Weights, and Interscapular Brown Adipose Tissue (IBAT) and Skeletal Muscle Weights

At the end of the whole experimental period, as expected, significantly lower body weights were observed in the groups submitted to energy restriction (R and RR) compared with the C group with no differences among them. In the case of the RSV group, body weight was similar to that found in the C group [29]. In the same line, significantly lower food intakes were found in both restricted groups (R and RR) compared with the C group, without differences between them [30]. When the weights of the four white adipose depots were pooled, a similar pattern to that found in the body weights, lower values in the restricted groups (R and RR) and no changes in the group treated with resveratrol (RSV) were noted (Table 1). Finally, IBAT and gastrocnemius weights did not show significant differences among the four experimental groups (Table 1).

Table 1. Weights of IBAT, gastrocnemius muscle and subcutaneous, perirenal, mesenteric and epididymal adipose tissues of rats fed on the experimental diets for 6 weeks.

	C	RSV	R	RR	ANOVA
IBAT (g)	0.76 ± 0.07	0.83 ± 0.03	0.83 ± 0.03	0.82 ± 0.06	NS
Gastrocnemius (g)	2.42 ± 0.03	2.65 ± 0.16	2.62 ± 0.10	2.60 ± 0.08	NS
Subcutaneous AT (g)	14.6 ± 1.1ab	15.2 ± 0.9a	12.0 ± 0.6bc	10.4 ± 0.6c	($p < 0.01$)
Perirenal AT (g)	14.6 ± 1.4a	13.6 ± 0.8a	8.7 ± 0.3b	9.3 ± 0.5b	($p < 0.05$)
Mesenteric AT (g)	3.9 ± 0.4ab	4.3 ± 0.1a	2.9 ± 0.3bc	268 ± 0.2c	($p < 0.05$)
Epididymal AT (g)	11.0 ± 0.9a	12.4 ± 0.2a	7.4 ± 0.5b	7.1 ± 0.5b	($p < 0.01$)

IBAT, interscapular brown adipose tissue; AT, adipose tissue. Values are mean ± standard error of the mean (SEM). Differences among groups were determined by using one-way analysis of variance (ANOVA) followed by Newman Keuls post-hoc test. Values not sharing a common letter are significantly different. NS: Not significant.

3.2. Enzyme Activities

Regarding CPT-1a in IBAT, significantly greater enzyme activities were observed in the three treated groups when compared with the C group ($p = 0.001$ in RSV, $p = 0.004$ in R and $p = 0.020$ in RR), with no differences among them (Figure 1A). As far as gastrocnemius muscle is concerned, a statistically significant increase in the activity of CPT-1b enzyme was observed in the groups supplemented with resveratrol (RSV and RR) when compared with the C group ($p = 0.017$ and $p = 0.023$, respectively), while in the case of the R group a non significant trend towards a greater activity ($+19.1\%$; $p = 0.065$) was observed (Figure 2A).

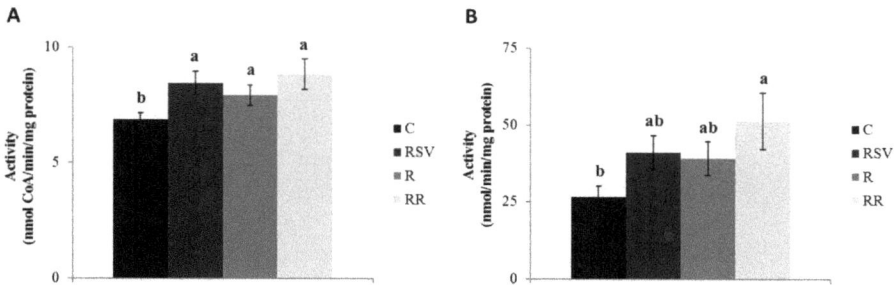

Figure 1. Activities of CPT-1a (**A**) and CS (**B**) in IBAT of rats fed an obesogenic diet for 6 weeks and then shifted to a standard diet (C), or standard diet supplemented with resveratrol (RSV), or submitted to energy restriction and fed a standard diet (R), or submitted to energy restriction and fed a standard diet supplemented with resveratrol (RR) ($n = 9$/group) for additional 6 weeks. Values are represented as means ± SEM. Differences among groups were determined by using one-way ANOVA followed by Newman–Keuls post hoc test. Values not sharing a common letter are significantly different ($p < 0.05$). CPT-1a: carnitine palmitoyltransferase-1a, CS: citrate synthase, IBAT: interscapular brown adipose tissue.

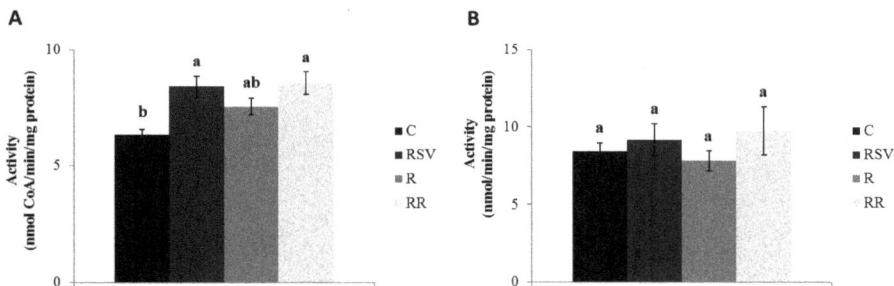

Figure 2. Activities of CPT-1b (**A**) and CS (**B**) in gastrocnemius muscle of rats fed an obesogenic diet for 6 weeks and then shifted to a standard diet (C), or standard diet supplemented with resveratrol (RSV), or submitted to energy restriction and fed a standard diet (R), or submitted to energy restriction and fed a standard diet supplemented with resveratrol (RR) ($n = 9$/group) for additional 6 weeks. Values are represented as means ± SEM. Differences among groups were determined by using one-way ANOVA followed by Newman–Keuls post hoc test. Values not sharing a common letter are significantly different ($p < 0.05$). CPT-1b: carnitine palmitoyltransferase-1b, CS: citrate synthase.

In the case of the CS, RSV and RR groups, these showed a significantly increased enzyme activity in IBAT when compared with the C group ($p = 0.05$ and $p = 0.04$, respectively) (Figure 1B). A trend towards greater enzyme activities was appreciated in R group when compared with the C group ($+47.9\%$; $p = 0.078$) (Figure 1B). In gastrocnemius muscle, no changes in the activity of this enzyme were found among the four experimental groups (Figure 2B).

3.3. Western Blot Analysis in IBAT and Skeletal Muscle

In order to analyze the effects induced by resveratrol administration, energy restriction and the combination on IBAT and skeletal muscle thermogenic capacities and fatty acid oxidation, the expression or the activation of different proteins was analyzed (Figure 3).

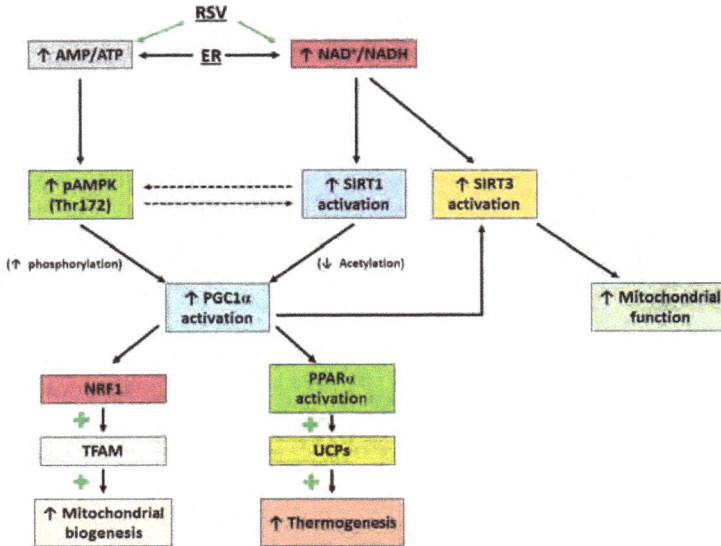

Figure 3. Effects of resveratrol and energy restriction in thermogenesis and mitochondrial synthesis pathways. RSV: resveratrol, ER: energy restriction, AMP: adenosine monophosphate, ATP: adenosine triphosphate, NAD$^+$: oxidized nicotinamide adenine dinucleotide, NADH: reduced nicotinamide adenine dinucleotide, AMPK: AMP activated protein kinase, SIRT1: sirtuin 1, SIRT3: sirtuin 3, PGC1α: peroxisome proliferator-activated receptor gamma coactivator 1-alpha, NRF1: nuclear respiratory factor 1, TFAM: mitochondrial transcription factor A, PPAR α: peroxisome proliferator-activated receptor alpha, UCP: uncoupling protein.

In IBAT, increased UCP1 protein expression was found in the group supplemented with resveratrol (RSV) in comparison with the C group ($p = 0.03$), as well as a tendency towards higher values in the RR group (+49.9%; $p = 0.10$) and no changes in the R group (Figure 4). In order to determine the molecular mechanisms underlying this effect, PGC1α, PPARα and SIRTs were studied. Decreased PGC1α acetylation, and thus greater activation of this protein, was found in the RSV and RR groups when compared with the C group ($p = 0.02$ and $p = 0.03$, respectively). In the case of R group, a tendency towards lower acetylation (-29.5%; $p = 0.06$) was observed (Figure 5). Regarding PPARα, although no differences in protein expression were found in the C group and the three treated groups, trends towards increased expressions were appreciated (+43.6%; $p = 0.055$ in the RSV group, +59.3%; $p = 0.073$ in the R group and +51.8%; $p = 0.053$ in the RR group) (Figure 5). Similarly, no significant changes were observed among the four groups in SIRT1 protein expression, but trends towards increased protein levels were found in the three treated groups when compared with the C group (+37.6%; $p = 0.057$ in the RSV group, +49.6%; $p = 0.094$ in the R group and +45.7%; $p = 0.065$ in the RR group) (Figure 4). As far as SIRT3 is concerned, greater protein levels were found in the three treated groups when compared with the C group ($p = 0.05$ in RSV, $p = 0.033$ in R and $p = 0.019$ in RR), with no differences among them (Figure 4). Finally, the phosphorylation ratio of threonine 172 residue was measured in AMPK to analyze its activation status. The groups supplemented with resveratrol (RSV and RR) showed greater phosphorylation ratios in comparison with the C group ($p = 0.022$ and

$p = 0.045$, respectively), without differences between them. In the case of the R group, no significant change in the phosphorylation ratio (and thus, in the activity) was found (Figure 4).

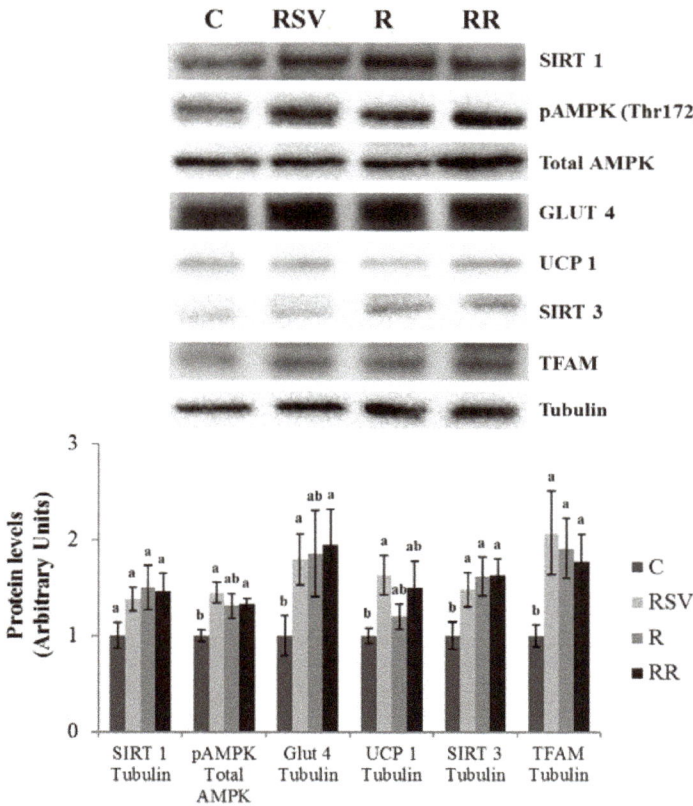

Figure 4. Protein levels of SIRT1, GLUT4, UCP1, SIRT3 and TFAM, and threonine 172 phosphorylation ratio of AMPK in IBAT of rats fed an obesogenic diet for 6 weeks and then shifted to a standard diet (C), or standard diet supplemented with resveratrol (RSV), or submitted to energy restriction and fed a standard diet (R), or submitted to energy restriction and fed a standard diet supplemented with resveratrol (RR) ($n = 9$/group) for additional 6 weeks. Values are represented as means ± SEM. Differences among groups were determined by using one-way ANOVA followed by Newman–Keuls post hoc test. Values not sharing a common letter are significantly different ($p < 0.05$). SIRT1: sirtuin 1, GLUT4: glucose transporter 4, UCP1: uncoupling protein 1, SIRT3: sirtuin 3, TFAM: mitochondrial transcription factor A, AMPK: AMP activated protein kinase, IBAT: interscapular brown adipose tissue.

Mitochondriogenesis is a process closely related to thermogenesis. Thus, proteins involved in this process were also analyzed. Increased protein expressions of NRF1 were found in the RSV, R and RR groups when compared with the C group ($p = 0.04$, $p = 0.01$ and $p = 0.02$, respectively), with no differences among them (Figure 5). A similar pattern of response was observed in TFAM protein levels ($p = 0.04$ in the RSV group, $p = 0.02$ in the R group and $p = 0.04$ in the RR group) (Figure 4). In addition, GLUT4 protein level, a glucose transporter that provides with this energy substrate to IBAT, was increased only in the groups supplemented with resveratrol (RSV and RR) ($p = 0.048$ and $p = 0.050$, respectively) (Figure 4).

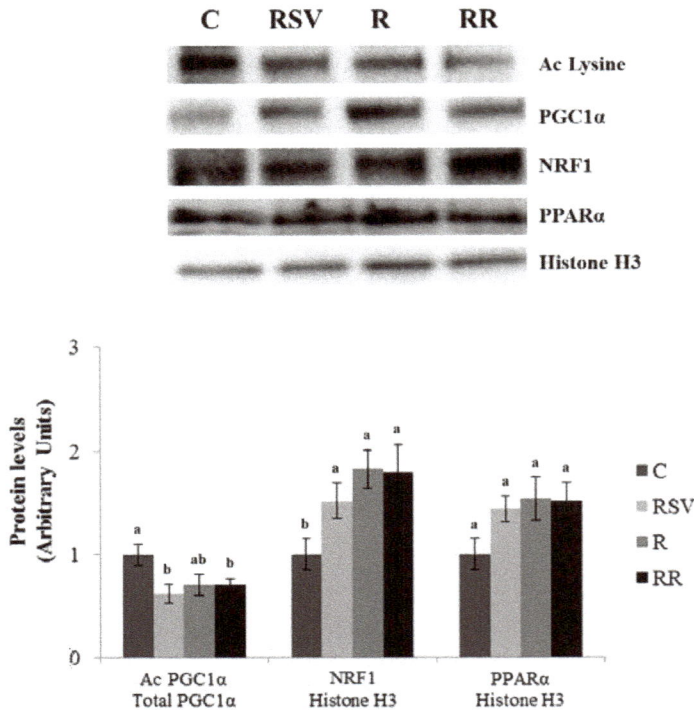

Figure 5. Acetylation ratio of PGC1α and protein levels of NRF1 and PPARα in IBAT of rats fed an obesogenic diet for 6 weeks and then shifted to a standard diet (C), or standard diet supplemented with resveratrol (RSV), or submitted to energy restriction and fed a standard diet (R), or submitted to energy restriction and fed a standard diet supplemented with resveratrol (RR) ($n = 9$/group) for additional 6 weeks. Values are represented as means ± SEM. Differences among groups were determined by using one-way ANOVA followed by Newman–Keuls post hoc test. Values not sharing a common letter are significantly different ($p < 0.05$). PGC1α: peroxisome proliferator-activated receptor gamma coactivator 1-alpha, NRF1: nuclear respiratory factor 1, PPARα: peroxisome proliferator-activated receptor alpha, IBAT: interscapular brown adipose tissue.

In the case of gastrocnemius muscle, no effects of the treatments were found in UCP3 protein expression (Figure 6). Regarding PGC1α, significantly lower acetylation, and thus greater activation of the protein, was observed in the RSV group in comparison to the C group ($p = 0.03$). In the case of restricted groups, only trends towards lower acetylation status were appreciated (-34.7%; $p = 0.053$ in R and -30.4%; $p = 0.10$ in RR) (Figure 7). Protein expressions of PPARβ/δ, SIRT1 and SIRT3 remained unchanged (Figures 6 and 7). Similarly, lack of change was also found in NRF1, although a trend towards increased protein expressions was appreciated in the groups submitted to energy restriction when compared to the C group ($+34.7\%$; $p = 0.065$ in the R group and $+25.5\%$; $p = 0.081$ in the RR group) (Figure 7). By contrast, greater protein expression of TFAM was observed in the three treated groups in comparison with the C group ($p = 0.04$ in RSV group, $p = 0.02$ in the R group and $p = 0.04$ in the RR group) (Figure 6). Finally, significantly greater activation of AMPK was only observed in the RR group when compared with the C group ($p = 0.024$). In the case of the RSV and R groups, tendencies towards an increased activation were found ($+50.9\%$; $p = 0.082$ and $+58.9\%$; $p = 0.054$, respectively) (Figure 6).

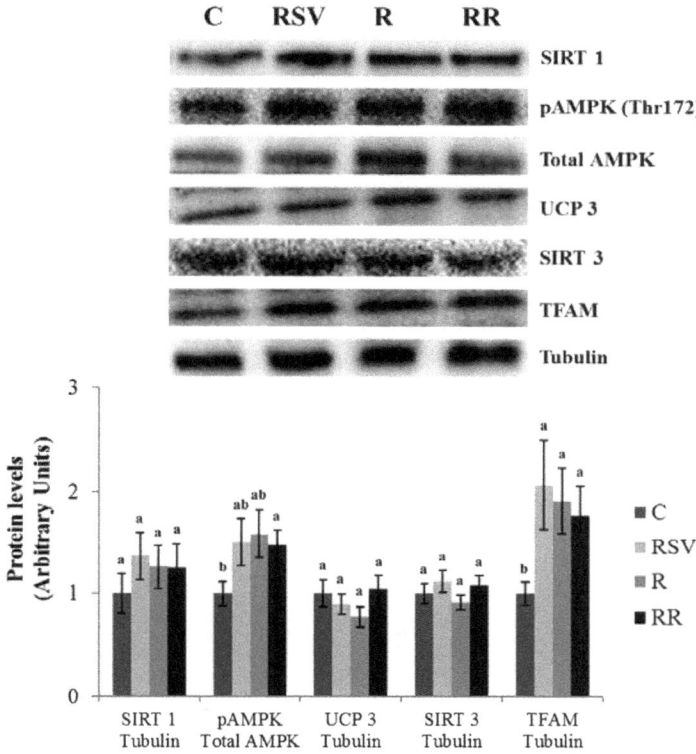

Figure 6. Protein levels of SIRT1, UCP3, SIRT3 and TFAM, and threonine 172 phosphorylation ratio of AMPK in gastrocnemius muscle of rats fed an obesogenic diet for 6 weeks and then shifted to a standard diet (C), or standard diet supplemented with resveratrol (RSV), or submitted to energy restriction and fed a standard diet (R), or submitted to energy restriction and fed a standard diet supplemented with resveratrol (RR) (n = 9/group) for additional 6 weeks. Values are represented as means ± SEM. Differences among groups were determined by using one-way ANOVA followed by Newman–Keuls post hoc test. Values not sharing a common letter are significantly different ($p < 0.05$). SIRT1: sirtuin 1, UCP3: uncoupling protein 3, SIRT3: sirtuin 3, TFAM: mitochondrial transcription factor 1, AMPK: AMP activated protein kinase.

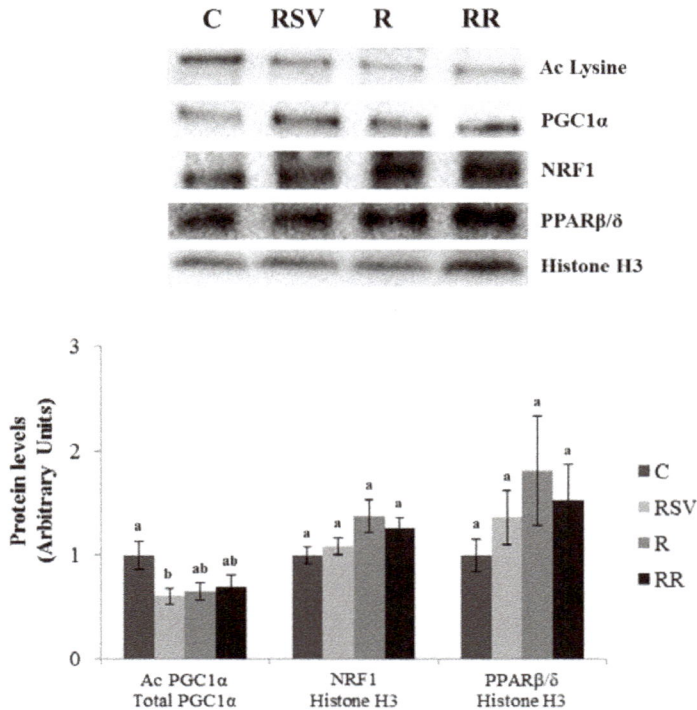

Figure 7. Acetylation ratio of PGC1α and protein levels of NRF1 and PPARβ/δ in gastrocnemius muscle of rats fed an obesogenic diet for 6 weeks and then shifted to a standard diet (C), or standard diet supplemented with resveratrol (RSV), or submitted to energy restriction and fed a standard diet (R), or submitted to energy restriction and fed a standard diet supplemented with resveratrol (RR) (*n* = 9/group) for additional 6 weeks. Values are represented as means ± SEM. Differences among groups were determined by using one-way ANOVA followed by Newman–Keuls post hoc test. Values not sharing a common letter are significantly different ($p < 0.05$). PGC1α: peroxisome proliferator-activated receptor gamma coactivator 1-alpha, NRF1: nuclear respiratory factor 1, PPAR β/δ: peroxisome proliferator-activated receptor beta/delta.

4. Discussion

As indicated in the introduction, the interest of the scientific community in natural bioactive compounds with beneficial health effects has been increasing in recent years. Regarding resveratrol, positive effects on several prevalent diseases have been reported both in animals and humans [19,31–34]. It is important to emphasize that, with regard to its effects on obesity and related co-morbilities such as insulin resistance and liver steatosis, the vast majority of the reported studies addressed in animal models have been carried out by using experimental designs in which resveratrol was administered together with an obesogenic diet. Consequently, the beneficial effects observed in these studies were related to the prevention of weight gain and metabolic alterations induced by this dietary pattern. However, the applicability of such experimental design in humans is unlikely. Indeed, for ethical reasons, it is not possible to recommend people to take resveratrol while they maintain an inappropriate dietary pattern.

Bearing this in mind, we focused our interest on the potential beneficial effects of resveratrol as a tool for obesity treatment. Thus, we assessed its effects on rats that had previously developed overweight/obesity (induced by diet). For this purpose, two approaches were designed. In the first, once obesity induction had stopped resveratrol was administered, as the single tool to treat obesity, together with a standard diet, while in the other resveratrol was combined with an energetically restricted diet, which is the most commonly strategy used in obesity treatment

It is important to point out that, in the vast majority of the reported studies, energy restriction ranges from 20% to 40%. In the present study a lower degree of restriction (15%) was chosen. The reason was based on a previous study from our group [35]. In that study we looked for synergistic effects between resveratrol, at a dose of 30 mg/kg of body weight/day, and 25% energy restriction. We observed that the addition of resveratrol to the restricted diet did not lead to additional reductions in fat mass or in serum insulin concentrations with regard to those produced by energy restriction alone. We believed that one of the reasons that could explain this situation was that the effects caused by energy restriction were strong enough to mask the potential positive effects ascribed to resveratrol. Consequently, a lower degree of energy restriction was preferred in the present study.

In IBAT, resveratrol administration increased UCP1 protein expression, suggesting a greater thermogenic capacity. In order to analyze the mechanism underlying this effect, we studied the regulation pathway described in Figure 3. Resveratrol induced deacetylation, and thus activation, of PGC1α, a co-activator of PPARα, which in turn regulates the expression of UCP1. It has been reported that SIRT1 is the main enzyme responsible for PGC1α deacetylation [36]. In the present study, a tendency towards increased protein expression of SIRT1 was observed. Although its activation was not directly measured, the deacetylation of PGC1α suggests that it was in fact activated. In addition, resveratrol increased the activity of AMPK, an enzyme that phosphorylates PGC1α, thus enhancing its activity. Furthermore, SIRT3 is activated by PGC1α, mediating the effects of this sirtuin on mitochondrial function and synthesis [37,38]. Moreover, the expression of this deacetylase has been reported to be positively correlated with a variety of mitochondrial proteins, UCP1 among them [39]. In the case of our study, significantly increased protein expression of SIRT3 was observed in resveratrol-treated rats. These results show that resveratrol increased the expression of UCP1 by activating the SIRT1/PGC1α/PPARα axis.

Fatty acid oxidation is an important part of the thermogenic program. It has been reported that the activation of PPARα by PGC1α leads to increased NRF1 and the subsequent increase in the synthesis of TFAM, which in turn results in enhanced duplication of mitochondrial DNA (Figure 3). Accordingly, in the present study PGC-1α activation was indeed accompanied by increases in NRF1 and TFAM expressions, suggesting that resveratrol, under the present experimental conditions, enhanced mitochondriogenesis. This is in good accordance with the increased activities of CPT1a and CS observed in rats treated with resveratrol. BAT can also use glucose as an energetic substrate. In the present study resveratrol induced a significant increase in GLUT4 protein expression, meaning that the capacity of IBAT to uptake glucose was greater in rats treated with this phenolic compound. Taken as a whole, these results show that resveratrol did not only increase the key factor for thermogenesis (UCP1) but also the availability of substrates to keep this process activated.

In previous studies from our laboratory we had already observed the induction of UCP1 by resveratrol in IBAT [22,40] and other authors had also reported similar results [41,42]. In all these studies the animals received the phenolic compound at the same time as an obesogenic diet, during the fattening period. By contrast, in this work the animals were fed a high-fat high sucrose diet to become obese and then they were shifted to a standard diet, and treated with resveratrol. Taken together, the present results and those reported previously demonstrate the ability of resveratrol to induce thermogenesis under both overfeeding and normal feeding conditions. This may represent a mechanism of action underlying the beneficial effect of resveratrol in obesity management.

As previously mentioned, a second approach in this study was to analyze the effects induced by resveratrol under energy restriction. In fact, the usefulness of this phenolic compound in combination with the most common strategy for obesity treatment was intended to analyze whether potential additive or synergistic effects could take place. This is an interesting approach because it would result in the same positive effect obtained by following a more restricted diet non supplemented with resveratrol, whose compliance is more difficult to achieve.

For this purpose, first of all we analyzed the effects of energy restriction on the parameters previously studied in the first approach. No change in UCP1 protein expression was observed in R group. By contrast, NRF1 and TFAM protein expressions, as well as the CPT1a activity were significantly increased in these animals, suggesting that mitochondrial synthesis and function were enhanced. The increased SIRT3 protein expression observed in this experimental group supports the idea of an ameliorated mitochondrial function, in good accordance with previous data describing the activation of this protein in different tissues under energy restriction conditions [43–45]. It is important to remember that resveratrol has been suggested as an energy restriction mimetic [20,21,46,47]. However, as shown by the present results, differential effects on thermogenic capacity are found between them.

When we analyzed the RR group, in general terms, the effects on the parameters studied were similar to those observed in the RSV group, although in this case only a trend towards higher values was observed in UCP1. These results demonstrate that the administration of resveratrol in combination with energy restriction does not provide any advantage.

In the case of skeletal muscle, the effects of resveratrol were not as clear as in IBAT. The administration of this polyphenol was not able to increase protein expression of UCP3, despite the activation of PGC-1α. Nevertheless, increased TFAM protein expression and CPT-1b activity suggest increased fatty acid oxidation, associated to enhanced mitochondrial synthesis. It has been reported that the activation of PGC-1α is based on sirtuin-mediated deacetylation and phosphorylation by AMPK [48,49]. In the case of skeletal muscle, the absence of any significant activation of AMPK by resveratrol may explain the lack of activation of every single step in mitochondriogenesis pathway, and consequently in CS activity.

In the studies reported by other authors there is no consensus regarding the effects of resveratrol on skeletal muscle mitochondrial biogenesis induction. Indeed, while an enhanced mitochondrial synthesis and/or function has been described in studies where the compound was administered in conditions of certain metabolic stress [41,50,51], this effect seems to disappear when the polyphenol is administered in healthy subjects [52–54]. Regarding UCP3, the lack of change found in this study is not in good accordance with data reported by other authors. In those studies, resveratrol effectively induced UCP3 mRNA or protein expression in the skeletal muscle of mice and rats fed in obesogenic diets [22,41]. Moreover, greater UCP3 protein expression was also described in this tissue in mice fed in a standard diet and supplemented with the polyphenol [55]. Nevertheless, the discrepancy between our results and those previously reported could result from significant differences in the experimental design (animal model, experimental period length, resveratrol dose and diet composition).

As far as energy restriction is concerned, no relevant significant changes were observed in the parameters analysed. By revising data reported in the literature concerning this issue we observed that some controversy exists. Thus, while some authors have reported that the maintenance of a 30% energy restriction for a period of 3 months effectively induces mitochondrial biogenesis and function (increased respiration and expression of genes important for oxidative function), others have found no such effects under similar experimental conditions [56,57]. In fact, in a study conducted in mice of different ages (6, 12 and 24 month old B6D2F1 mice) that underwent a lifelong energy restriction (40%), the authors concluded that energy restriction did not induce mitochondrial protein synthesis, but maintained this parameter while decreasing cellular proliferation [58]. Moreover, the authors point towards the techniques used by Nisoli et al., and Hancock et al. in determining the effects of energy restriction on mitochondrial synthesis (mRNA and protein expression of mitochondrial proteins) as being the cause of their contradictory results. Finally, when resveratrol was administered under energy restriction feeding conditions, the results were very similar to those observed when the compound was administered under standard feeding conditions.

We would like to point out that in previous studies conducted in this precise cohort of rats aimed at studying the effects of the aforementioned treatments on glucose homeostasis and hepatic steatosis ([29,30], respectively), resveratrol-induced effects were less marked than those produced by energy restriction. By contrast, when considering the effects on UCP expression and fatty acid oxidative capacity, as in the present study, resveratrol was more effective than a mild energy restriction.

In conclusion, in obese rats under standard feeding conditions, resveratrol is able to increase thermogenic and oxidative capacities in IBAT. This feature represents a mechanism by which this phenolic compound could show an anti-obesity action. Nevertheless, more research is needed in order to interpret the importance of this mechanism. In the case of skeletal muscle, oxidative capacity is increased by this polyphenol intake. The administration of resveratrol in combination with energy restriction apparently does not provide any advantage.

Supplementary Materials: The following are available online at http://www.mdpi.com/2072-6643/10/10/1446/s1, Figure S1: Timeline of the complete experimental period (12 weeks), Table S1: Composition of the experimental (A) High-fat High-sucrose and (B) Standard control diets, Table S2: References of the antibodies used for western blot analyses.

Author Contributions: Investigation, I.M.-L., U.E. and F.M.; Supervision, L.A.; Writing—original draft, M.P.P.; Writing—review and editing, A.M.

Funding: This research was funded by MINECO (AGL-2015-65719-R-MINECO/FEDER, UE), University of the Basque Country (ELDUNANOTEK UFI11/32), Instituto de Salud Carlos III (CIBERobn) and Basque Government (IT-572-13). Iñaki Milton-Laskibar is a recipient of a doctoral fellowship from the Gobierno Vasco.

Conflicts of Interest: The authors declare no conflict of interest.

References

1. Lowell, B.B.; Spiegelman, B.M. Towards a molecular understanding of adaptive thermogenesis. *Nature* **2000**, *404*, 652–660. [CrossRef] [PubMed]
2. Ricquier, D.; Casteilla, L.; Bouillaud, F. Molecular studies of the uncoupling protein. *FASEB J.* **1991**, *5*, 2237–2242. [CrossRef] [PubMed]
3. Cannon, B.; Nedergaard, J. The biochemistry of an inefficient tissue: Brown adipose tissue. *Essays Biochem.* **1985**, *20*, 110–164. [PubMed]
4. Palou, A.; Picó, C.; Bonet, M.L.; Oliver, P. The uncoupling protein, thermogenin. *Int. J. Biochem. Cell Biol.* **1998**, *30*, 7–11. [CrossRef]
5. Nedergaard, J.; Bengtsson, T.; Cannon, B. Unexpected evidence for active brown adipose tissue in adult humans. *Am. J. Physiol. Endocrinol. Metab.* **2007**, *293*, E444–E452. [CrossRef] [PubMed]
6. Saito, M.; Okamatsu-Ogura, Y.; Matsushita, M.; Watanabe, K.; Yoneshiro, T.; Nio-Kobayashi, J.; Iwanaga, T.; Miyagawa, M.; Kameya, T.; Nakada, K.; et al. High incidence of metabolically active brown adipose tissue in healthy adult humans: Effects of cold exposure and adiposity. *Diabetes* **2009**, *58*, 1526–1531. [CrossRef] [PubMed]
7. Lee, P.; Greenfield, J.R.; Ho, K.K.; Fulham, M.J. A critical appraisal of the prevalence and metabolic significance of brown adipose tissue in adult humans. *Am. J. Physiol. Endocrinol. Metab.* **2010**, *299*, E601–E606. [CrossRef] [PubMed]
8. Nedergaard, J.; Bengtsson, T.; Cannon, B. New powers of brown fat: Fighting the metabolic syndrome. *Cell Metab.* **2011**, *13*, 238–240. [CrossRef] [PubMed]
9. Bartelt, A.; Bruns, O.T.; Reimer, R.; Hohenberg, H.; Ittrich, H.; Peldschus, K.; Kaul, M.G.; Tromsdorf, U.I.; Weller, H.; Waurisch, C.; et al. Brown adipose tissue activity controls triglyceride clearance. *Nat. Med.* **2011**, *17*, 200–205. [CrossRef] [PubMed]
10. Zurlo, F.; Larson, K.; Bogardus, C.; Ravussin, E. Skeletal muscle metabolism is a major determinant of resting energy expenditure. *J. Clin. Investig.* **1990**, *86*, 1423–1427. [CrossRef] [PubMed]
11. Janssen, I.; Heymsfield, S.B.; Wang, Z.M.; Ross, R. Skeletal muscle mass and distribution in 468 men and women aged 18–88 yr. *J. Appl. Physiol.* **2000**, *89*, 81–88. [CrossRef] [PubMed]
12. Schrauwen, P. Skeletal muscle uncoupling protein 3 (UCP3): Mitochondrial uncoupling protein in search of a function. *Curr. Opin. Clin. Nutr. Metab. Care* **2002**, *5*, 265–270. [CrossRef] [PubMed]

13. Schrauwen, P.; Hardie, D.G.; Roorda, B.; Clapham, J.C.; Abuin, A.; Thomason-Hughes, M.; Green, K.; Frederik, P.M.; Hesselink, M.K. Improved glucose homeostasis in mice overexpressing human UCP3: A role for AMP-kinase? *Int. J. Obes.* **2004**, *28*, 824–828. [CrossRef] [PubMed]

14. Brand, M.D.; Esteves, T.C. Physiological functions of the mitochondrial uncoupling proteins UCP2 and UCP3. *Cell Metab.* **2005**, *2*, 85–93. [CrossRef] [PubMed]

15. Rodríguez, V.M.; Portillo, M.P.; Picó, C.; Macarulla, M.T.; Palou, A. Olive oil feeding up-regulates uncoupling protein genes in rat brown adipose tissue and skeletal muscle. *Am. J. Clin. Nutr.* **2002**, *75*, 213–220. [CrossRef] [PubMed]

16. Champigny, O.; Ricquier, D. Effects of fasting and refeeding on the level of uncoupling protein mRNA in rat brown adipose tissue: Evidence for diet-induced and cold-induced responses. *J. Nutr.* **1990**, *120*, 1730–1736. [CrossRef] [PubMed]

17. Markus, M.A.; Morris, B.J. Resveratrol in prevention and treatment of common clinical conditions of aging. *Clin. Interv. Aging* **2008**, *3*, 331–339. [PubMed]

18. Aguirre, L.; Fernandez-Quintela, A.; Arias, N.; Portillo, M.P. Resveratrol: Anti-obesity mechanisms of action. *Molecules* **2014**, *19*, 18632–18655. [CrossRef] [PubMed]

19. Fernández-Quintela, A.; Carpéné, C.; Fernández, M.; Aguirre, L.; Milton-Laskibar, I.; Contreras, J.; Portillo, M.P. Anti-obesity effects of resveratrol: Comparison between animal models and humans. *J. Physiol. Biochem.* **2016**, *73*, 417–429. [CrossRef] [PubMed]

20. Barger, J.L.; Kayo, T.; Vann, J.M.; Arias, E.B.; Wang, J.; Hacker, T.A.; Wang, Y.; Raederstorff, D.; Morrow, J.D.; Leeuwenburgh, C.; et al. A low dose of dietary resveratrol partially mimics caloric restriction and retards aging parameters in mice. *PLoS ONE* **2008**, *3*, e2264. [CrossRef]

21. Baur, J.A. Resveratrol, sirtuins, and the promise of a DR mimetic. *Mech. Ageing Dev.* **2010**, *131*, 261–269. [CrossRef] [PubMed]

22. Alberdi, G.; Rodríguez, V.M.; Miranda, J.; Macarulla, M.T.; Churruca, I.; Portillo, M.P. Thermogenesis is involved in the body-fat lowering effects of resveratrol in rats. *Food Chem.* **2013**, *141*, 1530–1535. [CrossRef] [PubMed]

23. Andrade, J.M.O.; Frade, A.C.M.; Guimarães, J.B.; Freitas, K.M.; Lopes, M.T.P.; Guimarães, A.L.S.; de Paula, A.M.B.; Coimbra, C.C.; Santos, S.H.S. Resveratrol increases brown adipose tissue thermogenesis markers by increasing SIRT1 and energy expenditure and decreasing fat accumulation in adipose tissue of mice fed a standard diet. *Eur. J. Nutr.* **2014**, *53*, 1503–1510. [CrossRef] [PubMed]

24. Macarulla, M.T.; Alberdi, G.; Gomez, S.; Tueros, I.; Bald, C.; Rodriguez, V.M.; Matinez, J.A.; Portillo, M.P. Effects of different doses of resveratrol on body fat and serum parameters in rats fed a hypercaloric diet. *J. Physiol. Biochem.* **2009**, *65*, 369–376. [CrossRef] [PubMed]

25. Bradford, M.M. A rapid and sensitive method for the quantitation of microgram quantities of protein utilizing the principle of protein-dye binding. *Anal. Biochem.* **1976**, *72*, 248–254. [CrossRef]

26. Bieber, L.L.; Abraham, T.; Helmrath, T. A rapid spectrophotometric assay for carnitine palmitoyltransferase. *Anal. Biochem.* **1972**, *50*, 509–518. [CrossRef]

27. Srere, P. Citrate synthase. In *Methods in Enzymology*; Elsevier: Amsterdam, The Netherlands, 1969; Volume 13, pp. 3–11.

28. Aguirre, L.; Hijona, E.; Macarulla, M.T.; Gracia, A.; Larrechi, I.; Bujanda, L.; Hijona, L.; Portillo, M.P. Several statins increase body and liver fat accumulation in a model of metabolic syndrome. *J. Physiol. Pharmacol.* **2013**, *64*, 281–288. [PubMed]

29. Milton-Laskibar, I.; Aguirre, L.; Macarulla, M.T.; Etxeberria, U.; Milagro, F.I.; Martínez, J.A.; Contreras, J.; Portillo, M.P. Comparative effects of energy restriction and resveratrol intake on glycemic control improvement. *Biofactors* **2017**, *43*, 371–378. [CrossRef] [PubMed]

30. Milton-Laskibar, I.; Aguirre, L.; Fernández-Quintela, A.; Rolo, A.P.; Soeiro Teodoro, J.; Palmeira, C.M.; Portillo, M.P. Lack of Additive Effects of Resveratrol and Energy Restriction in the Treatment of Hepatic Steatosis in Rats. *Nutrients* **2017**, *9*, 737. [CrossRef] [PubMed]

31. Smoliga, J.M.; Baur, J.A.; Hausenblas, H.A. Resveratrol and health–a comprehensive review of human clinical trials. *Mol. Nutr. Food Res.* **2011**, *55*, 1129–1141. [CrossRef] [PubMed]

32. Petrovski, G.; Gurusamy, N.; Das, D.K. Resveratrol in cardiovascular health and disease. *Ann. N. Y. Acad. Sci.* **2011**, *1215*, 22–33. [CrossRef] [PubMed]

33. Aguirre, L.; Portillo, M.P.; Hijona, E.; Bujanda, L. Effects of resveratrol and other polyphenols in hepatic steatosis. *World J. Gastroenterol.* **2014**, *20*, 7366–7380. [CrossRef] [PubMed]

34. Tellone, E.; Galtieri, A.; Russo, A.; Giardina, B.; Ficarra, S. Resveratrol: A Focus on Several Neurodegenerative Diseases. *Oxid. Med. Cell. Longev.* **2015**, *2015*, 392169. [CrossRef] [PubMed]

35. Alberdi, G.; Macarulla, M.T.; Portillo, M.P.; Rodriguez, V.M. Resveratrol does not increase body fat loss induced by energy restriction. *J. Physiol. Biochem.* **2014**, *70*, 639–646. [CrossRef] [PubMed]

36. Canto, C.; Auwerx, J. PGC-1alpha, SIRT1 and AMPK, an energy sensing network that controls energy expenditure. *Curr. Opin. Lipidol.* **2009**, *20*, 98–105. [CrossRef] [PubMed]

37. Kong, X.; Wang, R.; Xue, Y.; Liu, X.; Zhang, H.; Chen, Y.; Fang, F.; Chang, Y. Sirtuin 3, a new target of PGC-1alpha, plays an important role in the suppression of ROS and mitochondrial biogenesis. *PLoS ONE* **2010**, *5*, e11707. [CrossRef] [PubMed]

38. Teodoro, J.S.; Duarte, F.V.; Gomes, A.P.; Varela, A.T.; Peixoto, F.M.; Rolo, A.P.; Palmeira, C.M. Berberine reverts hepatic mitochondrial dysfunction in high-fat fed rats: A possible role for SirT3 activation. *Mitochondrion* **2013**, *13*, 637–646. [CrossRef] [PubMed]

39. Shi, T.; Wang, F.; Stieren, E.; Tong, Q. SIRT3, a mitochondrial sirtuin deacetylase, regulates mitochondrial function and thermogenesis in brown adipocytes. *J. Biol. Chem.* **2005**, *280*, 13560–13567. [CrossRef] [PubMed]

40. Arias, N.; Picó, C.; Teresa Macarulla, M.; Oliver, P.; Miranda, J.; Palou, A.; Portillo, M.P. A combination of resveratrol and quercetin induces browning in white adipose tissue of rats fed an obesogenic diet. *Obesity* **2017**, *25*, 111–121. [CrossRef] [PubMed]

41. Lagouge, M.; Argmann, C.; Gerhart-Hines, Z.; Meziane, H.; Lerin, C.; Daussin, F.; Messadeq, N.; Milne, J.; Lambert, P.; Elliott, P.; et al. Resveratrol improves mitochondrial function and protects against metabolic disease by activating SIRT1 and PGC-1alpha. *Cell* **2006**, *127*, 1109–1122. [CrossRef] [PubMed]

42. Wang, S.; Liang, X.; Yang, Q.; Fu, X.; Zhu, M.; Rodgers, B.D.; Jiang, Q.; Dodson, M.V.; Du, M. Resveratrol enhances brown adipocyte formation and function by activating AMP-activated protein kinase (AMPK) α1 in mice fed high-fat diet. *Mol. Nutr. Food Res.* **2017**, *61*, 1600746. [CrossRef] [PubMed]

43. Palacios, O.M.; Carmona, J.J.; Michan, S.; Chen, K.Y.; Manabe, Y.; Ward, J.L.; Goodyear, L.J.; Tong, Q. Diet and exercise signals regulate SIRT3 and activate AMPK and PGC-1alpha in skeletal muscle. *Aging (Albany NY)* **2009**, *1*, 771–783. [CrossRef] [PubMed]

44. Someya, S.; Yu, W.; Hallows, W.C.; Xu, J.; Vann, J.M.; Leeuwenburgh, C.; Tanokura, M.; Denu, J.M.; Prolla, T.A. Sirt3 mediates reduction of oxidative damage and prevention of age-related hearing loss under caloric restriction. *Cell* **2010**, *143*, 802–812. [CrossRef] [PubMed]

45. Tauriainen, E.; Luostarinen, M.; Martonen, E.; Finckenberg, P.; Kovalainen, M.; Huotari, A.; Herzig, K.H.; Lecklin, A.; Mervaala, E. Distinct effects of calorie restriction and resveratrol on diet-induced obesity and Fatty liver formation. *J. Nutr. Metabol.* **2011**, *2011*, 525094. [CrossRef] [PubMed]

46. Pearson, K.J.; Baur, J.A.; Lewis, K.N.; Peshkin, L.; Price, N.L.; Labinskyy, N.; Swindell, W.R.; Kamara, D.; Minor, R.K.; Perez, E.; et al. Resveratrol delays age-related deterioration and mimics transcriptional aspects of dietary restriction without extending life span. *Cell Metab.* **2008**, *8*, 157–168. [CrossRef] [PubMed]

47. Mercken, E.M.; Carboneau, B.A.; Krzysik-Walker, S.M.; de Cabo, R. Of mice and men: The benefits of caloric restriction, exercise, and mimetics. *Ageing Res. Rev.* **2012**, *11*, 390–398. [CrossRef] [PubMed]

48. Rodgers, J.T.; Lerin, C.; Haas, W.; Gygi, S.P.; Spiegelman, B.M.; Puigserver, P. Nutrient control of glucose homeostasis through a complex of PGC-1alpha and SIRT1. *Nature* **2005**, *434*, 113–118. [CrossRef] [PubMed]

49. Jäger, S.; Handschin, C.; St-Pierre, J.; Spiegelman, B.M. AMP-activated protein kinase (AMPK) action in skeletal muscle via direct phosphorylation of PGC-1alpha. *Proc. Natl. Acad. Sci. USA* **2007**, *104*, 12017–12022. [CrossRef] [PubMed]

50. Um, J.H.; Park, S.J.; Kang, H.; Yang, S.; Foretz, M.; McBurney, M.W.; Kim, M.K.; Viollet, B.; Chung, J.H. AMP-activated protein kinase-deficient mice are resistant to the metabolic effects of resveratrol. *Diabetes* **2010**, *59*, 554–563. [CrossRef] [PubMed]

51. Haohao, Z.; Guijun, Q.; Juan, Z.; Wen, K.; Lulu, C. Resveratrol improves high-fat diet induced insulin resistance by rebalancing subsarcolemmal mitochondrial oxidation and antioxidantion. *J. Physiol. Biochem.* **2015**, *71*, 121–131. [CrossRef] [PubMed]

52. Yoshino, J.; Conte, C.; Fontana, L.; Mittendorfer, B.; Imai, S.; Schechtman, K.B.; Gu, C.; Kunz, I.; Rossi Fanelli, F.; Patterson, B.W.; et al. Resveratrol supplementation does not improve metabolic function in nonobese women with normal glucose tolerance. *Cell Metab.* **2012**, *16*, 658–664. [CrossRef] [PubMed]

53. Higashida, K.; Kim, S.H.; Jung, S.R.; Asaka, M.; Holloszy, J.O.; Han, D.H. Effects of resveratrol and SIRT1 on PGC-1α activity and mitochondrial biogenesis: A reevaluation. *PLoS Biol.* **2013**, *11*, e1001603. [CrossRef] [PubMed]

54. Olesen, J.; Gliemann, L.; Biensø, R.; Schmidt, J.; Hellsten, Y.; Pilegaard, H. Exercise training, but not resveratrol, improves metabolic and inflammatory status in skeletal muscle of aged men. *J. Physiol.* **2014**, *592*, 1873–1886. [CrossRef] [PubMed]

55. Do, G.M.; Jung, U.J.; Park, H.J.; Kwon, E.Y.; Jeon, S.M.; McGregor, R.A.; Choi, M.S. Resveratrol ameliorates diabetes-related metabolic changes via activation of AMP-activated protein kinase and its downstream targets in db/db mice. *Mol. Nutr. Food Res.* **2012**, *56*, 1282–1291. [CrossRef] [PubMed]

56. Nisoli, E.; Tonello, C.; Cardile, A.; Cozzi, V.; Bracale, R.; Tedesco, L.; Falcone, S.; Valerio, A.; Cantoni, O.; Clementi, E.; et al. Calorie restriction promotes mitochondrial biogenesis by inducing the expression of eNOS. *Science* **2005**, *310*, 314–317. [CrossRef] [PubMed]

57. Hancock, C.R.; Han, D.H.; Higashida, K.; Kim, S.H.; Holloszy, J.O. Does calorie restriction induce mitochondrial biogenesis? A reevaluation. *FASEB J.* **2011**, *25*, 785–791. [CrossRef] [PubMed]

58. Miller, B.F.; Robinson, M.M.; Bruss, M.D.; Hellerstein, M.; Hamilton, K.L. A comprehensive assessment of mitochondrial protein synthesis and cellular proliferation with age and caloric restriction. *Aging Cell* **2012**, *11*, 150–161. [CrossRef] [PubMed]

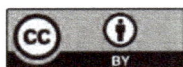

nutrients

MDPI

Review

Resveratrol, Metabolic Syndrome, and Gut Microbiota

Alice Chaplin [1],*, Christian Carpéné [2] and Josep Mercader [3,4,*

[1] Cardiovascular Research Institute, School of Medicine, Case Western Reserve University, Cleveland, OH 44106, USA

[2] INSERM U1048, Institute of Metabolic and Cardiovascular Diseases (I2MC) and University Paul Sabatier, 31432 Toulouse, France; christian.carpene@inserm.fr

[3] Department of Fundamental Biology and Health Sciences, University of the Balearic Islands, 07122 Palma, Spain

[4] Balearic Islands Health Research Institute (IdISBa), 07122 Palma, Spain

* Correspondence: amc315@case.edu (A.C.); josep.mercader@uib.es (J.M.); Tel: +1-216-258-8385 (A.C.); +34-971-172-009 (J.M.)

Received: 15 October 2018; Accepted: 29 October 2018; Published: 3 November 2018

Abstract: Resveratrol is a polyphenol which has been shown to have beneficial effects on metabolic syndrome-related alterations in experimental animals, including glucose and lipid homeostasis improvement and a reduction in fat mass, blood pressure, low-grade inflammation, and oxidative stress. Clinical trials have been carried out to address its potential; however, results are still inconclusive. Even though resveratrol is partly metabolized by gut microbiota, the relevance of this "forgotten organ" had not been widely considered. However, in the past few years, data has emerged suggesting that the therapeutic potential of this compound may be due to its interaction with gut microbiota, reporting changes in bacterial composition associated with beneficial metabolic outcomes. Even though data is still scarce and for the most part observational, it is promising nevertheless, suggesting that resveratrol supplementation could be a useful tool for the treatment of metabolic syndrome and its associated conditions.

Keywords: resveratrol; gut microbiota; metabolic syndrome

---

1. Introduction

In obese states, insulin resistance and inflammation are the underlying causes of the metabolic syndrome, and together with high blood triglycerides, altered cholesterol levels, glucose intolerance and hypertension, they greatly increase the risk of type 2 diabetes and cardiovascular disease [1]. Currently, the main treatments for metabolic syndrome are weight loss and physical activity; however, there is also evidence that pharmacotherapy (insulin sensitizers, statins, angiotensin-converting enzyme inhibitors) and, more recently, nutritional strategies could be beneficial [2]. Within this context, resveratrol, a natural phytochemical widely found in plants, fruits, and red wine, presents itself as a potential candidate, due to the recent observations in various animal models and human studies of its beneficial effects in terms of glucose and lipid homeostasis and reduced body fat accumulation [3–6]. It is known as a phytoalexin because of its ability to inhibit the progress of certain infections, and is one of the components of red wine believed to contribute to the French Paradox, which refers to a low prevalence of ischemic heart disease in populations with high intakes of saturated fat [7]. Furthermore, it has been demonstrated that resveratrol mimics calorie restriction effects through sirtuin 1 (SIRT1) activation, and thus extends the lifespan in simple organisms and prevents the deleterious effects of excess caloric intake in rodents, such as insulin resistance and body fat accumulation [4,8]. In humans, however, the effectiveness towards the treatment of metabolic syndrome has been reported to be in some cases lower than in experimental animals [9]. In addition, discrepancies and inconsistencies have been observed in clinical trials, which can be explained by differences regarding the form of supplementation and the characteristics of the treated individuals, such as age, sex, presence of single nucleotide polymorphisms, presence of metabolic disturbances, and gut microbiota composition. Considering resveratrol is metabolized by gut microbiota [10,11] and that it can influence its composition [12], the interplay between this stilbenoid and the host microbiota may strongly influence treatment efficiency, by either increasing its bioavailability, producing certain metabolites, or even by promoting the growth of specific bacteria. Thus, the resveratrol/microbiota interaction is a key element in the effectiveness of the treatment of metabolic syndrome. In this review, we aim to discuss the current knowledge regarding the effects of resveratrol on metabolic syndrome alterations and on gut microbiota and also try to determine how such interactions could modulate the beneficial effects of this phytochemical.

2. Resveratrol Occurrence, Absorption, Metabolism, and Bioavailability

Resveratrol (3,5,4'-trihydroxy-*trans*-stilbene) is a natural phytochemical widely found in its *trans* isomer form in various plants, such as *Polygonum cuspidatum*, in fruits, including grapes and berries, peanuts, and in red wine [13,14]. It is a polyphenolic compound of low molecular weight that belongs to the stilbenoid family of polyphenolic compounds (hydroxylated derivatives of stilbene based on a C_6-C_2-C_6 polyphenolic structure). Resveratrol naturally occurs in these sources mainly in its glycosylated form, known as piceid and polydatin (3,4',5-trihydroxy-stilbene-3-β-mono-D-glucoside). Its use as a nutraceutical has been studied in both animal and human models, including clinical trials, in the context of obesity, metabolic syndrome, heart disease, and cancer, among others; however, to date, there are no specific recommendations concerning dosage and length of supplementation.

Upon ingestion, resveratrol or its precursors travel through the gastrointestinal tract, and it is estimated that around 70% of the intake of resveratrol is absorbed [13]. In the intestine, resveratrol binds to several nutrients, such as proteins, and the solubility of these will influence its absorption or elimination in feces [13]. Resveratrol absorption occurs by passive diffusion or by forming complexes with intestinal membrane transporters, including integrins. Free resveratrol circulates in the bloodstream bound to lipoproteins and albumin. However, the free form of resveratrol is found at very low levels in the bloodstream due to extensive glucuronidation in the liver and intestine and sulfation in the liver, thereby decreasing its bioavailability [14]. Hence, the major circulating forms of resveratrol are glucuronide (*trans*-resveratrol-3-glucoronide, *trans*-resveratrol-4'-glucuronide) and sulfate (*trans*-resveratrol-3-sulfate, *trans*-resveratrol-3,4'-disulfate, *trans*-resveratrol-3,5-disulfate) conjugate metabolites [13]. Likewise, resveratrol-3-sulfate and resveratrol-3-glucuronide are detected in target organs, such as in the liver, adipose tissue or the heart, after oral administration [15,16].

Besides resveratrol conjugates, other resveratrol derivatives are also detected in target tissues, such as piceatannol and dihydroresveratrol [17,18]. The occurrence of piceatannol (3,3',4,5'-tetrahydroxy-*trans*-stilbene) results from resveratrol hydroxylation in the liver by cytochrome P450 [18] and stands out due to its potentially beneficial effect on the metabolic syndrome [19]. It is a more stable stilbenoid that also naturally occurs in diverse plants. Dihydroresveratrol, synthesized by gut bacteria, together with free resveratrol, are detected in tissues after sustained resveratrol administration, whereas glucuronide and sulfate are the main resveratrol metabolites detected in tissues after an acute administration of resveratrol [17]. Therefore, the bioavailability of resveratrol and its metabolites largely differs on whether the administration is acute or sustained. In addition, the bioavailability of resveratrol and its metabolites is dose-dependent [15,16].

In turn, free resveratrol can be synthesized back from its sulfate and glucuronide derivatives by ubiquitously expressed sulfatase and β-glucuronidase [13]. Moreover, resveratrol metabolites can return to the small intestine through the bile enterohepatic transport. So far, up to 21 resveratrol metabolites have been identified in human urine after moderate consumption of red wine for

Nutrients **2018**, *10*, 1651

28 days [20], and it has been observed that some of these metabolites are by-products of gut microbial metabolism.

Impact of Gut Microbiota on Resveratrol Metabolism

The fact that the gut microbiota is highly responsible for metabolizing resveratrol has been known for some time; however, the importance of this process and of the metabolites and other by-products derived from this is only starting to gain relevance. As illustrated in Figure 1, the gut microbiota actively participates in resveratrol metabolism by increasing its availability from resveratrol precursors and producing resveratrol derivatives.

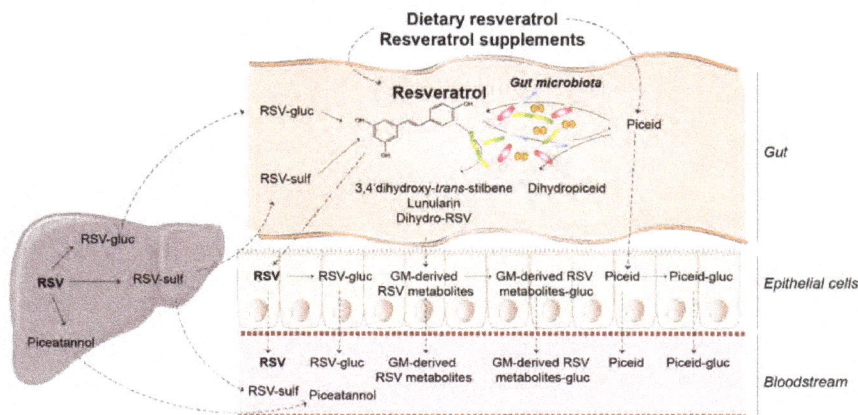

Figure 1. Overview of the metabolism of resveratrol and the impact of gut microbiota. Upon intake, RSV and RSV precursors enter the gut and are partly metabolised by gut microbiota to produce particular RSV derivatives and RSV. Free RSV, RSV precursors and microbiota-derived RSV metabolites are conjugated in the intestine and liver, from where conjugated forms can return to the intestine. In the liver, RSV is metabolised to piceatannol, which can be released into the bloodstream, and delivered to target tissues together with RSV, RSV precursors, microbiota-derived RSV metabolites and their respective conjugate forms. RSV, resveratrol; gluc, glucuronides; sulf, sulfates.

Gut bacteria metabolize resveratrol precursors to resveratrol, thereby increasing its bioavailability [14,21]. In particular, gut bacteria hydrolyze the glucoside moieties of plant glycosydes, such as the resveratrol precursor piceid, and thus externalize their aglycones. *Bifidobacteria infantis* and *Lactobacillus acidophilus* are two bacteria responsible for resveratrol production from piceid [11,21,22]. In turn, resveratrol can be glycosylated in the gut to produce piceid again. Piceid is conjugated to piceid glucuronide, and can be absorbed in both its free form, and most abundantly, in its conjugated form [23].

On the other hand, gut bacteria metabolize resveratrol and its precursors, resulting in certain resveratrol derivatives. Dihydroresveratrol was the first derivative identified, which is produced by *Slackia equolifaciens* and *Adlercreutzia equolifaciens*, followed by two other bacterial *trans*-resveratrol metabolites, 3,4'-dihydroxy-*trans*-stilbene and 3,4'-dihydroxybibenzyl (lunularin) [10]. Gut bacteria also metabolize piceid to produce dihydropiceid and dihydroresveratrol [22]. As resveratrol, gut bacteria-derived resveratrol derivatives are also conjugated to its glucuronide forms.

Furthermore, higher concentrations of dihydroresveratrol glucuronides than resveratrol glucuronides and glucosides have been found in human plasma and urine after the intake of a grape extract or red wine [23]. In tissues of rats receiving resveratrol, dihydroresveratrol glucuronide is also detected in the liver, whereas dihydroresveratrol sulfate is detected in the liver and adipose tissue [16].

The amount of dihydroresveratrol sulfate in the liver is remarkably higher than that of resveratrol sulfate. These observations highlight the importance of gut microbiota in resveratrol metabolism, particularly in producing specific resveratrol derivatives in significant amounts.

3. Effect of Resveratrol on Metabolic Syndrome

Metabolic syndrome is a cluster of a least three of the five following metabolic alterations: Central obesity, high blood glucose, high blood pressure, high serum triglycerides, and low serum high-density lipoprotein (HDL), the presence of which increases the risk of developing cardiovascular disease and type 2 diabetes [1]. Here, we describe the potential effect of resveratrol supplementation on each metabolic alteration and review the clinical trials that analyze the effects on them. It is important to note that there are still many discrepant and inconsistent results in human studies and it is clear that further research needs to be carried out to further understand the effect of resveratrol on metabolic syndrome.

3.1. Fat Accumulation

Over a decade ago, it was discovered that resveratrol can reduce diet-induced obesity through SIRT1 activation, generating high expectations as a potential anti-obesity molecule; since then, this effect has been shown in both mice and rats [4,8,24–26]. SIRT1 activation is of interest because it deacetylates and activates peroxisome proliferator-activated receptor (PPAR) γ coactivator 1α [4], which controls mitochondrial biogenesis and function. Furthermore, it triggers lipolysis and loss of fat by repressing PPARγ in adipocytes [27]. Resveratrol also acts by inhibiting cAMP-specific phosphodiesterases, leading to elevated cyclic adenosine monophosphate levels, which in turn activate adenosine monophosphate-activated protein kinase (AMPK) [28]. Other anti-lipogenic mechanisms of action have been described, including the upregulation of certain microRNAs by resveratrol, which leads to the inhibition of lipogenesis in white adipose tissue [29].

3.1.1. Resveratrol and Adipose Depot Extension

Since the discovery of its actions on SIRT1, many other studies have been carried out to determine the potential of resveratrol in the treatment of obesity. Studies carried out in cell systems so far have shown that the anti-obesity effect of resveratrol is attributed to its actions on (1) pre-adipocytes, including the induction of apoptosis and the inhibition of proliferation and differentiation [30,31]; (2) mature white adipocytes, including the activation of lipolysis, inhibition of *de novo* lipogenesis, and promotion of brown adipocyte features [30,32–35]; and (3) brown adipocytes, in which the expression of the uncoupling protein-1 and typical brown-phenotype genes are induced [36]. Studies in rodents show that the resveratrol-induced reduction in fat mass is partly explained by both the activation of lipolysis through the adipose triglyceride lipase, and the inhibition of *de novo* lipogenesis by controlling the expression of the lipogenic enzymes mediated by the transcription factor, sterol regulatory element-binding protein-1c [25,29,37,38]. Moreover, the activation of brown adipose tissue and the induction of brown-like adipocytes in white adipose tissue (browning) seem to contribute to body fat reduction in resveratrol-treated rodents [34,36,39].

In humans, however, most of the research published until now shows a lack of effect on body adiposity and body weight. *Trans*-resveratrol supplementation at doses between 100 and 500 mg for a 4-week to 6-month period did not affect fat mass or body weight in obese healthy individuals [32,40,41]. Despite this, adipocyte size was reduced, meaning that adipose tissue was modified by resveratrol intake, even if to a small degree [42]. Furthermore, two studies looking into the effect of resveratrol supplementation in patients with metabolic syndrome showed discrepant results; while Kjœr et al. [43] reported no effects on body composition with doses of 150 mg and 1000 mg, Méndez del Villar et al. [44] showed a reduction in fat mass, waist circumference, body mass index, and body weight after receiving 500 mg three times a day. However, patients with non-alcoholic fatty liver disease (NAFLD) or type 2 diabetes showed no changes regarding fat mass or body weight after resveratrol intake [45–48]. Moreover, other studies looking into the effect of resveratrol combined with other molecules, such as the intestinal lipase inhibitor orlistat [32] or epigallocatechin-3-gallate (EGCC) [49], did not show significant changes in fat mass.

3.1.2. Resveratrol and Hepatic Fat Accumulation

A lifestyle pattern including unbalanced diets and sedentary behavior promotes the accumulation of ectopic fat, particularly in the liver. As in metabolic syndrome, visceral adiposity and the pro-inflammatory state are also key in the development of NAFLD. In view of the inhibitory effects of resveratrol on fat accumulation, many studies have addressed its effect on hepatic fat and the management of NAFLD. Interestingly, hepatic triacylglycerol and cholesterol content is reduced by resveratrol supplementation in rodents fed a high-fat diet [26,50–55]. An increased number of mitochondria and fatty acid oxidation activity and a decreased lipogenic activity seem to be involved in normalizing hepatic steatosis in rodents [50,51,55], in addition to the anti-oxidant and anti-inflammatory action of the polyphenol [53,54]. In humans, resveratrol supplementation was also shown to reduce intrahepatic lipid content in one study involving obese individuals [41], but not in another [40]. Furthermore, when considering patients with NAFLD, clinical trials are still insufficient to demonstrate a clear positive effect of resveratrol according to the conclusions of two meta-analyses, which show a lack of effect on NAFLD features [56,57]. Likewise, hepatic lipid deposition is unaffected in individuals with type 2 diabetes [58] or metabolic syndrome [43].

3.2. Resveratrol and Glucose Intolerance and Insulin Resistance

As it was demonstrated that resveratrol improves insulin sensitivity by activating AMPK [4], many later studies have evaluated the use of the polyphenol in the management of glucose control and in type 2 diabetes mellitus, the risk of which is increased under the persistence of glucose intolerance. Studies in cultured cells and animals have further contributed to the understanding of the mechanism of action of resveratrol on glycemic control and insulin resistance. Resveratrol activates the insulin-signaling components insulin receptor substrate-1 and Akt [59,60] and reduces the expression of adipokines that influence insulin sensitivity, including adiponectin [61], resistin, and retinol-binding protein 4 [33]. Resveratrol enhances insulin-stimulated glucose uptake in cultured cells [30] and, in vivo, reduces glycemia, insulinemia, and improves insulin resistance in diet-induced insulin-resistant mice [4,60,62]. Furthermore, the polyphenol protects from diabetic complications, such as diabetic nephropathy, diabetic retinopathy, and diabetes-induced hypertension [63–66].

When looking at the effects of resveratrol in a human setting, clinical trials have been conducted to elucidate its potential action on glucose homeostasis in individuals with different degrees of alteration in glucose homeostasis, from normoglycemia to type 2 diabetes. In non-diabetic individuals, four studies reported no changes in insulin sensitivity and insulin and glucose levels after resveratrol supplementation at doses between 75 and 2000 mg [40,67–69]. However, in other studies, a decrease in circulating glucose, an improved homeostatic model assessment–insulin resistance (HOMA-IR) score and a suppression in postprandial glucagon response were observed after supplementation with a 150-mg resveratrol dose for 30 days in obese non-diabetic individuals [41,70]. However, in type 2 diabetic patients, it was ineffective in improving insulin sensitivity following the same supplementation protocol. It was speculated that the lack of effect could be due to the interaction found between metformin and dihydroresveratrol levels [58]. The intake of higher doses of resveratrol did not affect the circulating levels of glucose, insulin, glycosylated hemoglobin, and glucagon-like peptide-1 in type 2 diabetic patients [47,48], as well as glucose tolerance and insulin sensitivity in older glucose-intolerant adults [71]. A beneficial effect in glucose intolerant or type 2 diabetic patients is, on the other hand, described in other studies [72–75], even at low doses (10 mg) [73]. Furthermore, in individuals with NAFLD, no changes in insulin resistance were observed in several studies [45,46,57], whereas glucose levels and insulin resistance were improved in one study [76]. Likewise, mixed outcomes are also reported in individuals with metabolic syndrome; while Méndez del Villar et al. [44] reported a decreased insulin response to glucose and total insulin secretion without affecting glucose levels, Kjær et al. [43] reported no beneficial effects and actually found an increase in circulating fructosamine levels. Several meta-analyses have been carried out to shed light on the inconsistency of the above-mentioned results. In an early meta-analysis of 11 studies, Liu et al. concluded that there was no effect on glycemic measures in nondiabetic participants [77]. Among type 2 diabetic patients, Hausenblas et al. [78] identified a beneficial effect on hemoglobin A1c, but not on glucose, insulin, and HOMA-IR. More recently, a meta-analysis that included nine studies showed a beneficial effect on glucose and insulin levels and HOMA-IR, which was particularly more favorable for doses ≥100 mg/day [6]. Despite the discrepant results, the sample size, and the duration of the trials, it concluded that resveratrol might be used for treating diabetes, alone or in combination with current anti-diabetic therapies [66,79].

3.3. Resveratrol and High Blood Pressure

Excessive weight is linked to high blood pressure, which is a major risk factor for cardiovascular disease. Resveratrol supplementation reduces blood pressure in animal models of hypertension, including plexiglas clip- [80], angiotensin II- [81], or hypoxia-induced hypertensive rats, and in fructose-fed rats [82]. Several mechanisms are involved in the modulation of blood pressure by resveratrol, including AMPK phosphorylation, increased nitric oxide (NO) levels, SIRT1 activation, and decreased reactive oxygen species (ROS) production by regulating nicotinamide adenine dinucleotide phosphate oxidase, superoxide dismutase 2, and glutathione reductase [80–83]. In clinical trials, a reduction in blood pressure by resveratrol supplementation has been reported in individuals with obesity [41], NAFLD [84], or type 2 diabetes [72,85]; however, such an effect has not been found in other studies involving subjects with obesity [40,86], NAFLD [46], or metabolic syndrome [43]. Furthermore, several meta-analyses of randomized controlled trials show no significant effect of resveratrol supplementation on systolic and diastolic blood pressure [5,87], even though subgroup and meta-regression analyses indicate that resveratrol intake reduces systolic blood pressure and diastolic blood pressure at doses higher than 150–300 mg/day [5,88,89]. According to these analyses, a beneficial effect of resveratrol supplementation on blood pressure is observed when the effect is analyzed among diabetic patients [89] or overweight and obese individuals [88]. Moreover, despite reporting no changes in blood pressure, resveratrol supplementation improves endothelial dysfunction in obese subjects [86], which is also seen in hypertensive patients [90] and individuals with mild hypertension [91].

3.4. Hypertriglyceridemia

Excessive fat intake and the persistence of increased adiposity can lead to dyslipidemia, which increases cardiovascular risk. Studies have been carried out evaluating the effect of resveratrol on circulating lipids, particularly triacylglycerides and cholesterol, offering interesting results. Resveratrol supplementation reduces triglyceridemia in diet-induced obese rodents [25,26,54,55], which can be partly explained by the inhibition of hepatocyte fatty acid and triacylglycerol synthesis described in rat hepatocytes [92]. In humans, a reduction in triglyceridemia is observed when resveratrol is provided within a grape extract [93], mixed in a nutraceutical formula [94], or combined with other molecules, such as epigallocatechin-3-gallate (EGCC) [49] or orlistat [32]. When resveratrol is provided alone, it reduces plasma triglyceride levels in individuals with dyslipidemia [95] or obesity [58]. However, in other studies carried out in individuals with obesity [67], type 2 diabetes [74], NAFLD [46] or hypertriglyceridemia [68], resveratrol does not influence triglyceridemia, which is confirmed by Sahebkar's meta-analysis [87]. Furthermore, other studies actually report an increase in triglyceridemia, including Haghighatdosst's meta-analysis of 20 studies [3,48].

3.5. Altered Cholesterolemia

The effect of resveratrol on circulating levels of total, low-density lipoprotein (LDL), and HDL cholesterol has been evaluated. It is thought resveratrol may affect cholesterolemia by increasing the synthesis and efflux of bile acids, decreasing the synthesis of hepatic cholesterol, and increasing the efflux of cholesterol [96–98]. In this context, it has been shown that resveratrol supplementation reduces total cholesterol levels in diet-induced obese rodents [25,26,54,55,97], whereas mixed results are reported in humans, showing either a lack of effect [67] toward the reduction [72,88,95], and even an increase in total cholesterol levels [43,48], as described for triglyceridemia. A lowering effect of resveratrol supplementation on plasma LDL and total cholesterol concentrations has been reported in studies in which the compound is given within a plant extract or when combined with a nutraceutical formula [93,94,99], in which it was concluded that the presence of resveratrol is necessary to achieve this effect [99]. A recent meta-analysis of randomized clinical trials that used resveratrol as a mono food supplement concluded that the compound had no effect on the circulating levels of total, LDL, or HDL cholesterol [3]. In addition to its potential ability to influence cholesterol levels, resveratrol has been shown to inhibit LDL and HDL oxidation in vitro [98] and to reduce plasma oxidized LDL cholesterol levels [99].

3.6. Inflammation and Oxidative Stress

3.6.1. Inflammation

Studies have shown that resveratrol exerts an anti-inflammatory activity, and have demonstrated its capacity to inhibit the production of pro-inflammatory cytokines, as well as the activity of cyclooxygenases (COX)-1 and -2 and inducible NO synthase. This anti-inflammatory effect is mainly mediated by the ability to inhibit the transcriptional activity of nuclear factor kappa beta (NF-κβ) and activator protein-1 [100], and can also be attributed to the modulatory effect of microRNAs expression with either an anti-inflammatory or a pro-inflammatory role [101]. Within this context, it has been revealed that resveratrol can decrease chronic low-grade inflammation, which is characterized by adipose tissue macrophage accumulation and abnormal cytokine production. For example, in murine adipocytes and human adipose tissue explants it decreases the secretion of monocyte chemoattractant protein-1 [102], tumor necrosis factor-α (TNF-α), and interleukins (Il)-1β, -6, and -8 [30,103,104], as well as the production of prostaglandin E2 [105], and the expression of vascular endothelial growth factor [106]. These effects are observed in cells treated with TNF-α or Il-1β, exposed to hypoxic conditions, or treated with the microbial product lipopolysaccharide (LPS) [59,107]. In vivo, resveratrol intake reverses obesity-associated inflammation in genetically-induced obese rats [108] and diet-induced obese rodents and monkeys [25,54,55,109–112]. Furthermore, several human studies have reported that resveratrol can even have an acute anti-inflammatory effect in healthy subjects. For example, the intake of a single grape extract reduces plasma IL-1β levels induced by a high-fat and high-carbohydrate meal and, interestingly, plasma endotoxin levels [113]. In type 2 diabetic and hypertensive patients, long-term grape extract supplementation reduces serum Il-6 and alkaline phosphatase levels and alters the expression of pro-inflammatory genes and microRNAs in peripheral blood mononuclear cells [114]. However, in a study involving type 2 diabetic patients, 800 mg/day resveratrol supplementation did not change plasma levels of inflammatory cytokines [115]. Meta-analyses of randomized controlled trials indicate that resveratrol treatment reduces the levels of C-reactive protein and that of TNF-α among obese subjects, confirming the anti-inflammatory action of resveratrol [116]. Interestingly, the pro-inflammatory status which occurs in diabetic complications, such as diabetic neuropathy and nephropathy, seems to also be inhibited by resveratrol [64,117].

3.6.2. Oxidative Stress

Resveratrol exerts an anti-oxidant action, which underlies the beneficial effect of this polyphenol on several metabolic disturbances, such as glucose intolerance, insulin resistance, and hepatic fat accumulation. The mechanisms of action of its anti-oxidant effects include direct mechanisms, such as neutralizing ROS and reactive nitrogen species, and indirect mechanisms such as the ability to increase the transcriptional activity of nuclear factor-E(2)-related factor-2 (Nrf2) and forkhead box

O [118]. Experiments on cell cultures designed to study the effect of resveratrol on metabolic syndrome alterations, particularly by exposing cells to a high glucose concentration or to pro-inflammatory cytokines, show a reduction in ROS levels in many cell types, including in vascular endothelial cells [119,120], adipocytes [104], monocytes [121], and cardiomyocytes [122]. In obese and/or diabetic rodents, a reduction in oxidative stress accompanies the improvement of inflammation [55,110,112], hyperglycemia and insulin resistance [62,112], diabetic nephropathy [63], fat mass accumulation [112], hepatic steatosis [52,53,55,123], hypertriglyceridemia [55], hypercholesterolemia [55], endothelial function [124,125], ventricular diastolic relaxation [126], and hypertension [123]. In humans, the intake of resveratrol reduces oxidative stress in both healthy individuals and patients with metabolic diseases that are characterized by a high oxidative stress degree. The intake of a resveratrol supplement or resveratrol-containing extract increases the total antioxidant capacity and reduces oxidative stress in healthy individuals [93,94,127], as well as oxidative stress generated by the intake of a meal rich in fat [113]. In type 2 diabetic patients, resveratrol supplementation reduces markers of oxidative stress, which are accompanied by an improvement of insulin sensitivity, blood pressure, and cardiovascular function [73,85]. The improvement in insulin sensitivity and diabetic complications caused by resveratrol is explained by its ability to reduce oxidative stress [64,65,73]. Since resveratrol is a relatively unstable molecule, strategies aimed at increasing its stability and thus enhancing its inhibitory action on oxidative stress have been developed. In this context, an enhanced reduction in oxidative stress in obese individuals has been achieved by the intake of a more stable resveratrol derivative [128].

4. Role of Resveratrol Metabolites in Metabolic Syndrome

Most of the studies dealing with the potential beneficial effects of resveratrol on metabolic syndrome use *trans*-resveratrol. However, in vivo effects cannot be solely attributed to this molecule, as it is likely that resveratrol metabolites are also involved. As detailed above, upon intake, several resveratrol metabolites can be produced in the body, including piceid, glucuronide, and sulfate resveratrol conjugates, dihydroresveratrol and other derivatives produced by gut microbiota, and piceatannol, among others. One of the most studied resveratrol metabolites is piceid, which shows a higher bioavailability than resveratrol. As described for resveratrol, piceid shows anti-oxidant and anti-inflammatory activities and shares with resveratrol many of the described molecular targets, including SIRT1, NF-κβ, and NRF2. Interestingly, its anti-oxidant activity is higher than that of resveratrol [129]. In vivo, piceid treatment reduces insulin resistance, steatosis, and dyslipidemia [130–132]. Regarding resveratrol conjugates, there are little data on their potential metabolic effects. Resveratrol glucuronides and sulfates inhibit triacylglycerol accumulation in differentiating adipocytes and adipokine expression in mature adipocytes [133,134]. Additionally, resveratrol glucuronides seem to have a greater potential to lowering the effect of cholesterol [96] compared to resveratrol, whereas resveratrol sulfates inhibit NO production and exert a differentiated effect when compared to glucuronides on free radical scavenging and COX activity, NF-κβ induction, and pro-inflammatory cytokine expression inhibition [135,136]. It would be interesting to elucidate whether the resveratrol metabolites produced by gut bacteria are able to trigger beneficial effects, particularly bearing in mind the high concentrations of dihydroresveratrol and its derivatives detected in plasma and tissues [16,23]. Only limited data exist regarding the effects of dihydroresveratrol, 3,4′-dihydroxy-*trans*-stilbene, and lunularin in parameters related to metabolic syndrome. Dihydroresveratrol exhibits significant antioxidant activity [137], reduces fatty acid-binding protein-4 expression, involved in fatty acid uptake in human macrophages treated with oxidized LDL [138] and stimulates fatty acid oxidation in human fibroblasts [139]. Lunularin reduces the expression of pro-inflammatory mediators in endothelial cells in response to LPS [140], and 3,4′-dihydroxy-*trans*-stilbene activates AMPK, induces glucose uptake in C2C12 myotubes, and reduces PPARg and resistin expression in 3T3-L1 adipocytes, showing a larger effect than resveratrol [141]. Collectively, these results suggest that gut bacteria-derived resveratrol metabolites could be involved in the effect of resveratrol supplementation on metabolic syndrome alterations, and consequently, gut bacteria amount and composition may be determinant. A resveratrol-related stilbenoid with reported effects against metabolic syndrome alterations is piceatannol, which inhibits fatty acid-induced inflammation and oxidative stress and reduces hyperlipidemia, hyperglycemia, and insulin resistance [19,100,142–144]. Research has thus focused on this stilbenoid due to its higher stability and absorption compared to resveratrol [145], which is associated with a higher anti-inflammatory activity versus resveratrol [146]. Moreover, differential effects between these stilbene derivatives have been shown regarding their anti-lipolytic activity, being stronger for piceatannol, which was linked to its inhibitory action on lipotoxicity [143]. Overall, it seems that resveratrol metabolites could be involved in some of the beneficial effects attributed to resveratrol with regards to the metabolic syndrome alterations. The fact that the gut microbiota plays an important role in the conversion and/or production of some of these resveratrol-related metabolites has led to the idea that it could actually be modulating such described effects.

5. The Role of Gut Microbiota in Health and Disease

The gut microbiota, including its role in health and disease, is currently one of the topics of highest interest in biomedical research, due to its potential key role in the aetiology and development of many diseases [147,148]. In the last decade, it has been associated with conditions such as obesity, diabetes, cardiovascular disease, and cancer, which are among the leading causes of mortality and morbidity worldwide [149–153]. More recently, the hypothesis that the gut microbiota is one of the key modulators that influence disease risk due to its close links to metabolism and the immune system has been posed [154]. It was even coined as "the forgotten organ" initially [155], due to the vast amount of processes it is involved in, including the processing of non-digestible polysaccharides from the diet into short-chain fatty acids (SCFA) [156], synthesis of vitamins, and regulation of energy balance and immune functions [147,157]. The term "gut microbiota" refers to the bacteria, archaea, and eukarya found in the gastrointestinal tract [158]. It is widely thought that the number of microorganisms greatly outnumber human cells (with a suggested ratio of 1:10) [159], and 100 times the amount of genomic content ("gut microbiome") [158], which inevitably leads to the assumption that they carry out a major role in the body; interestingly, this calculation was recently challenged and the idea that the ratio may be closer to 1:1 was put forward [160], without underestimating their impact on human health. This new focus on the role of gut microbiota on health and disease has led to large studies worldwide, including the Human Microbiome Project [161], which was essentially an extension of the Human Genome Project, and the MyNewGut project, which is currently ongoing and focuses on the role of the microbiome in the development of diet and brain-related disorders, among others. The ultimate goal of this new "gut microbiota era" is to understand what bacterial composition defines a healthy gut, and how this knowledge can be translated into efficient and targeted therapies for diseases in which it seems to be playing a main role.

Initially, it was thought that humans could be divided into three main enterotypes based on the make-up of their gut microbiota composition, focusing on one of three dominating genera: Bacteroides, Prevotella, and Ruminococcus [162]; since then it has been shown that gut bacteria are easily modified by many factors, including delivery method, diet, lifestyle, medication use, and infections [148,163–165], making an individual´s enterotype variable throughout their lifespan and hence the use of bacterial clusters as biomarkers for disease not as effective as previously thought [166]. Although it is still being debated what constitutes a "healthy" gut microbiota composition, it has been widely established that dysbiosis, which refers to a disturbance in the amount and/or composition of an individual's "normal" gut microbiota, is strongly associated to many common diseases [150,152,154,163]. People presenting certain conditions, such as obesity and metabolic syndrome particularly, consistently present a lower bacterial diversity and composition compared to their healthy counterparts [153,163,167–171]. Furthermore, it was recently hypothesized that since a more diverse microbiota translates into carrying more genes and is involved in more metabolic pathways, it is better prepared to adapt to changes in diet and thus the host could respond better to dietary treatment [172].

5.1. The Impact of Gut Microbiota on Energy Metabolism

As previously discussed, the potential modulation of energy homeostasis by the gut microbiota has been of great interest, with studies indicating significant differences between the gut microbiota of obese versus lean subjects. Many animal studies are offering potential mechanistic views on how the gut microbiota operates, and although this proves to be more challenging in a human setting [173], evidence continues to point to the "forgotten organ" as one of the key players.

Over a decade ago, the first data emerged showing that germ-free mice weighed significantly less and had a lower amount of body fat [174–176]. Since then, numerous studies have shown that the gut microbiota composition in obesity is different compared to lean subjects, characterized by increased levels of Firmicutes and less Bacteroidetes [177,178], increased capacity in energy harvesting from dietary polysaccharides [175,179], and is associated with increased adiposity and insulin resistance [180,181] and lower levels of short-chain fatty acids in the caecum [173].

Furthermore, more and more evidence points towards the significant role of systemic and adipose tissue inflammation in the development of obesity, diabetes, and metabolic syndrome, thus many studies soon began to investigate whether gut microbiota could be contributing to it [182–185]. It has been shown that LPS, found on the outer membrane of Gram-negative bacteria, triggers inflammatory pathways by binding the CD14/Toll-like receptor-4 complex and that chronic high levels in plasma lead to insulin resistance and diabetes [185–187]. Hence, it is hypothesized that certain factors (such as diet) can promote Gram-negative bacteria in the gut, promoting leakage of LPS through the gut epithelium and thus leading to an increase in plasma LPS levels, inducing insulin resistance and what is known as metabolic endotoxaemia [172,188].

Thus, it seems that the gut microbiota has a big impact at both the peripheral and the central level with regard to overall energy regulation, and hence it is being considered as a potential therapeutic strategy for subjects who present obesity, diabetes and/or metabolic syndrome. One of the key ways to manipulate gut microbiota is through the diet, as discussed in the next section, with a focus on the influence of natural polyphenols.

5.2. Diet as a Key Modulator of the Gut Microbiota

Data so far point to the gut microbiota and its metabolic products as a key player in obesity and metabolic syndrome [149,150,152], hence the next step at present is to determine plausible ways in which to manipulate bacterial composition in order to impact host physiology in a beneficial manner. Evidence suggests that gut microbiota may be the link between diet and obesity development, due to its capacity for changing microbial composition and activity in the gut, as seen in both mice and humans [149,150,152]. Therefore, it is essential to consider diet as an important factor when designing new therapies and prevention strategies regarding obesity [189–191].

Dietary habits on the whole have a significant role in shaping the gut microbiota–this is evidenced by the fact that individuals of different countries have distinct bacterial populations [192]. One of the first studies to publish this was carried out by De Filippo et al., which showed that children in a rural African village had low levels of Firmicutes and high levels of Bacteroidetes in fecal samples compared to Italian children, who presented high levels of Enterobacteriaceae [193].

Furthermore, even though gut microbiota is relatively stable throughout adulthood in humans [194], studies have shown that it can be rapidly modified by diet [195], with composition changes seen in as little as a few days of dietary intervention [174]. However, it seems this can be rapidly reversed, hence it has been suggested that a long-term (dietary) intervention may be needed in order to observe a significant shift in the enterotype of an individual [196].

Research has mainly focused on the effect of certain dietary patterns, such as high-fat and/or "Western" diets, which lead to decreased bacterial diversity, high numbers of Firmicutes and Proteobacteria, and low Bifidobacteria levels, which in turn are associated to a wide array of conditions, particularly obesity [196–198]. Other dietary interventions, such as the use of fructans, high-fiber, specific nutrients or prebiotics have been shown to promote bacterial diversity and increase

Bifidobacteria in the gut, and thus having an overall beneficial effect on the host, such as decreasing low-grade inflammation [167,195,198,199].

Within the study of specific macro and micronutrients, we find an increased interest in the effects of molecules such as polyphenols, which have the ability to cause a significant shift in gut microbiota [12]. Here we will focus particularly on the effect of resveratrol has on the gut microbiota and how this knowledge could be used in the context of obesity and the metabolic syndrome.

5.3. Resveratrol and Gut Microbiota

Owing to the low bioavailability of resveratrol, it has been postulated that one of its mechanisms of action is through its interaction with the gut [200]. Recent studies have shown that resveratrol induces changes in the gut microbiota, which could lead to lower body weight and body fat, together with improved glucose homeostasis and obesity-related parameters. It seems this could be either by directly modulating bacterial populations to promote a composition associated with a healthy phenotype, or by the action of its by-products, which could be having an impact on genes and pathways involved in energy regulation. A summary of the studies discussed in this section can be found in Table 1.

Table 1. Review of studies analyzing the effect of resveratrol on gut microbiota composition.

Species	Resveratrol Dose	Duration	Modulation of Gut Microbiota	Effects on Metabolic Syndrome Alterations	
C57Bl/6N mice	0.4% resveratrol (+FMT)	2–8 weeks	↑ *Bacteroides* and *Parabacteroides* ↓ *Turicibacteraceae, Moryella, Lachnospiraceae* and *Akkermansia*	FMT from resveratrol-fed mice improved glucose homeostasis and lowered blood pressure.	[201,202]
C57Bl/6J and ApoE−/− mice	0.4% resveratrol	1 or 2 months	↑ *Lactobacillus* and *Bifidobacterium*	Inhibition of TMAO synthesis and reduced atherosclerosis.	[203]
C57Bl/6N mice	450 mg/kg/day	2 weeks	↓ Bacteriodetes-to-Firmicutes ratio ↑ *Parabacteroides, Bilophila* and *Akkermansia* ↓ *Lachnospiraceae*	Increased skeletal muscle insulin sensitivity, glucose utilization and metabolic rate.	[204]
C57Bl/6J mice	200 mg/kg/day	8 weeks	↓ *Lactococcus, Clostridium XI, Oscillibacter* & *Hydrogenoanaerobacterium*	Reduced fat deposition and body weight gain.	[205]
C57Bl/6 mice	0.1% resveratrol, 0.1% piceatannol or 0.25% piceatannol	18 weeks	Piceatannol: ↑ Firmicutes, Clostridiales, Shpingobacteriales, Blautia, *P. kwangyangensis* & *Lactobacillus* ↓ Bacteroidetes	Piceatannol: Reduced body weight, perigonadal adipose tissue, adipocyte size, plasma glucose and cholesterol Resveratrol: Reduced perigonadal adipose tissue, adipocyte size	[206]
Kunming mice	200 mg/kg/day	12 weeks	↑ Bacteroidetes, *Lactobacillus* & *Bifidobacterium* ↓ Firmicutes and *Enterococcus faecalis*	Decreased body and visceral adipose weight. Lower plasma glucose and lipid levels.	[207]
C57Bl/6J and Glp1r− mice	60 mg/kg/day	5 weeks	Restored bacterial composition of animals fed a high-fat diet. ↓ *Parabacteroides jonsonii DMS 18315* (a), *Alistipes putredinis DMS 17216* (b) and *Bacteroides vulgatus ATCC 8482*	Reduced glucose intolerance in diabetic mice without affecting fasting glycemia.	[208]

Table 1. *Cont.*

Species	Resveratrol Dose	Duration	Modulation of Gut Microbiota	Effects on Metabolic Syndrome Alterations	
Wistar rats	Quercetin (30 mg/kg/day) and resveratrol (15 mg/kg/day)	10 weeks	↑ *Bacteroidales S24-7 group, Christensenellaceae, Akkermansia muciniphila, Ruminococcaceae, Ruminococcaceae UCG-014 & Ruminococcaceae UCG-005* ↓Firmicutes & Firmicutes-to-Bacteroidetes ratio	Lower body weight gain and adipose tissue weight.	[209]
Zucker rat (*fa/fa*)	Piceatannol (15 and 45 mg/kg/day)	6 weeks	↓ *Clostridium hathewayi*	No impact on body weight and body fat, glucose, and lipid metabolic parameters.	[210]
Wistar rats	*Trans*-resveratrol (15 mg/kg/day) or *trans*-resveratrol + quercetin (30 mg/kg/day)	6 weeks	*Trans*-resveratrol & quercetin: ↓Firmicutes-to-Bacteroidetes ratio ↓*Erysipelotrichaceae, Bacillus, Eubacterium cylindroides*	Improved HOMA-IR and insulin sensitivity.	[211]
Sprague Dawley rats	50 mg/L of resveratrol 50 mg/L	3 months	↑ Firmicutes-to-Proteobacteria ratio	Restored systolic and diastolic blood pressure.	[212]
Humans	EGCG (282 mg/day) + resveratrol (80 mg/day)	12 weeks	Men: ↓ Bacteroidetes	Increased fat oxidation and skeletal muscle mitochondrial oxidative capacity.	[213]

FMT, fecal microbiota transplant; TMAO, trimethylamine N-oxide; HOMA-IR, homeostatic model assessment–insulin resistance; HF, high-fat; ND, normal-diet; EGCC, epigallocatechin-3-gallate; ↑, increase; ↓, decrease.

5.3.1. Effects of Resveratrol on Body Weight and Fat Metabolism

As previously discussed in this review, resveratrol could have a beneficial effect on body weight and body fat regulation based on evidence obtained in experimental animals, and studies are starting to point towards a potential implication of the gut microbiota as reviewed in Table 1. One study showed that C57Bl/6J mice on a high-fat diet and receiving 200 mg/kg/day of resveratrol supplementation through oral gavage five times a week (for a total of eight weeks) presented reduced fat deposition and body weight gain compared to controls receiving a high-fat diet alone [205]. In order to understand the potential mechanism through which resveratrol acts, the authors show that resveratrol activated the mammalian target of the rapamycin (mTOR) complex 2 (mTORC2) signalling pathway and inhibited mTORC1, a key player in energy regulation, suggesting that this suppresses the presence of obesity-associated gut microbiota, including *Lactococcus, Clostridium XI, Oscillibacter*, and *Hydrogenoanaerobacterium*.

In tune with these results, Kunming mice on a high-fat diet supplemented with the same amount of resveratrol (200 mg/kg/day) for 12 weeks also showed decreased body fat and weight by the end of the experiment [207]. These parameters were correlated with changes in gut microbiota, since resveratrol significantly increased *Lactobacillus* and *Bifidobacterium* (negatively correlated with body weight), and decreased *Enterococcus faecalis* (positively correlated with body weight). Furthermore, they showed a higher abundance of Bacteroidetes and a lower amount of Firmicutes bacteria (a ratio which was negatively correlated with body weight). Although the authors suggest that resveratrol could be having a prebiotic effect on bacteria, and that this could be having a positive effect on body weight and fat mass, further studies are needed to identify the potential mechanisms through which resveratrol acts.

Other studies have looked at the effect of resveratrol supplementation together with other compounds of interest. For example, one group administered a combination of quercetin (30 mg/kg body weight) and resveratrol (15 mg/kg body weight) by oral gavage per day to Wistar rats on a high-fat diet for 10 weeks [209]. By the end of the experiment, animals receiving supplementation presented lower body weight gain and adipose tissue weight compared to animals on a high-fat diet alone. Interestingly, they also had decreased Firmicutes and a lower Firmicutes to Bacteroidetes ratio, as well as increased levels of *Bacteroidales S24-7 group, Christensenellaceae, Akkermansia muciniphila, Ruminococcaceae, Ruminococcaceae UCG-014*, and *Ruminococcaceae UCG-005*, which have all been associated with reducing high-fat-diet-induced obesity.

In line with these results, it seems resveratrol could be a promising compound for use in promoting a healthy gut microbiota, which is known to have a wide array of beneficial effects. However, to the best of our knowledge, very few studies have been carried out which investigate the effects of resveratrol supplementation on gut microbiota in humans and the results obtained were slightly milder than those observed in animals. A recent study gave both males and females a combination of epigallocatechin-3-gallate (282 mg/day) and resveratrol (80 mg/day) supplements for 12 weeks; by the end of the experiment, they observed only slight differences in the gut microbiota composition of men only, with a minor reduction in Bacteroidetes and *Faecalibacterium prausnitzii* [213]. However, an increase in fat oxidation and skeletal muscle mitochondrial oxidative capacity was observed associated with supplementation and, interestingly, the Bacteroidetes level was correlated with fat oxidation in men.

5.3.2. Resveratrol Potentially Improves Glucose Homeostasis through the Gut Microbiota

Recent studies have focused on whether the beneficial effect of resveratrol supplementation on glucose homeostasis may be mediated, at least in part, by alterations in the gut microbiota. Two recent studies carried out by the same group using a fecal microbiota transplant (FMT) show that obese mice receiving a resveratrol (0.4%)-fed mice-FMT present less Proteobacteria [201,202]; considering the association of Proteobacteria with inflammation, the authors postulated that the reduction observed could be indicative of the benefits seen in treated animals. Furthermore, they also reported decreased inflammation in the colon of FMT-recipients and suggested that bacterial metabolites or by-products of the polyphenol may be responsible for these benefits. In contrast, the authors reported decreased levels of *Akkermansia muciniphila*, a species that has been associated to improved body weight and glucose management. An interesting observation however was that resveratrol-FMT is actually more efficient than oral supplementation *per se* for the regulation of glucose homeostasis once obesity and insulin resistance are already present [201,202]. Decreased intestinal inflammation linked to resveratrol supplementation and improved glucose homeostasis has also been reported [208], in which C57Bl/6J and glucagon-like peptide-1 (GLP-1) receptor knock-out (Glp1r$^{-/-}$) mice on a high-fat diet supplemented with 60 mg/kg/day of resveratrol for five weeks showed an increase in glucose-induced glucagon-like peptide-1 (GLP-1) and insulin secretion. This was accompanied by changes in gut microbiota composition, which suggest to be linked to the decreased intestinal inflammation in these animals. It is hypothesised that animals on a high-fat diet have increased inflammation, which leads to decreased glucose-induced insulin secretion and ultimately insulin resistance [185]. Thus, it seems that resveratrol may potentially mitigate intestinal inflammation caused by high-fat feeding via gut microbiota modulation, which could in turn increase incretin actions such as insulin and GLP-1 secretion and ameliorate glycemic control. Hence, based on the in vivo demonstration of the influence of resveratrol on the enteroendocrine axis in mice [208], a novel therapeutic action of this polyphenol should be considered.

In another study, C57Bl/6N mice with induced heart failure were administered a high dose of resveratrol (450 mg/kg/day) together with a high-fat diet for two weeks and reported a decreased Bacteroidetes-to-Firmicutes ratio in the gut microbiota and an increase in the genus Akkermansia [204]. This latter one, as previously mentioned, has been linked to improved glucose homeostasis in insulin-resistant and obese animal models, and is in contrast with what was observed in the above-discussed studies. This was accompanied by a higher abundance of the genera Parabacteroides and Bilophila, and a decrease in the Lachnospiraceae family, changes which are associated to an increased metagenomics capacity for carbohydrate metabolism, indicating a potential mechanism by which resveratrol improves insulin signaling and glucose homeostasis.

Rats under a high-fat, high-sucrose diet were supplemented with either *trans*-resveratrol (15mg/kg body weight/day) or with a combination of *trans*-resveratrol and quercetin (30mg/kg/day) for six weeks [211]. Besides a reduced weight gain, animals receiving the polyphenols exhibited lower serum insulin levels and improved insulin sensitivity. Treatments did not alter bacteria at the phylum level, however *trans*-resveratrol did reduce significantly the *Graciibacteraceae* family, the *Parabacteroides* genus, and the species *Clostridium aldenense, Clostridium hathewayi, Clostridium sp. C9, Clostridium sp. MLG661, Gracilibacter thermotolerans* and *Parabacteroides distasonis*, as well as increasing significantly the relative abundance of *Clostridium sp. XB90* versus animals on a high-fat, high-sucrose diet alone. Even though these changes were accompanied by a decrease in HOMA-IR, the authors could not conclude a direct association between the changes observed in gut microbiota and the beneficial effects seen in insulin resistance.

5.3.3. Effects on Cardiovascular Health

Cardiovascular health is closely related to metabolic syndrome, which, as described above, is characterized by abdominal fat, high glucose, and triglyceride levels, low high-density lipoprotein cholesterol levels, and hypertension [214]. Thus, determining therapies to promote a healthy cardiovascular system will inevitably lead to an improvement of the metabolic syndrome outcome. Within this context, one group showed a protective effect of resveratrol on atherosclerosis by supplementing C57BL/6J and ApoE$^{-/-}$ mice with 0.4% resveratrol. Supplementation increased levels of the genera Lactobacillus and Bifidobacterium, and decreased gut microbial trimethylamine production through changes in the gut microbiota, hence leading to inhibited trimethylamine-n-oxide synthesis and reduced atherosclerosis [203]. Interestingly, another study investigated the effect of supplementing Sprague Dawley rats with 50 mg/L of resveratrol in their drinking water during pregnancy and lactation whilst on a high-fructose diet [212]. They observed that the offspring from animals receiving resveratrol presented a restored systolic and diastolic blood pressure versus animals not receiving supplementation, which was elevated compared to control rats. This was accompanied by changes in gut microbiota since animals receiving a high-fructose diet presented a decreased Firmicutes-to-Proteobacteria ratio, which was normalized by resveratrol intake. Furthermore, it seems that supplementation increased the relative abundance of *Lactobacillus* and *Bifidobacterium* species, which was in accordance with that observed by Chen et al. [203], thus counteracting the impact of the high-fructose diet [212]. However, further studies are needed to determine whether such changes can be directly attributed to the beneficial impact of resveratrol on hypertension.

5.3.4. Resveratrol Analogues and Gut Microbiota

Due to the reported low bioavailability of resveratrol, a few studies have been carried out to explore the potential effects of analogs such as piceatannol [215], a polyphenol that presents better bioavailability. However, the studies published so far present differing results. On the one hand, one group showed that the administration of piceatannol (15 or 45 mg/kg/day for six weeks) to Zucker (*fa/fa*) rats has little effect on gut microbiota, as well as no major impact on body weight, body fat, and glucose and lipid metabolic parameters, other than a decrease in circulating non-esterified fatty acids and in fecal *Clostridium hathewayi*, belonging to the butyrate-produce cluster Clostridium XIVa [210]. On the other hand, another study showed that 0.25% piceatannol supplementation under a high-fat diet reduced the body weight of C57Bl/6N mice, and that both 0.1% resveratrol and 0.1% and 0.25% piceatannol were able to partially prevent the increase of body fat content and adipocyte size compared to a high-fat diet alone [206]. This was accompanied by significant changes in gut microbiota, where animals supplemented with piceatannol particularly recovered from the alterations caused by a high-fat diet, which intriguingly consisted of a decreased Firmicutes abundance and increased Bacteroidetes [206]. The differences in the results between these two studies could be due to a variety of reasons, such as different concentrations and length of supplementation, together with different metagenomic workflow. Furthermore, the results of the latter study, reporting a piceatannol-induced increase in Firmicutes versus animals on a high-fat diet deserves further confirmation, since it has been well documented that this dietary intervention, revealing an obese phenotype, is generally associated to dysbiosis and lower bacterial diversity [197]. Otherwise, the rapid action of piceatannol, which results in lowering blood glucose 1 h after acute oral administration in *db/db* mice (50 mg/kg body weight), indicates that not all the beneficial effects of stilbenoids are mediated by a modulatory action effect on gut microbiota [144]. Together with the interactions between stilbenoids and bacteria, changes at the intestinal level and even in other targets, warrant further study regarding the potential of polyphenols for the chronic treatment of metabolic syndrome. However, such future investigations should not consider these metabolites as inactive; as mentioned above and as illustrated by the case of urolithin A, a major ellagitannin metabolite, they are endowed with noticeable health benefits [216].

6. Future Directions

When reflecting on the impact a certain compound has on health, in this case, resveratrol, and whether its effects may be mediated by gut microbiota, many questions appear: Is gut microbiota at the base of energy regulation? Could resveratrol be having a significant impact on it, making it relevant to consider it a prebiotic in the future? Thus, there are still many issues to consider and investigate in the near future.

As recently reviewed [217], the modulation of gut microbiota is being considered as a key method to treat obesity. However, it is seen that the efficiency of this strategy is inconsistent due to inherent differences in gut microbiota among individuals. Furthermore, it is yet to be determined what an "ideal" gut microbiota composition is and how to effectively manipulate it.

Although the results so far are promising, further studies are warranted in both animals and humans. It seems that resveratrol does have an effect on gut microbiota that was initially unsuspected when, more than a decade ago, the stilbenoid was found to modulate energy balance. Now, resveratrol is considered as a potential prebiotic candidate to promote changes in bacterial composition associated with a healthy phenotype. However, whether this interaction is involved in several of the beneficial health effects attributed to this polyphenol is yet to be elucidated. At present, and to the best of our knowledge, most studies are still observational, and nearly all in animal models, presenting interesting correlations but few mechanistic clues as to how the resveratrol-gut microbiota-metabolism axis could be functioning. As discussed above, it seems that in the past 10 years most studies have shown associations between gut microbiota and health and disease, but they have failed to prove a direct causal relationship [154]. One of the potential mechanisms put forward by Nohr et al. [218] could be that resveratrol reverses or inhibits the effects of Gram-negative bacteria-derived LPS in the gut, thereby preventing an alteration of the intestinal epithelium permeability, and consequently decreasing endotoxemia of intestinal origin, low-grade inflammation, and obesity. However, more studies are needed in order to confirm this interesting hypothesis. Another future route of study could be to analyze the potential effects of resveratrol on SCFA in the gut since recent studies seem to be pointing to the by-products of resveratrol as the key actors, including SCFA, already known to play a regulatory role in energy homeostasis.

At this stage, and considering the observations made in different models, we hypothesize two putative mechanisms of action of resveratrol on the interactions between bacteria and intestinal mucosa.

First, resveratrol may influence the turnover of SCFA and various intraluminal lipids by modulating both bacterial production and handling in the intestine. Indeed, resveratrol has been reported to exert an important anti-lipogenic effect on an in vitro model of the human small intestinal mucosa, in which epithelial cells were treated with LPS with or without prior challenge with resveratrol [219]. Among the genes found to be regulated by LPS but repressed by resveratrol were endothelial lipase, acyl-CoA synthetase, and many others involved in lipid synthesis and/or cholesterol handling. Furthermore, resveratrol has been reported to inhibit lipogenesis in rodent fat cells too, in an acute, short-term manner. Taking together these observations, it could be suggested that resveratrol can directly reduce the activity of enzymes involved in lipogenic pathways, in a concerted manner with the down-regulatory role it plays on their expression [143]. All these integrated actions of resveratrol limit LPS bacterial production and its consequences on epithelial transcript factors, reshape intestinal lipid metabolism, and lead to a reinforcement of the intestinal barrier when challenged by an excess of lipids. As a consequence of such modulation, the beneficial effects of ingested resveratrol or its metabolites before and after trans-epithelial absorption seemingly include changes in the intraluminal microbiota and SCFA levels, gut barrier integrity, and blood cholesterol and triglycerides.

Our second hypothesis is that the antioxidant properties of polyphenols can trigger pleiotropic responses in both the microbiota and the host. It is worthy to note that NADPH oxidase was upregulated by LPS but down-regulated by resveratrol in epithelial cells used in the abovementioned study [219]. NADPH oxidase is a complex membrane-bound enzyme implicated in the immune response, but it is also recognized as generating superoxides and ROS. Because of their antioxidant properties, resveratrol and its derivatives can potentially counteract the consequences of ROS produced by NADPH oxidase and other ROS-generating enzymes. In this sense, we recently confirmed that resveratrol impairs not only the fate of hydrogen peroxide generated by monoamide oxidase in fat cells but also the catalytic activity of the oxidase itself [143]. In bacteria, there are amine oxidases equivalent to those found in mammalian cells. Although their roles are not completely defined, it has been proposed that they are useful for survival in harsh culture conditions, allowing for diversification of the sources of nitrogen and provide a growth advantage over competing species (via the hydrogen peroxide they produce). Noteworthy, the deletion of the *Escherichia coli* copper amine oxidase (ECAO) has been demonstrated to alter the growth abilities of its associated strain, with significant metabolic changes [220]. Many other alterations have been reported among strains expressing (or not) ECAO and have led to this enzyme being characterized as capable of influencing bacterial growth and adhesion [220]. Thus, in addition to its well-known antimicrobial properties, resveratrol might reshape gut bacteria composition by counteracting ROS actions and inhibiting amine oxidase activities, thereby selecting given bacterial species. However, whether this potential mechanism is different from other dietary antioxidants and contributes to the specificity of the stilbenoid in reversing gut microbial dysbiosis remains to be elucidated.

As a final note, it is important to mention that differences in results among the studies discussed may be due to a variety of reasons: Species (mice vs. rats vs. humans) and disease model (knock-out, obese, etc.); a wide variety in dosage of resveratrol and duration of supplementation; the administration route (mixed in diet or drinking water, oral gavage); and the combination with other compounds (e.g. quercetin), making it difficult to dissect the effects of each. Furthermore, studies also differ in how they report the changes observed in gut microbiota composition, where differences are seen in either species, genus, and/or the phylum level, making it tricky to elucidate the impact of polyphenol-microbiota interactions in the first instance.

7. Conclusions

It is becoming clear that we are moving towards an era in which treatments and strategies, particularly nutritional interventions such as resveratrol supplementation, to counteract obesity and metabolic syndrome will need a personalized approach tailored to the individual in order to be as effective as possible. The gut microbiota composition is an important factor to consider in this equation. Further studies, together with growing knowledge on the role of gut microbiota composition, will inevitably provide exciting future directions, as in the case of resveratrol-based supplementations.

Author Contributions: Conceptualization, A.C. and J.M.; writing—original draft preparation, A.C. and J.M.; writing—review and editing, A.C., C.C. and J.M.

Funding: This research received no external funding.

Conflicts of Interest: The authors declare no conflict of interest.

References

1. Huang, P.L. A comprehensive definition for metabolic syndrome. *Dis. Model Mech.* **2009**, *2*, 231–237. [CrossRef] [PubMed]

2. Deedwania, P.C.; Gupta, R. Management issues in the metabolic syndrome. *J. Assoc. Physic. India* **2006**, *54*, 797–810.

3. Haghighatdoost, F.; Hariri, M. Effect of resveratrol on lipid profile: An updated systematic review and meta-analysis on randomized clinical trials. *Pharmacol. Res.* **2018**, *129*, 141–150. [CrossRef] [PubMed]

4. Lagouge, M.; Argmann, C.; Gerhart-Hines, Z.; Meziane, H.; Lerin, C.; Daussin, F.; Messadeq, N.; Milne, J.; Lambert, P.; Elliott, P.; et al. Resveratrol improves mitochondrial function and protects against metabolic disease by activating SIRT1 and PGC-1alpha. *Cell* **2006**, *127*, 1109–1122. [CrossRef] [PubMed]

5. Liu, Y.; Ma, W.; Zhang, P.; He, S.; Huang, D. Effect of resveratrol on blood pressure: A meta-analysis of randomized controlled trials. *Clin. Nutr.* **2015**, *34*, 27–34. [CrossRef] [PubMed]

6. Zhu, X.; Wu, C.; Qiu, S.; Yuan, X.; Li, L. Effects of resveratrol on glucose control and insulin sensitivity in subjects with type 2 diabetes: Systematic review and meta-analysis. *Nutr. Metab.* **2017**, *14*, 60. [CrossRef] [PubMed]

7. Haseeb, S.; Alexander, B.; Baranchuk, A. Wine and Cardiovascular Health: A Comprehensive Review. *Circulation* **2017**, *136*, 1434–1448. [CrossRef] [PubMed]

8. Baur, J.A.; Pearson, K.J.; Price, N.L.; Jamieson, H.A.; Lerin, C.; Kalra, A.; Prabhu, V.V.; Allard, J.S.; Lopez-Lluch, G.; Lewis, K.; et al. Resveratrol improves health and survival of mice on a high-calorie diet. *Nature* **2006**, *444*, 337–342. [CrossRef] [PubMed]

9. Fernández-Quintela, A.; Carpéné, C.; Fernández, M.; Aguirre, L.; Milton-Laskibar, I.; Contreras, J.; Portillo, M.P. Anti-obesity effects of resveratrol: Comparison between animal models and humans. *J. Physiol. Biochem.* **2016**, *73*, 417–429. [CrossRef] [PubMed]

10. Bode, L.M.; Bunzel, D.; Huch, M.; Cho, G.S.; Ruhland, D.; Bunzel, M.; Bub, A.; Franz, C.M.; Kulling, S.E. *In vivo* and *in vitro* metabolism of trans-resveratrol by human gut microbiota. *Am. J. Clin. Nutr.* **2013**, *97*, 295–309. [CrossRef] [PubMed]

11. Theilmann, M.C.; Goh, Y.J.; Nielsen, K.F.; Klaenhammer, T.R.; Barrangou, R.; Abou Hachem, M. Metabolizes dietary plant glucosides and externalizes their bioactive phytochemicals. *MBio* **2017**. [CrossRef] [PubMed]

12. Carrera-Quintanar, L.; López Roa, R.I.; Quintero-Fabián, S.; Sánchez-Sánchez, M.A.; Vizmanos, B.; Ortuño-Sahagún, D. Phytochemicals that influence gut microbiota as prophylactics and for the treatment of obesity and inflammatory diseases. *Mediators Inflamm.* **2018**, *2018*, 9734845. [CrossRef] [PubMed]

13. Gambini, J.; Inglés, M.; Olaso, G.; Lopez-Grueso, R.; Bonet-Costa, V.; Gimeno-Mallench, L.; Mas-Bargues, C.; Abdelaziz, K.M.; Gomez-Cabrera, M.C.; Vina, J.; et al. Properties of resveratrol: *In vitro* and *in vivo* studies about metabolism, bioavailability, and biological effects in animal models and humans. *Oxid. Med. Cell Longev.* **2015**, *2015*, 837042. [CrossRef] [PubMed]

14. Walle, T. Bioavailability of resveratrol. *Ann. N. Y. Acad. Sci.* **2011**, *1215*, 9–15. [CrossRef] [PubMed]

15. Bresciani, L.; Calani, L.; Bocchi, L.; Delucchi, F.; Savi, M.; Ray, S.; Brighenti, F.; Stilli, D.; Del Rio, D. Bioaccumulation of resveratrol metabolites in myocardial tissue is dose-time dependent and related to cardiac hemodynamics in diabetic rats. *Nutr. Metab. Cardiovasc. Dis.* **2014**, *24*, 408–415. [CrossRef] [PubMed]

16. Andres-Lacueva, C.; Macarulla, M.T.; Rotches-Ribalta, M.; Boto-Ordóñez, M.; Urpi-Sarda, M.; Rodríguez, V.M.; Portillo, M.P. Distribution of resveratrol metabolites in liver, adipose tissue, and skeletal muscle in rats fed different doses of this polyphenol. *J. Agric. Food Chem.* **2012**, *60*, 4833–4840. [CrossRef] [PubMed]

17. Menet, M.C.; Baron, S.; Taghi, M.; Diestra, R.; Dargère, D.; Laprévote, O.; Nivet-Antoine, V.; Beaudeux, J.L.; Bédarida, T.; Cottart, C.H. Distribution of trans-resveratrol and its metabolites after acute or sustained administration in mouse heart, brain, and liver. *Mol. Nutr. Food Res.* **2017**. [CrossRef] [PubMed]

18. Potter, G.A.; Patterson, L.H.; Wanogho, E.; Perry, P.J.; Butler, P.C.; Ijaz, T.; Ruparelia, K.C.; Lamb, J.H.; Farmer, P.B.; Stanley, L.A.; et al. The cancer preventative agent resveratrol is converted to the anticancer agent piceatannol by the cytochrome P450 enzyme CYP1B1. *Br. J. Cancer* **2002**, *86*, 774–778. [CrossRef] [PubMed]

19. Kershaw, J.; Kim, K.H. The Therapeutic Potential of Piceatannol, a Natural Stilbene, in Metabolic Diseases: A Review. *J. Med. Food* **2017**, *20*, 427–438. [CrossRef] [PubMed]

20. Rotches-Ribalta, M.; Urpi-Sarda, M.; Llorach, R.; Boto-Ordoñez, M.; Jauregui, O.; Chiva-Blanch, G.; Perez-Garcia, L.; Jaeger, W.; Guillen, M.; Corella, D.; et al. Gut and microbial resveratrol metabolite profiling after moderate long-term consumption of red wine versus dealcoholized red wine in humans by an optimized ultra-high-pressure liquid chromatography tandem mass spectrometry method. *J. Chromatogr. A* **2012**, *1265*, 105–113. [CrossRef] [PubMed]

21. Basholli-Salihu, M.; Schuster, R.; Mulla, D.; Praznik, W.; Viernstein, H.; Mueller, M. Bioconversion of piceid to resveratrol by selected probiotic cell extracts. *Bioprocess Biosyst. Eng.* **2016**, *39*, 1879–1885. [CrossRef] [PubMed]

22. Wang, D.; Zhang, Z.; Ju, J.; Wang, X.; Qiu, W. Investigation of piceid metabolites in rat by liquid chromatography tandem mass spectrometry. *J. Chromatogr. B. Anal. Technol. Biomed. Life Sci.* **2011**, *879*, 69–74. [CrossRef] [PubMed]

23. Rotches-Ribalta, M.; Andres-Lacueva, C.; Estruch, R.; Escribano, E.; Urpi-Sarda, M. Pharmacokinetics of resveratrol metabolic profile in healthy humans after moderate consumption of red wine and grape extract tablets. *Pharmacol. Res.* **2012**, *66*, 375–382. [CrossRef] [PubMed]

24. Macarulla, M.T.; Alberdi, G.; Gómez, S.; Tueros, I.; Bald, C.; Rodríguez, V.M.; Martínez, J.A.; Portillo, M.P. Effects of different doses of resveratrol on body fat and serum parameters in rats fed a hypercaloric diet. *J. Physiol. Biochem.* **2009**, *65*, 369–376. [CrossRef] [PubMed]

25. Kim, S.; Jin, Y.; Choi, Y.; Park, T. Resveratrol exerts anti-obesity effects via mechanisms involving down-regulation of adipogenic and inflammatory processes in mice. *Biochem. Pharmacol.* **2011**, *81*, 1343–1351. [CrossRef] [PubMed]

26. Cho, S.J.; Jung, U.J.; Choi, M.S. Differential effects of low-dose resveratrol on adiposity and hepatic steatosis in diet-induced obese mice. *Br. J. Nutr.* **2012**, *108*, 2166–2175. [CrossRef] [PubMed]

27. Picard, F.; Kurtev, M.; Chung, N.; Topark-Ngarm, A.; Senawong, T.; Machado De Oliveira, R.; Leid, M.; McBurney, M.W.; Guarente, L. Sirt1 promotes fat mobilization in white adipocytes by repressing PPAR-gamma. *Nature* **2004**, *429*, 771–776. [CrossRef] [PubMed]

28. Park, S.J.; Ahmad, F.; Philp, A.; Baar, K.; Williams, T.; Luo, H.; Ke, H.; Rehmann, H.; Taussig, R.; Brown, A.L.; et al. Resveratrol ameliorates aging-related metabolic phenotypes by inhibiting cAMP phosphodiesterases. *Cell* **2012**, *148*, 421–433. [CrossRef] [PubMed]

29. Gracia, A.; Miranda, J.; Fernández-Quintela, A.; Eseberri, I.; Garcia-Lacarte, M.; Milagro, F.I.; Martínez, J.A.; Aguirre, L.; Portillo, M.P. Involvement of miR-539-5p in the inhibition of de novo lipogenesis induced by resveratrol in white adipose tissue. *Food Funct.* **2016**, *7*, 1680–1688. [CrossRef] [PubMed]

30. Fischer-Posovszky, P.; Kukulus, V.; Tews, D.; Unterkircher, T.; Debatin, K.M.; Fulda, S.; Wabitsch, M. Resveratrol regulates human adipocyte number and function in a Sirt1-dependent manner. *Am. J. Clin. Nutr.* **2010**, *92*, 5–15. [CrossRef] [PubMed]

31. Hsu, C.L.; Yen, G.C. Induction of cell apoptosis in 3T3-L1 pre-adipocytes by flavonoids is associated with their antioxidant activity. *Mol. Nutr. Food Res.* **2006**, *50*, 1072–1079. [CrossRef] [PubMed]

32. Arzola-Paniagua, M.A.; García-Salgado López, E.R.; Calvo-Vargas, C.G.; Guevara-Cruz, M. Efficacy of an orlistat-resveratrol combination for weight loss in subjects with obesity: A randomized controlled trial. *Obesity* **2016**, *24*, 1454–1463. [CrossRef] [PubMed]

33. Mercader, J.; Palou, A.; Bonet, M.L. Resveratrol enhances fatty acid oxidation capacity and reduces resistin and Retinol-Binding Protein 4 expression in white adipocytes. *J. Nutr. Biochem.* **2011**, *22*, 828–834. [CrossRef] [PubMed]

34. Wang, S.; Liang, X.; Yang, Q.; Fu, X.; Rogers, C.J.; Zhu, M.; Rodgers, B.D.; Jiang, Q.; Dodson, M.V.; Du, M. Resveratrol induces brown-like adipocyte formation in white fat through activation of AMP-activated protein kinase (AMPK) α1. *Int. J. Obes.* **2015**, *39*, 967–976. [CrossRef] [PubMed]

35. Gomez-Zorita, S.; Tréguer, K.; Mercader, J.; Carpéné, C. Resveratrol directly affects in vitro lipolysis and glucose transport in human fat cells. *J. Physiol. Biochem.* **2013**, *69*, 585–593. [CrossRef] [PubMed]

36. Wang, S.; Liang, X.; Yang, Q.; Fu, X.; Zhu, M.; Rodgers, B.D.; Jiang, Q.; Dodson, M.V.; Du, M. Resveratrol enhances brown adipocyte formation and function by activating AMP-activated protein kinase (AMPK) α1 in mice fed high-fat diet. *Mol. Nutr. Food Res.* **2017**. [CrossRef] [PubMed]

37. Lasa, A.; Schweiger, M.; Kotzbeck, P.; Churruca, I.; Simón, E.; Zechner, R.; Portillo, M.P. Resveratrol regulates lipolysis via adipose triglyceride lipase. *J. Nutr. Biochem.* **2012**, *23*, 379–384. [CrossRef] [PubMed]

38. Alberdi, G.; Rodríguez, V.M.; Miranda, J.; Macarulla, M.T.; Arias, N.; Andrés-Lacueva, C.; Portillo, M.P. Changes in white adipose tissue metabolism induced by resveratrol in rats. *Nutr. Metab.* **2011**, *8*, 29. [CrossRef] [PubMed]

39. Alberdi, G.; Rodríguez, V.M.; Miranda, J.; Macarulla, M.T.; Churruca, I.; Portillo, M.P. Thermogenesis is involved in the body-fat lowering effects of resveratrol in rats. *Food Chem.* **2013**, *141*, 1530–1535. [CrossRef] [PubMed]

40. Poulsen, M.M.; Vestergaard, P.F.; Clasen, B.F.; Radko, Y.; Christensen, L.P.; Stødkilde-Jørgensen, H.; Møller, N.; Jessen, N.; Pedersen, S.B.; Jørgensen, J.O. High-dose resveratrol supplementation in obese men: An investigator-initiated, randomized, placebo-controlled clinical trial of substrate metabolism, insulin sensitivity, and body composition. *Diabetes* **2013**, *62*, 1186–1195. [CrossRef] [PubMed]

41. Timmers, S.; Konings, E.; Bilet, L.; Houtkooper, R.H.; van de Weijer, T.; Goossens, G.H.; Hoeks, J.; van der Krieken, S.; Ryu, D.; Kersten, S.; et al. Calorie restriction-like effects of 30 days of resveratrol supplementation on energy metabolism and metabolic profile in obese humans. *Cell Metab.* **2011**, *14*, 612–622. [CrossRef] [PubMed]

42. Konings, E.; Timmers, S.; Boekschoten, M.V.; Goossens, G.H.; Jocken, J.W.; Afman, L.A.; Müller, M.; Schrauwen, P.; Mariman, E.C.; Blaak, E.E. The effects of 30 days resveratrol supplementation on adipose tissue morphology and gene expression patterns in obese men. *Int. J. Obes.* **2014**, *38*, 470–473. [CrossRef] [PubMed]

43. Kjær, T.N.; Ornstrup, M.J.; Poulsen, M.M.; Stødkilde-Jørgensen, H.; Jessen, N.; Jørgensen, J.O.L.; Richelsen, B.; Pedersen, S.B. No Beneficial Effects of Resveratrol on the Metabolic Syndrome: A Randomized Placebo-Controlled Clinical Trial. *J. Clin. Endocrinol. Metab.* **2017**, *102*, 1642–1651. [CrossRef] [PubMed]

44. Méndez-del Villar, M.; González-Ortiz, M.; Martínez-Abundis, E.; Pérez-Rubio, K.G.; Lizárraga-Valdez, R. Effect of resveratrol administration on metabolic syndrome, insulin sensitivity, and insulin secretion. *Metab. Syndr. Relat. Disord.* **2014**, *12*, 497–501. [CrossRef] [PubMed]

45. Chachay, V.S.; Macdonald, G.A.; Martin, J.H.; Whitehead, J.P.; O'Moore-Sullivan, T.M.; Lee, P.; Franklin, M.; Klein, K.; Taylor, P.J.; Ferguson, M.; et al. Resveratrol does not benefit patients with nonalcoholic fatty liver disease. *Clin. Gastroenterol. Hepatol.* **2014**, *12*, 2092–2103. [CrossRef] [PubMed]

46. Faghihzadeh, F.; Adibi, P.; Hekmatdoost, A. The effects of resveratrol supplementation on cardiovascular risk factors in patients with non-alcoholic fatty liver disease: A randomised, double-blind, placebo-controlled study. *Br. J. Nutr.* **2015**, *114*, 796–803. [CrossRef] [PubMed]

47. Thazhath, S.S.; Wu, T.; Bound, M.J.; Checklin, H.L.; Standfield, S.; Jones, K.L.; Horowitz, M.; Rayner, C.K. Administration of resveratrol for 5 wk has no effect on glucagon-like peptide 1 secretion, gastric emptying, or glycemic control in type 2 diabetes: A randomized controlled trial. *Am. J. Clin. Nutr.* **2016**, *103*, 66–70. [CrossRef] [PubMed]

48. Bo, S.; Ponzo, V.; Ciccone, G.; Evangelista, A.; Saba, F.; Goitre, I.; Procopio, M.; Pagano, G.F.; Cassader, M.; Gambino, R. Six months of resveratrol supplementation has no measurable effect in type 2 diabetic patients. A randomized, double blind, placebo-controlled trial. *Pharmacol. Res.* **2016**, *111*, 896–905. [CrossRef] [PubMed]

49. Most, J.; Timmers, S.; Warnke, I.; Jocken, J.W.; van Boekschoten, M.; de Groot, P.; Bendik, I.; Schrauwen, P.; Goossens, G.H.; Blaak, E.E. Combined epigallocatechin-3-gallate and resveratrol supplementation for 12 wk increases mitochondrial capacity and fat oxidation, but not insulin sensitivity, in obese humans: A randomized controlled trial. *Am. J. Clin. Nutr.* **2016**, *104*, 215–227. [CrossRef] [PubMed]

50. Poulsen, M.M.; Larsen, J.; Hamilton-Dutoit, S.; Clasen, B.F.; Jessen, N.; Paulsen, S.K.; Kjær, T.N.; Richelsen, B.; Pedersen, S.B. Resveratrol up-regulates hepatic uncoupling protein 2 and prevents development of nonalcoholic fatty liver disease in rats fed a high-fat diet. *Nutr. Res.* **2012**, *32*, 701–708. [CrossRef] [PubMed]

51. Alberdi, G.; Rodríguez, V.M.; Macarulla, M.T.; Miranda, J.; Churruca, I.; Portillo, M.P. Hepatic lipid metabolic pathways modified by resveratrol in rats fed an obesogenic diet. *Nutrition* **2013**, *29*, 562–567. [CrossRef] [PubMed]

52. Bujanda, L.; Hijona, E.; Larzabal, M.; Beraza, M.; Aldazabal, P.; García-Urkia, N.; Sarasqueta, C.; Cosme, A.; Irastorza, B.; González, A.; et al. Resveratrol inhibits nonalcoholic fatty liver disease in rats. *BMC Gastroenterol.* **2008**, *8*, 40. [CrossRef] [PubMed]

53. Gómez-Zorita, S.; Fernández-Quintela, A.; Macarulla, M.T.; Aguirre, L.; Hijona, E.; Bujanda, L.; Milagro, F.; Martínez, J.A.; Portillo, M.P. Resveratrol attenuates steatosis in obese Zucker rats by decreasing fatty acid availability and reducing oxidative stress. *Br. J. Nutr.* **2012**, *107*, 202–210. [CrossRef] [PubMed]

54. Andrade, J.M.; Paraíso, A.F.; de Oliveira, M.V.; Martins, A.M.; Neto, J.F.; Guimarães, A.L.; de Paula, A.M.; Qureshi, M.; Santos, S.H. Resveratrol attenuates hepatic steatosis in high-fat fed mice by decreasing lipogenesis and inflammation. *Nutrition* **2014**, *30*, 915–919. [CrossRef] [PubMed]

55. Pan, Q.R.; Ren, Y.L.; Liu, W.X.; Hu, Y.J.; Zheng, J.S.; Xu, Y.; Wang, G. Resveratrol prevents hepatic steatosis and endoplasmic reticulum stress and regulates the expression of genes involved in lipid metabolism, insulin resistance, and inflammation in rats. *Nutr. Res.* **2015**, *35*, 576–584. [CrossRef] [PubMed]

56. Elgebaly, A.; Radwan, I.A.; AboElnas, M.M.; Ibrahim, H.H.; Eltoomy, M.F.; Atta, A.A.; Mesalam, H.A.; Sayed, A.A.; Othman, A.A. Resveratrol supplementation in patients with non-alcoholic fatty liver disease: systematic review and meta-analysis. *J. Gastrointestin. Liver Dis.* **2017**, *26*, 59–67. [PubMed]

57. Zhang, C.; Yuan, W.; Fang, J.; Wang, W.; He, P.; Lei, J.; Wang, C. Efficacy of Resveratrol Supplementation against Non-Alcoholic Fatty Liver Disease: A Meta-Analysis of Placebo-Controlled Clinical Trials. *PLoS ONE* **2016**, *11*, e0161792. [CrossRef] [PubMed]

58. Timmers, S.; de Ligt, M.; Phielix, E.; van de Weijer, T.; Hansen, J.; Moonen-Kornips, E.; Schaart, G.; Kunz, I.; Hesselink, M.K.; Schrauwen-Hinderling, V.B.; et al. Resveratrol as Add-on Therapy in Subjects With Well-Controlled Type 2 Diabetes: A Randomized Controlled Trial. *Diabetes Care* **2016**, *39*, 2211–2217. [CrossRef] [PubMed]

59. Kang, L.; Heng, W.; Yuan, A.; Baolin, L.; Fang, H. Resveratrol modulates adipokine expression and improves insulin sensitivity in adipocytes: Relative to inhibition of inflammatory responses. *Biochimie* **2010**, *92*, 789–796. [CrossRef] [PubMed]

60. Kang, W.; Hong, H.J.; Guan, J.; Kim, D.G.; Yang, E.J.; Koh, G.; Park, D.; Han, C.H.; Lee, Y.J.; Lee, D.H. Resveratrol improves insulin signaling in a tissue-specific manner under insulin-resistant conditions only: In vitro and in vivo experiments in rodents. *Metabolism* **2012**, *61*, 424–433. [CrossRef] [PubMed]

61. Costa, C.o.S.; Rohden, F.; Hammes, T.O.; Margis, R.; Bortolotto, J.W.; Padoin, A.V.; Mottin, C.C.; Guaragna, R.M. Resveratrol upregulated SIRT1, FOXO1, and adiponectin and downregulated PPARγ1-3 mRNA expression in human visceral adipocytes. *Obes. Surg.* **2011**, *21*, 356–361. [CrossRef] [PubMed]

62. Bagul, P.K.; Middela, H.; Matapally, S.; Padiya, R.; Bastia, T.; Madhusudana, K.; Reddy, B.R.; Chakravarty, S.; Banerjee, S.K. Attenuation of insulin resistance, metabolic syndrome and hepatic oxidative stress by resveratrol in fructose-fed rats. *Pharmacol. Res.* **2012**, *66*, 260–268. [CrossRef] [PubMed]

63. Kitada, M.; Kume, S.; Imaizumi, N.; Koya, D. Resveratrol improves oxidative stress and protects against diabetic nephropathy through normalization of Mn-SOD dysfunction in AMPK/SIRT1-independent pathway. *Diabetes* **2011**, *60*, 634–643. [CrossRef] [PubMed]

64. Palsamy, P.; Subramanian, S. Resveratrol protects diabetic kidney by attenuating hyperglycemia-mediated oxidative stress and renal inflammatory cytokines via Nrf2-Keap1 signaling. *Biochim. Biophys. Acta* **2011**, *1812*, 719–731. [CrossRef] [PubMed]

65. Chang, C.C.; Chang, C.Y.; Wu, Y.T.; Huang, J.P.; Yen, T.H.; Hung, L.M. Resveratrol retards progression of diabetic nephropathy through modulations of oxidative stress, proinflammatory cytokines, and AMP-activated protein kinase. *J. Biomed. Sci.* **2011**, *18*, 47. [CrossRef] [PubMed]

66. Öztürk, E.; Arslan, A.K.K.; Yerer, M.B.; Bishayee, A. Resveratrol and diabetes: A critical review of clinical studies. *Biomed. Pharmacother.* **2017**, *95*, 230–234. [CrossRef] [PubMed]

67. Van der Made, S.M.; Plat, J.; Mensink, R.P. Resveratrol does not influence metabolic risk markers related to cardiovascular health in overweight and slightly obese subjects: A randomized, placebo-controlled crossover trial. *PLoS ONE* **2015**, *10*, e0118393. [CrossRef] [PubMed]

68. Dash, S.; Xiao, C.; Morgantini, C.; Szeto, L.; Lewis, G.F. High-dose resveratrol treatment for 2 weeks inhibits intestinal and hepatic lipoprotein production in overweight/obese men. *Arterioscler. Thromb. Vasc. Biol.* **2013**, *33*, 2895–2901. [CrossRef] [PubMed]

69. Yoshino, J.; Conte, C.; Fontana, L.; Mittendorfer, B.; Imai, S.; Schechtman, K.B.; Gu, C.; Kunz, I.; Rossi Fanelli, F.; Patterson, B.W.; et al. Resveratrol supplementation does not improve metabolic function in nonobese women with normal glucose tolerance. *Cell Metab.* **2012**, *16*, 658–664. [CrossRef] [PubMed]

70. Knop, F.K.; Konings, E.; Timmers, S.; Schrauwen, P.; Holst, J.J.; Blaak, E.E. Thirty days of resveratrol supplementation does not affect postprandial incretin hormone responses, but suppresses postprandial glucagon in obese subjects. *Diabet. Med.* **2013**, *30*, 1214–1218. [CrossRef] [PubMed]

71. Pollack, R.M.; Barzilai, N.; Anghel, V.; Kulkarni, A.S.; Golden, A.; O'Broin, P.; Sinclair, D.A.; Bonkowski, M.S.; Coleville, A.J.; Powell, D.; et al. Resveratrol improves vascular function and mitochondrial number but not glucose metabolism in older adults. *J. Gerontol. A Biol. Sci. Med. Sci.* **2017**, *72*, 1703–1709. [CrossRef] [PubMed]

72. Bhatt, J.K.; Thomas, S.; Nanjan, M.J. Resveratrol supplementation improves glycemic control in type 2 diabetes mellitus. *Nutr. Res.* **2012**, *32*, 537–541. [CrossRef] [PubMed]

73. Brasnyó, P.; Molnár, G.A.; Mohás, M.; Markó, L.; Laczy, B.; Cseh, J.; Mikolás, E.; Szijártó, I.A.; Mérei, A.; Halmai, R.; et al. Resveratrol improves insulin sensitivity, reduces oxidative stress and activates the Akt pathway in type 2 diabetic patients. *Br. J. Nutr.* **2011**, *106*, 383–389. [CrossRef] [PubMed]

74. Zare Javid, A.; Hormoznejad, R.; Yousefimanesh, H.A.; Zakerkish, M.; Haghighi-Zadeh, M.H.; Dehghan, P.; Ravanbakhsh, M. The impact of resveratrol supplementation on blood glucose, insulin, insulin resistance, triglyceride, and periodontal markers in type 2 diabetic patients with chronic periodontitis. *Phytother. Res.* **2017**, *31*, 108–114. [CrossRef] [PubMed]

75. Crandall, J.P.; Oram, V.; Trandafirescu, G.; Reid, M.; Kishore, P.; Hawkins, M.; Cohen, H.W.; Barzilai, N. Pilot study of resveratrol in older adults with impaired glucose tolerance. *J. Gerontol. A Biol. Sci. Med. Sci.* **2012**, *67*, 1307–1312. [CrossRef] [PubMed]

76. Chen, S.; Zhao, X.; Ran, L.; Wan, J.; Wang, X.; Qin, Y.; Shu, F.; Gao, Y.; Yuan, L.; Zhang, Q.; et al. Resveratrol improves insulin resistance, glucose and lipid metabolism in patients with non-alcoholic fatty liver disease: A randomized controlled trial. *Dig. Liver Dis.* **2015**, *47*, 226–232. [CrossRef] [PubMed]

77. Liu, K.; Zhou, R.; Wang, B.; Mi, M.T. Effect of resveratrol on glucose control and insulin sensitivity: A meta-analysis of 11 randomized controlled trials. *Am. J. Clin. Nutr.* **2014**, *99*, 1510–1519. [CrossRef] [PubMed]

78. Hausenblas, H.A.; Schoulda, J.A.; Smoliga, J.M. Resveratrol treatment as an adjunct to pharmacological management in type 2 diabetes mellitus–systematic review and meta-analysis. *Mol. Nutr. Food Res.* **2015**, *59*, 147–159. [CrossRef] [PubMed]

79. Szkudelski, T.; Szkudelska, K. Resveratrol and diabetes: From animal to human studies. *Biochim. Biophys. Acta.* **2015**, *1852*, 1145–1154. [CrossRef] [PubMed]

80. Mozafari, M.; Nekooeian, A.A.; Panjeshahin, M.R.; Zare, H.R. The effects of resveratrol in rats with simultaneous type 2 diabetes and renal hypertension: A study of antihypertensive mechanisms. *Iran. J. Med. Sci.* **2015**, *40*, 152–160. [PubMed]

81. Gordish, K.L.; Beierwaltes, W.H. Chronic resveratrol reverses a mild angiotensin II-induced pressor effect in a rat model. *Integr. Blood Press Control* **2016**, *9*, 23–31. [PubMed]

82. Cheng, P.W.; Ho, W.Y.; Su, Y.T.; Lu, P.J.; Chen, B.Z.; Cheng, W.H.; Lu, W.H.; Sun, G.C.; Yeh, T.C.; Hsiao, M.; et al. Resveratrol decreases fructose-induced oxidative stress, mediated by NADPH oxidase via an AMPK-dependent mechanism. *Br. J. Pharmacol.* **2014**, *171*, 2739–2750. [CrossRef] [PubMed]

83. Yu, L.; Tu, Y.; Jia, X.; Fang, K.; Liu, L.; Wan, L.; Xiang, C.; Wang, Y.; Sun, X.; Liu, T.; et al. Resveratrol protects against pulmonary arterial hypertension in rats via activation of silent information regulator 1. *Cell Physiol. Biochem.* **2017**, *42*, 55–67. [CrossRef] [PubMed]

84. Heebøll, S.; Kreuzfeldt, M.; Hamilton-Dutoit, S.; Kjær Poulsen, M.; Stødkilde-Jørgensen, H.; Møller, H.J.; Jessen, N.; Thorsen, K.; Kristina Hellberg, Y.; Bønløkke Pedersen, S.; et al. Placebo-controlled, randomised clinical trial: High-dose resveratrol treatment for non-alcoholic fatty liver disease. *Scand. J. Gastroenterol.* **2016**, *51*, 456–464. [CrossRef] [PubMed]

85. Imamura, H.; Yamaguchi, T.; Nagayama, D.; Saiki, A.; Shirai, K.; Tatsuno, I. Resveratrol ameliorates arterial stiffness assessed by cardio-ankle vascular index in patients with type 2 diabetes mellitus. *Int. Heart J.* **2017**, *58*, 577–583. [CrossRef] [PubMed]

86. Wong, R.H.; Berry, N.M.; Coates, A.M.; Buckley, J.D.; Bryan, J.; Kunz, I.; Howe, P.R. Chronic resveratrol consumption improves brachial flow-mediated dilatation in healthy obese adults. *J. Hypertens.* **2013**, *31*, 1819–1827. [CrossRef] [PubMed]

87. Sahebkar, A.; Serban, C.; Ursoniu, S.; Wong, N.D.; Muntner, P.; Graham, I.M.; Mikhailidis, D.P.; Rizzo, M.; Rysz, J.; Sperling, L.S.; et al. Lack of efficacy of resveratrol on C-reactive protein and selected cardiovascular risk factors–Results from a systematic review and meta-analysis of randomized controlled trials. *Int. J. Cardiol.* **2015**, *189*, 47–55. [CrossRef] [PubMed]

88. Huang, H.; Chen, G.; Liao, D.; Zhu, Y.; Pu, R.; Xue, X. The effects of resveratrol intervention on risk markers of cardiovascular health in overweight and obese subjects: A pooled analysis of randomized controlled trials. *Obes. Rev.* **2016**, *17*, 1329–1340. [CrossRef] [PubMed]

89. Fogacci, F.; Tocci, G.; Presta, V.; Fratter, A.; Borghi, C.; Cicero, A.F.G. Effect of resveratrol on blood pressure: A systematic review and meta-analysis of randomized, controlled, clinical trials. *Crit. Rev. Food Sci. Nutr.* **2018**. [CrossRef] [PubMed]

90. Marques, B.C.A.A.; Trindade, M.; Aquino, J.C.F.; Cunha, A.R.; Gismondi, R.O.; Neves, M.F.; Oigman, W. Beneficial effects of acute trans-resveratrol supplementation in treated hypertensive patients with endothelial dysfunction. *Clin. Exp. Hypertens.* **2018**, *40*, 218–223. [CrossRef] [PubMed]

91. Wong, R.H.; Howe, P.R.; Buckley, J.D.; Coates, A.M.; Kunz, I.; Berry, N.M. Acute resveratrol supplementation improves flow-mediated dilatation in overweight/obese individuals with mildly elevated blood pressure. *Nutr. Metab. Cardiovasc. Dis.* **2011**, *21*, 851–856. [CrossRef] [PubMed]

92. Gnoni, G.V.; Paglialonga, G. Resveratrol inhibits fatty acid and triacylglycerol synthesis in rat hepatocytes. *Eur. J. Clin. Invest.* **2009**, *39*, 211–218. [CrossRef] [PubMed]

93. Zern, T.L.; Wood, R.J.; Greene, C.; West, K.L.; Liu, Y.; Aggarwal, D.; Shachter, N.S.; Fernandez, M.L. Grape polyphenols exert a cardioprotective effect in pre- and postmenopausal women by lowering plasma lipids and reducing oxidative stress. *J. Nutr.* **2005**, *135*, 1911–1917. [CrossRef] [PubMed]

94. Qureshi, A.A.; Khan, D.A.; Mahjabeen, W.; Papasian, C.J.; Qureshi, N. Suppression of nitric oxide production and cardiovascular risk factors in healthy seniors and hypercholesterolemic subjects by a combination of polyphenols and vitamins. *J. Clin. Exp. Cardiolog.* **2012**. [CrossRef]

95. Simental-Mendía, L.E.; Guerrero-Romero, F. Effect of resveratrol supplementation on lipid profile in subjects with dyslipidemia: A randomized double-blind, placebo-controlled trial. *Nutrition* **2018**, *58*, 7–10. [CrossRef] [PubMed]

96. Shao, D.; Wang, Y.; Huang, Q.; Shi, J.; Yang, H.; Pan, Z.; Jin, M.; Zhao, H.; Xu, X. Cholesterol-lowering effects and mechanisms in view of bile acid pathway of resveratrol and resveratrol glucuronides. *J. Food Sci.* **2016**, *81*, H2841–H2848. [CrossRef] [PubMed]

97. Chen, Q.; Wang, E.; Ma, L.; Zhai, P. Dietary resveratrol increases the expression of hepatic 7α-hydroxylase and ameliorates hypercholesterolemia in high-fat fed C57BL/6J mice. *Lipids Health Dis.* **2012**, *11*, 56. [CrossRef] [PubMed]

98. Berrougui, H.; Grenier, G.; Loued, S.; Drouin, G.; Khalil, A. A new insight into resveratrol as an atheroprotective compound: Inhibition of lipid peroxidation and enhancement of cholesterol efflux. *Atherosclerosis* **2009**, *207*, 420–427. [CrossRef] [PubMed]

99. Tomé-Carneiro, J.; Gonzálvez, M.; Larrosa, M.; García-Almagro, F.J.; Avilés-Plaza, F.; Parra, S.; Yáñez-Gascón, M.J.; Ruiz-Ros, J.A.; García-Conesa, M.T.; Tomás-Barberán, F.A.; et al. Consumption of a grape extract supplement containing resveratrol decreases oxidized LDL and ApoB in patients undergoing primary prevention of cardiovascular disease: A triple-blind, 6-month follow-up, placebo-controlled, randomized trial. *Mol. Nutr. Food Res.* **2012**, *56*, 810–821. [CrossRef] [PubMed]

100. Dvorakova, M.; Landa, P. Anti-inflammatory activity of natural stilbenoids: A review. *Pharmacol. Res.* **2017**, *124*, 126–145. [CrossRef] [PubMed]

101. Latruffe, N.; Lançon, A.; Frazzi, R.; Aires, V.; Delmas, D.; Michaille, J.J.; Djouadi, F.; Bastin, J.; Cherkaoui-Malki, M. Exploring new ways of regulation by resveratrol involving miRNAs, with emphasis on inflammation. *Ann. N. Y. Acad. Sci.* **2015**, *1348*, 97–106. [CrossRef] [PubMed]

102. Zhu, J.; Yong, W.; Wu, X.; Yu, Y.; Lv, J.; Liu, C.; Mao, X.; Zhu, Y.; Xu, K.; Han, X. Anti-inflammatory effect of resveratrol on TNF-alpha-induced MCP-1 expression in adipocytes. *Biochem. Biophys. Res. Commun.* **2008**, *369*, 471–477. [CrossRef] [PubMed]

103. Olholm, J.; Paulsen, S.K.; Cullberg, K.B.; Richelsen, B.; Pedersen, S.B. Anti-inflammatory effect of resveratrol on adipokine expression and secretion in human adipose tissue explants. *Int. J. Obes.* **2010**, *34*, 1546–1553. [CrossRef] [PubMed]

104. Yen, G.C.; Chen, Y.C.; Chang, W.T.; Hsu, C.L. Effects of polyphenolic compounds on tumor necrosis factor-α (TNF-α)-induced changes of adipokines and oxidative stress in 3T3-L1 adipocytes. *J. Agric. Food Chem.* **2011**, *59*, 546–551. [CrossRef] [PubMed]

105. Gonzales, A.M.; Orlando, R.A. Curcumin and resveratrol inhibit nuclear factor-kappaB-mediated cytokine expression in adipocytes. *Nutr. Metab.* **2008**, *5*, 17. [CrossRef] [PubMed]

106. Cullberg, K.B.; Olholm, J.; Paulsen, S.K.; Foldager, C.B.; Lind, M.; Richelsen, B.; Pedersen, S.B. Resveratrol has inhibitory effects on the hypoxia-induced inflammation and angiogenesis in human adipose tissue *in vitro*. *Eur. J. Pharm. Sci.* **2013**, *49*, 251–257. [CrossRef] [PubMed]

107. Tran, H.T.; Liong, S.; Lim, R.; Barker, G.; Lappas, M. Resveratrol ameliorates the chemical and microbial induction of inflammation and insulin resistance in human placenta, adipose tissue and skeletal muscle. *PLoS ONE* **2017**, *12*, e0173373. [CrossRef] [PubMed]

108. Gómez-Zorita, S.; Fernández-Quintela, A.; Lasa, A.; Hijona, E.; Bujanda, L.; Portillo, M.P. Effects of resveratrol on obesity-related inflammation markers in adipose tissue of genetically obese rats. *Nutrition* **2013**, *29*, 1374–1380. [CrossRef] [PubMed]

109. Jeon, B.T.; Jeong, E.A.; Shin, H.J.; Lee, Y.; Lee, D.H.; Kim, H.J.; Kang, S.S.; Cho, G.J.; Choi, W.S.; Roh, G.S. Resveratrol attenuates obesity-associated peripheral and central inflammation and improves memory deficit in mice fed a high-fat diet. *Diabetes* **2012**, *61*, 1444–1454. [CrossRef] [PubMed]

110. Wang, B.; Sun, J.; Li, X.; Zhou, Q.; Bai, J.; Shi, Y.; Le, G. Resveratrol prevents suppression of regulatory T-cell production, oxidative stress, and inflammation of mice prone or resistant to high-fat diet-induced obesity. *Nutr. Res.* **2013**, *33*, 971–981. [CrossRef] [PubMed]

111. Jimenez-Gomez, Y.; Mattison, J.A.; Pearson, K.J.; Martin-Montalvo, A.; Palacios, H.H.; Sossong, A.M.; Ward, T.M.; Younts, C.M.; Lewis, K.; Allard, J.S.; et al. Resveratrol improves adipose insulin signaling and reduces the inflammatory response in adipose tissue of rhesus monkeys on high-fat, high-sugar diet. *Cell Metab.* **2013**, *18*, 533–545. [CrossRef] [PubMed]

112. Wang, B.; Sun, J.; Li, L.; Zheng, J.; Shi, Y.; Le, G. Regulatory effects of resveratrol on glucose metabolism and T-lymphocyte subsets in the development of high-fat diet-induced obesity in C57BL/6 mice. *Food Funct.* **2014**, *5*, 1452–1463. [CrossRef] [PubMed]

113. Ghanim, H.; Sia, C.L.; Korzeniewski, K.; Lohano, T.; Abuaysheh, S.; Marumganti, A.; Chaudhuri, A.; Dandona, P. A resveratrol and polyphenol preparation suppresses oxidative and inflammatory stress response to a high-fat, high-carbohydrate meal. *J. Clin. Endocrinol. Metab.* **2011**, *96*, 1409–1414. [CrossRef] [PubMed]

114. Tomé-Carneiro, J.; Larrosa, M.; Yáñez-Gascón, M.J.; Dávalos, A.; Gil-Zamorano, J.; Gonzálvez, M.; García-Almagro, F.J.; Ruiz Ros, J.A.; Tomás-Barberán, F.A.; Espín, J.C.; et al. One-year supplementation with a grape extract containing resveratrol modulates inflammatory-related microRNAs and cytokines expression in peripheral blood mononuclear cells of type 2 diabetes and hypertensive patients with coronary artery disease. *Pharmacol. Res.* **2013**, *72*, 69–82. [CrossRef] [PubMed]

115. Khodabandehloo, H.; Seyyedebrahimi, S.; Esfahani, E.N.; Razi, F.; Meshkani, R. Resveratrol supplementation decreases blood glucose without changing the circulating CD14. *Nutr. Res.* **2018**, *54*, 40–51. [CrossRef] [PubMed]

116. Haghighatdoost, F.; Hariri, M. Can resveratrol supplement change inflammatory mediators? A systematic review and meta-analysis on randomized clinical trials. *Eur. J. Clin. Nutr.* **2018**. [CrossRef] [PubMed]

117. Kumar, A.; Sharma, S.S. NF-kappaB inhibitory action of resveratrol: A probable mechanism of neuroprotection in experimental diabetic neuropathy. *Biochem. Biophys. Res. Commun.* **2010**, *394*, 360–365. [CrossRef] [PubMed]

118. Truong, V.L.; Jun, M.; Jeong, W.S. Role of resveratrol in regulation of cellular defense systems against oxidative stress. *Biofactors* **2018**, *44*, 36–49. [CrossRef] [PubMed]

119. Ungvari, Z.; Labinskyy, N.; Mukhopadhyay, P.; Pinto, J.T.; Bagi, Z.; Ballabh, P.; Zhang, C.; Pacher, P.; Csiszar, A. Resveratrol attenuates mitochondrial oxidative stress in coronary arterial endothelial cells. *Am. J. Physiol. Heart Circ. Physiol.* **2009**, *297*, H1876–H1881. [CrossRef] [PubMed]

120. Chen, F.; Qian, L.H.; Deng, B.; Liu, Z.M.; Zhao, Y.; Le, Y.Y. Resveratrol protects vascular endothelial cells from high glucose-induced apoptosis through inhibition of NADPH oxidase activation-driven oxidative stress. *CNS Neurosci. Ther.* **2013**, *19*, 675–681. [CrossRef] [PubMed]

121. Yun, J.M.; Chien, A.; Jialal, I.; Devaraj, S. Resveratrol up-regulates SIRT1 and inhibits cellular oxidative stress in the diabetic milieu: Mechanistic insights. *J. Nutr. Biochem.* **2012**, *23*, 699–705. [CrossRef] [PubMed]

122. Guo, S.; Yao, Q.; Ke, Z.; Chen, H.; Wu, J.; Liu, C. Resveratrol attenuates high glucose-induced oxidative stress and cardiomyocyte apoptosis through AMPK. *Mol. Cell Endocrinol.* **2015**, *412*, 85–94. [CrossRef] [PubMed]

123. Franco, J.G.; Lisboa, P.C.; Lima, N.S.; Amaral, T.A.; Peixoto-Silva, N.; Resende, A.C.; Oliveira, E.; Passos, M.C.; Moura, E.G. Resveratrol attenuates oxidative stress and prevents steatosis and hypertension in obese rats programmed by early weaning. *J. Nutr. Biochem.* **2013**, *24*, 960–966. [CrossRef] [PubMed]

124. Zhang, H.; Zhang, J.; Ungvari, Z.; Zhang, C. Resveratrol improves endothelial function: Role of TNFα and vascular oxidative stress. *Arterioscler. Thromb. Vasc. Biol.* **2009**, *29*, 1164–1171. [CrossRef] [PubMed]

125. Ungvari, Z.; Bagi, Z.; Feher, A.; Recchia, F.A.; Sonntag, W.E.; Pearson, K.; de Cabo, R.; Csiszar, A. Resveratrol confers endothelial protection via activation of the antioxidant transcription factor Nrf2. *Am. J. Physiol. Heart Circ. Physiol.* **2010**, *299*, H18–H24. [CrossRef] [PubMed]

126. Zhang, H.; Morgan, B.; Potter, B.J.; Ma, L.; Dellsperger, K.C.; Ungvari, Z.; Zhang, C. Resveratrol improves left ventricular diastolic relaxation in type 2 diabetes by inhibiting oxidative/nitrative stress: *In vivo* demonstration with magnetic resonance imaging. *Am. J. Physiol. Heart Circ. Physiol.* **2010**, *299*, H985–H994. [CrossRef] [PubMed]

127. Apostolidou, C.; Adamopoulos, K.; Iliadis, S.; Kourtidou-Papadeli, C. Alterations of antioxidant status in asymptomatic hypercholesterolemic individuals after resveratrol intake. *Int. J. Food Sci. Nutr.* **2015**, *67*, 541–552. [CrossRef] [PubMed]

128. De Groote, D.; Van Belleghem, K.; Devière, J.; Van Brussel, W.; Mukaneza, A.; Amininejad, L. Effect of the intake of resveratrol, resveratrol phosphate, and catechin-rich grape seed extract on markers of oxidative stress and gene expression in adult obese subjects. *Ann. Nutr. Metab.* **2012**, *61*, 15–24. [CrossRef] [PubMed]

129. Wang, H.L.; Gao, J.P.; Han, Y.L.; Xu, X.; Wu, R.; Gao, Y.; Cui, X.H. Comparative studies of polydatin and resveratrol on mutual transformation and antioxidative effect in vivo. *Phytomedicine* **2015**, *22*, 553–559. [CrossRef] [PubMed]

130. Hao, J.; Chen, C.; Huang, K.; Huang, J.; Li, J.; Liu, P.; Huang, H. Polydatin improves glucose and lipid metabolism in experimental diabetes through activating the Akt signaling pathway. *Eur. J. Pharmacol.* **2014**, *745*, 152–165. [CrossRef] [PubMed]

131. Wang, Y.; Ye, J.; Li, J.; Chen, C.; Huang, J.; Liu, P.; Huang, H. Polydatin ameliorates lipid and glucose metabolism in type 2 diabetes mellitus by downregulating proprotein convertase subtilisin/kexin type 9 (PCSK9). *Cardiovasc. Diabetol.* **2016**, *15*, 19. [CrossRef] [PubMed]

132. Zhao, X.J.; Yu, H.W.; Yang, Y.Z.; Wu, W.Y.; Chen, T.Y.; Jia, K.K.; Kang, L.L.; Jiao, R.Q.; Kong, L.D. Polydatin prevents fructose-induced liver inflammation and lipid deposition through increasing miR-200a to regulate Keap1/Nrf2 pathway. *Redox. Biol.* **2018**, *18*, 124–137. [CrossRef] [PubMed]

133. Eseberri, I.; Lasa, A.; Churruca, I.; Portillo, M.P. Resveratrol metabolites modify adipokine expression and secretion in 3T3-L1 pre-adipocytes and mature adipocytes. *PLoS ONE* **2013**, *8*, e63918. [CrossRef] [PubMed]

134. Lasa, A.; Churruca, I.; Eseberri, I.; Andrés-Lacueva, C.; Portillo, M.P. Delipidating effect of resveratrol metabolites in 3T3-L1 adipocytes. *Mol. Nutr. Food Res.* **2012**, *56*, 1559–1568. [CrossRef] [PubMed]

135. Hoshino, J.; Park, E.J.; Kondratyuk, T.P.; Marler, L.; Pezzuto, J.M.; van Breemen, R.B.; Mo, S.; Li, Y.; Cushman, M. Selective synthesis and biological evaluation of sulfate-conjugated resveratrol metabolites. *J. Med. Chem.* **2010**, *53*, 5033–5043. [CrossRef] [PubMed]

136. Schueller, K.; Pignitter, M.; Somoza, V. Sulfated and glucuronated trans-resveratrol metabolites regulate chemokines and sirtuin-1 expression in u-937 macrophages. *J. Agric. Food Chem.* **2015**, *63*, 6535–6545. [CrossRef] [PubMed]

137. Stivala, L.A.; Savio, M.; Carafoli, F.; Perucca, P.; Bianchi, L.; Maga, G.; Forti, L.; Pagnoni, U.M.; Albini, A.; Prosperi, E.; et al. Specific structural determinants are responsible for the antioxidant activity and the cell cycle effects of resveratrol. *J. Biol. Chem.* **2001**, *276*, 22586–22594. [CrossRef] [PubMed]

138. Azorín-Ortuño, M.; Yáñez-Gascón, M.J.; González-Sarrías, A.; Larrosa, M.; Vallejo, F.; Pallarés, F.J.; Lucas, R.; Morales, J.C.; Tomás-Barberán, F.A.; García-Conesa, M.T.; et al. Effects of long-term consumption of low doses of resveratrol on diet-induced mild hypercholesterolemia in pigs: A transcriptomic approach to disease prevention. *J. Nutr. Biochem.* **2012**, *23*, 829–837. [CrossRef] [PubMed]

139. Aires, V.; Delmas, D.; Le Bachelier, C.; Latruffe, N.; Schlemmer, D.; Benoist, J.F.; Djouadi, F.; Bastin, J. Stilbenes and resveratrol metabolites improve mitochondrial fatty acid oxidation defects in human fibroblasts. *Orphanet. J. Rare. Dis.* **2014**, *9*, 79. [CrossRef] [PubMed]

140. Vogl, S.; Atanasov, A.G.; Binder, M.; Bulusu, M.; Zehl, M.; Fakhrudin, N.; Heiss, E.H.; Picker, P.; Wawrosch, C.; Saukel, J.; et al. The herbal drug melampyrum pratense l. (koch): isolation and identification of its bioactive compounds targeting mediators of inflammation. *Evid. Based Complem. Alternat. Med.* **2013**, *2013*, 395316. [CrossRef] [PubMed]

141. Ito-Nagahata, T.; Kurihara, C.; Hasebe, M.; Ishii, A.; Yamashita, K.; Iwabuchi, M.; Sonoda, M.; Fukuhara, K.; Sawada, R.; Matsuoka, A.; et al. Stilbene analogs of resveratrol improve insulin resistance through activation of AMPK. *Biosci. Biotechnol. Biochem.* **2013**, *77*, 1229–1235. [CrossRef] [PubMed]

142. Carpéné, C.; Pejenaute, H.; Del Moral, R.; Boulet, N.; Hijona, E.; Andrade, F.; Villanueva-Millán, M.J.; Aguirre, L.; Arbones-Mainar, J.M. The dietary antioxidant piceatannol inhibits adipogenesis of human adipose mesenchymal stem cells and limits glucose transport and lipogenic activities in adipocytes. *Int. J. Mol. Sci.* **2018**. [CrossRef] [PubMed]

143. Les, F.; Deleruyelle, S.; Cassagnes, L.E.; Boutin, J.A.; Balogh, B.; Arbones-Mainar, J.M.; Biron, S.; Marceau, P.; Richard, D.; Nepveu, F.; et al. Piceatannol and resveratrol share inhibitory effects on hydrogen peroxide release, monoamine oxidase and lipogenic activities in adipose tissue, but differ in their antilipolytic properties. *Chem. Biol. Interact.* **2016**, *258*, 115–125. [CrossRef] [PubMed]

144. Uchida-Maruki, H.; Inagaki, H.; Ito, R.; Kurita, I.; Sai, M.; Ito, T. Piceatannol lowers the blood glucose level in diabetic mice. *Biol. Pharm. Bull.* **2015**, *38*, 629–633. [CrossRef] [PubMed]

145. Setoguchi, Y.; Oritani, Y.; Ito, R.; Inagaki, H.; Maruki-Uchida, H.; Ichiyanagi, T.; Ito, T. Absorption and metabolism of piceatannol in rats. *J. Agric. Food Chem.* **2014**, *62*, 2541–2548. [CrossRef] [PubMed]

146. Eräsalo, H.; Hämäläinen, M.; Leppänen, T.; Mäki-Opas, I.; Laavola, M.; Haavikko, R.; Yli-Kauhaluoma, J.; Moilanen, E. Natural stilbenoids have anti-inflammatory properties in vivo and down-regulate the production of inflammatory mediators no, il6, and mcp1 possibly in a pi3k/akt-dependent manner. *J. Nat. Prod.* **2018**, *81*, 1131–1142. [CrossRef] [PubMed]

147. Clemente, J.C.; Ursell, L.K.; Parfrey, L.W.; Knight, R. The impact of the gut microbiota on human health: An integrative view. *Cell* **2012**, *148*, 1258–1270. [CrossRef] [PubMed]

148. Lankelma, J.M.; Nieuwdorp, M.; de Vos, W.M.; Wiersinga, W.J. The gut microbiota in internal medicine: Implications for health and disease. *Neth. J. Med.* **2015**, *73*, 61–68. [PubMed]

149. Zhao, L. The gut microbiota and obesity: From correlation to causality. *Nat. Rev. Microbiol.* **2013**, *11*, 639–647. [CrossRef] [PubMed]

150. De Vos, W.M.; de Vos, E.A. Role of the intestinal microbiome in health and disease: From correlation to causation. *Nutr. Rev.* **2012**. [CrossRef] [PubMed]

151. Tilg, H.; Adolph, T.E.; Gerner, R.R.; Moschen, A.R. The intestinal microbiota in colorectal cancer. *Cancer Cell* **2018**, *33*, 954–964. [CrossRef] [PubMed]

152. Li, J.; Zhao, F.; Wang, Y.; Chen, J.; Tao, J.; Tian, G.; Wu, S.; Liu, W.; Cui, Q.; Geng, B.; et al. Gut microbiota dysbiosis contributes to the development of hypertension. *Microbiome* **2017**, *5*, 14. [CrossRef] [PubMed]

153. Tilg, H.; Moschen, A.R. Microbiota and diabetes: An evolving relationship. *Gut* **2014**, *63*, 1513–1521. [CrossRef] [PubMed]

154. Cani, P.D. Gut microbiota-At the intersection of everything? *Nat. Rev. Gastroenterol. Hepatol.* **2017**, *14*, 321–322. [CrossRef] [PubMed]

155. O'Hara, A.M.; Shanahan, F. The gut flora as a forgotten organ. *EMBO Rep.* **2006**, *7*, 688–693. [CrossRef] [PubMed]

156. Den Besten, G.; van Eunen, K.; Groen, A.K.; Venema, K.; Reijngoud, D.J.; Bakker, B.M. The role of short-chain fatty acids in the interplay between diet, gut microbiota, and host energy metabolism. *J. Lipid Res.* **2013**, *54*, 2325–2340. [CrossRef] [PubMed]

157. Remely, M.; Aumueller, E.; Merold, C.; Dworzak, S.; Hippe, B.; Zanner, J.; Pointner, A.; Brath, H.; Haslberger, A.G. Effects of short chain fatty acid producing bacteria on epigenetic regulation of FFAR3 in type 2 diabetes and obesity. *Gene* **2014**, *537*, 85–92. [CrossRef] [PubMed]

158. Thursby, E.; Juge, N. Introduction to the human gut microbiota. *Biochem. J.* **2017**, *474*, 1823–1836. [CrossRef] [PubMed]

159. Luckey, T.D. Introduction to intestinal microecology. *Am. J. Clin. Nutr.* **1972**, *25*, 1292–1294. [CrossRef] [PubMed]
160. Sender, R.; Fuchs, S.; Milo, R. Are we really vastly outnumbered? revisiting the ratio of bacterial to host cells in humans. *Cell* **2016**, *164*, 337–340. [CrossRef] [PubMed]
161. Integrative HMP (iHMP) Research Network Consortium. The Integrative Human Microbiome Project: Dynamic analysis of microbiome-host omics profiles during periods of human health and disease. *Cell Host. Microbe.* **2014**, *16*, 276–289. [CrossRef] [PubMed]
162. Arumugam, M.; Raes, J.; Pelletier, E.; Le Paslier, D.; Yamada, T.; Mende, D.R.; Fernandes, G.R.; Tap, J.; Bruls, T.; Batto, J.M.; et al. Enterotypes of the human gut microbiome. *Nature* **2011**, *473*, 174–180. [CrossRef] [PubMed]
163. Le Chatelier, E.; Nielsen, T.; Qin, J.; Prifti, E.; Hildebrand, F.; Falony, G.; Almeida, M.; Arumugam, M.; Batto, J.M.; Kennedy, S.; et al. Richness of human gut microbiome correlates with metabolic markers. *Nature* **2013**, *500*, 541–546. [CrossRef] [PubMed]
164. Wen, L.; Duffy, A. Factors influencing the gut microbiota, inflammation, and type 2 diabetes. *J. Nutr.* **2017**, *147*, 1468S–1475S. [CrossRef] [PubMed]
165. Dethlefsen, L.; Relman, D.A. Incomplete recovery and individualized responses of the human distal gut microbiota to repeated antibiotic perturbation. *Proc. Natl. Acad. Sci. USA* **2011**, *108*, 4554–4561. [CrossRef] [PubMed]
166. Knights, D.; Ward, T.L.; McKinlay, C.E.; Miller, H.; Gonzalez, A.; McDonald, D.; Knight, R. Rethinking "enterotypes". *Cell Host. Microbe.* **2014**, *16*, 433–437. [CrossRef] [PubMed]
167. Cani, P.D.; Delzenne, N.M. The role of the gut microbiota in energy metabolism and metabolic disease. *Curr. Pharm. Des.* **2009**, *15*, 1546–1558. [CrossRef] [PubMed]
168. Scheithauer, T.P.; Dallinga-Thie, G.M.; de Vos, W.M.; Nieuwdorp, M.; van Raalte, D.H. Causality of small and large intestinal microbiota in weight regulation and insulin resistance. *Mol. Metab.* **2016**, *5*, 759–770. [CrossRef] [PubMed]
169. Larsen, N.; Vogensen, F.K.; van den Berg, F.W.; Nielsen, D.S.; Andreasen, A.S.; Pedersen, B.K.; Al-Soud, W.A.; Sorensen, S.J.; Hansen, L.H.; Jakobsen, M. Gut microbiota in human adults with type 2 diabetes differs from non-diabetic adults. *PLoS ONE* **2010**, *5*, e9085. [CrossRef] [PubMed]
170. Million, M.; Lagier, J.C.; Yahav, D.; Paul, M. Gut bacterial microbiota and obesity. *Clin. Microbiol. Infect.* **2013**, *19*, 305–313. [CrossRef] [PubMed]
171. Turnbaugh, P.J.; Hamady, M.; Yatsunenko, T.; Cantarel, B.L.; Duncan, A.; Ley, R.E.; Sogin, M.L.; Jones, W.J.; Roe, B.A.; Affourtit, J.P.; et al. A core gut microbiome in obese and lean twins. *Nature* **2009**, *457*, 480–484. [CrossRef] [PubMed]
172. Plovier, H.; Cani, P.D. Microbial impact on host metabolism: Opportunities for novel treatments of nutritional disorders? *Microbiol. Spectr.* **2017**. [CrossRef] [PubMed]
173. Karlsson, F.H.; Tremaroli, V.; Nookaew, I.; Bergstrom, G.; Behre, C.J.; Fagerberg, B.; Nielsen, J.; Backhed, F. Gut metagenome in European women with normal, impaired and diabetic glucose control. *Nature* **2013**, *498*, 99–103. [CrossRef] [PubMed]
174. Turnbaugh, P.J.; Ridaura, V.K.; Faith, J.J.; Rey, F.E.; Knight, R.; Gordon, J.I. The effect of diet on the human gut microbiome: A metagenomic analysis in humanized gnotobiotic mice. *Sci. Transl. Med.* **2009**. [CrossRef] [PubMed]
175. Turnbaugh, P.J.; Gordon, J.I. The core gut microbiome, energy balance and obesity. *J. Physiol.* **2009**, *587*, 4153–4158. [CrossRef] [PubMed]
176. Mahowald, M.A.; Rey, F.E.; Seedorf, H.; Turnbaugh, P.J.; Fulton, R.S.; Wollam, A.; Shah, N.; Wang, C.; Magrini, V.; Wilson, R.K.; et al. Characterizing a model human gut microbiota composed of members of its two dominant bacterial phyla. *Proc. Natl. Acad. Sci. USA* **2009**, *106*, 5859–5864. [CrossRef] [PubMed]
177. Ley, R.E.; Backhed, F.; Turnbaugh, P.; Lozupone, C.A.; Knight, R.D.; Gordon, J.I. Obesity alters gut microbial ecology. *Proc. Natl. Acad. Sci. USA* **2005**, *102*, 11070–11075. [CrossRef] [PubMed]
178. Ley, R.E.; Turnbaugh, P.J.; Klein, S.; Gordon, J.I. Microbial ecology: Human gut microbes associated with obesity. *Nature* **2006**, *444*, 1022–1023. [CrossRef] [PubMed]
179. Rawls, J.F.; Mahowald, M.A.; Ley, R.E.; Gordon, J.I. Reciprocal gut microbiota transplants from zebrafish and mice to germ-free recipients reveal host habitat selection. *Cell* **2006**, *127*, 423–433. [CrossRef] [PubMed]

180. Rabot, S.; Membrez, M.; Bruneau, A.; Gerard, P.; Harach, T.; Moser, M.; Raymond, F.; Mansourian, R.; Chou, C.J. Germ-free C57BL/6J mice are resistant to high-fat-diet-induced insulin resistance and have altered cholesterol metabolism. *FASEB J.* **2010**, *24*, 4948–4959. [CrossRef] [PubMed]

181. Caricilli, A.M.; Picardi, P.K.; de Abreu, L.L.; Ueno, M.; Prada, P.O.; Ropelle, E.R.; Hirabara, S.M.; Castoldi, A.; Vieira, P.; Camara, N.O.; et al. Gut microbiota is a key modulator of insulin resistance in TLR 2 knockout mice. *PLoS Biol.* **2011**, *9*, e1001212. [CrossRef] [PubMed]

182. Olefsky, J.M.; Glass, C.K. Macrophages, inflammation, and insulin resistance. *Annu. Rev. Physiol.* **2010**, *72*, 219–246. [CrossRef] [PubMed]

183. Osborn, O.; Olefsky, J.M. The cellular and signaling networks linking the immune system and metabolism in disease. *Nat. Med.* **2012**, *18*, 363–374. [CrossRef] [PubMed]

184. Cani, P.D.; Delzenne, N.M. Involvement of the gut microbiota in the development of low grade inflammation associated with obesity: Focus on this neglected partner. *Acta. Gastroenterol. Belg.* **2010**, *73*, 267–269. [PubMed]

185. Cani, P.D.; Amar, J.; Iglesias, M.A.; Poggi, M.; Knauf, C.; Bastelica, D.; Neyrinck, A.M.; Fava, F.; Tuohy, K.M.; Chabo, C.; et al. Metabolic endotoxemia initiates obesity and insulin resistance. *Diabetes* **2007**, *56*, 1761–1772. [CrossRef] [PubMed]

186. Luche, E.; Cousin, B.; Garidou, L.; Serino, M.; Waget, A.; Barreau, C.; Andre, M.; Valet, P.; Courtney, M.; Casteilla, L.; et al. Metabolic endotoxemia directly increases the proliferation of adipocyte precursors at the onset of metabolic diseases through a CD14-dependent mechanism. *Mol. Metab.* **2013**, *2*, 281–291. [CrossRef] [PubMed]

187. Pussinen, P.J.; Havulinna, A.S.; Lehto, M.; Sundvall, J.; Salomaa, V. Endotoxemia is associated with an increased risk of incident diabetes. *Diabetes Care* **2011**, *34*, 392–397. [CrossRef] [PubMed]

188. Cani, P.D.; Osto, M.; Geurts, L.; Everard, A. Involvement of gut microbiota in the development of low-grade inflammation and type 2 diabetes associated with obesity. *Gut Microbes* **2012**, *3*, 279–288. [CrossRef] [PubMed]

189. Salonen, A.; de Vos, W.M. Impact of diet on human intestinal microbiota and health. *Annu. Rev. Food Sci. Technol.* **2014**, *5*, 239–262. [CrossRef] [PubMed]

190. Sonnenburg, J.L.; Backhed, F. Diet-microbiota interactions as moderators of human metabolism. *Nature* **2016**, *535*, 56–64. [CrossRef] [PubMed]

191. Cani, P.D.; Everard, A. Talking microbes: When gut bacteria interact with diet and host organs. *Mol. Nutr. Food Res.* **2016**, *60*, 58–66. [CrossRef] [PubMed]

192. Yatsunenko, T.; Rey, F.E.; Manary, M.J.; Trehan, I.; Dominguez-Bello, M.G.; Contreras, M.; Magris, M.; Hidalgo, G.; Baldassano, R.N.; Anokhin, A.P.; et al. Human gut microbiome viewed across age and geography. *Nature* **2012**, *486*, 222–227. [CrossRef] [PubMed]

193. De Filippo, C.; Cavalieri, D.; Di Paola, M.; Ramazzotti, M.; Poullet, J.B.; Massart, S.; Collini, S.; Pieraccini, G.; Lionetti, P. Impact of diet in shaping gut microbiota revealed by a comparative study in children from Europe and rural Africa. *Proc. Natl. Acad. Sci. USA* **2010**, *107*, 14691–14696. [CrossRef] [PubMed]

194. Faith, J.J.; Guruge, J.L.; Charbonneau, M.; Subramanian, S.; Seedorf, H.; Goodman, A.L.; Clemente, J.C.; Knight, R.; Heath, A.C.; Leibel, R.L.; et al. The long-term stability of the human gut microbiota. *Science* **2013**, *341*, 1237439. [CrossRef] [PubMed]

195. David, L.A.; Maurice, C.F.; Carmody, R.N.; Gootenberg, D.B.; Button, J.E.; Wolfe, B.E.; Ling, A.V.; Devlin, A.S.; Varma, Y.; Fischbach, M.A.; et al. Diet rapidly and reproducibly alters the human gut microbiome. *Nature* **2014**, *505*, 559–563. [CrossRef] [PubMed]

196. Wu, G.D.; Chen, J.; Hoffmann, C.; Bittinger, K.; Chen, Y.Y.; Keilbaugh, S.A.; Bewtra, M.; Knights, D.; Walters, W.A.; Knight, R.; et al. Linking long-term dietary patterns with gut microbial enterotypes. *Science* **2011**, *334*, 105–108. [CrossRef] [PubMed]

197. Rabot, S.; Membrez, M.; Blancher, F.; Berger, B.; Moine, D.; Krause, L.; Bibiloni, R.; Bruneau, A.; Gerard, P.; Siddharth, J.; et al. High fat diet drives obesity regardless the composition of gut microbiota in mice. *Sci. Rep.* **2016**, *6*, 32484. [CrossRef] [PubMed]

198. Ramirez-Farias, C.; Slezak, K.; Fuller, Z.; Duncan, A.; Holtrop, G.; Louis, P. Effect of inulin on the human gut microbiota: Stimulation of Bifidobacterium adolescentis and Faecalibacterium prausnitzii. *Br. J. Nutr.* **2009**, *101*, 541–550. [CrossRef] [PubMed]

199. Chaplin, A.; Parra, P.; Laraichi, S.; Serra, F.; Palou, A. Calcium supplementation modulates gut microbiota in a prebiotic manner in dietary obese mice. *Mol. Nutr. Food Res.* **2016**, *60*, 468–480. [CrossRef] [PubMed]

200. Cote, C.D.; Rasmussen, B.A.; Duca, F.A.; Zadeh-Tahmasebi, M.; Baur, J.A.; Daljeet, M.; Breen, D.M.; Filippi, B.M.; Lam, T.K. Resveratrol activates duodenal Sirt1 to reverse insulin resistance in rats through a neuronal network. *Nat. Med.* **2015**, *21*, 498–505. [CrossRef] [PubMed]

201. Sung, M.M.; Kim, T.T.; Denou, E.; Soltys, C.M.; Hamza, S.M.; Byrne, N.J.; Masson, G.; Park, H.; Wishart, D.S.; Madsen, K.L.; et al. Improved glucose homeostasis in obese mice treated with resveratrol is associated with alterations in the gut microbiome. *Diabetes* **2017**, *66*, 418–425. [CrossRef] [PubMed]

202. Kim, T.T.; Parajuli, N.; Sung, M.M.; Bairwa, S.C.; Levasseur, J.; Soltys, C.M.; Wishart, D.S.; Madsen, K.; Schertzer, J.D.; Dyck, J.R.B. Fecal transplant from resveratrol-fed donors improves glycaemia and cardiovascular features of the metabolic syndrome in mice. *Am. J. Physiol. Endocrinol. Metab.* **2018**. [CrossRef] [PubMed]

203. Chen, M.L.; Yi, L.; Zhang, Y.; Zhou, X.; Ran, L.; Yang, J.; Zhu, J.D.; Zhang, Q.Y.; Mi, M.T. Resveratrol Attenuates Trimethylamine-N-Oxide (TMAO)-Induced Atherosclerosis by Regulating TMAO Synthesis and Bile Acid Metabolism via Remodeling of the Gut Microbiota. *MBio* **2016**, *7*, e02210-15. [CrossRef] [PubMed]

204. Sung, M.M.; Byrne, N.J.; Robertson, I.M.; Kim, T.T.; Samokhvalov, V.; Levasseur, J.; Soltys, C.L.; Fung, D.; Tyreman, N.; Denou, E.; et al. Resveratrol improves exercise performance and skeletal muscle oxidative capacity in heart failure. *Am. J. Physiol. Heart Circ. Physiol.* **2017**, *312*, H842–H853. [CrossRef] [PubMed]

205. Jung, M.J.; Lee, J.; Shin, N.R.; Kim, M.S.; Hyun, D.W.; Yun, J.H.; Kim, P.S.; Whon, T.W.; Bae, J.W. Chronic repression of mtor complex 2 induces changes in the gut microbiota of diet-induced obese mice. *Sci. Rep.* **2016**, *6*, 30887. [CrossRef] [PubMed]

206. Tung, Y.C.; Lin, Y.H.; Chen, H.J.; Chou, S.C.; Cheng, A.C.; Kalyanam, N.; Ho, C.T.; Pan, M.H. Piceatannol Exerts Anti-Obesity Effects in C57BL/6 Mice through Modulating Adipogenic Proteins and Gut Microbiota. *Molecules* **2016**. [CrossRef] [PubMed]

207. Qiao, Y.; Sun, J.; Xia, S.; Tang, X.; Shi, Y.; Le, G. Effects of resveratrol on gut microbiota and fat storage in a mouse model with high-fat-induced obesity. *Food Funct.* **2014**, *5*, 1241–1249. [CrossRef] [PubMed]

208. Dao, T.M.; Waget, A.; Klopp, P.; Serino, M.; Vachoux, C.; Pechere, L.; Drucker, D.J.; Champion, S.; Barthelemy, S.; Barra, Y.; et al. Resveratrol increases glucose induced GLP-1 secretion in mice: A mechanism which contributes to the glycemic control. *PLoS ONE* **2011**, *6*, e20700. [CrossRef] [PubMed]

209. Zhao, L.; Zhang, Q.; Ma, W.; Tian, F.; Shen, H.; Zhou, M. A combination of quercetin and resveratrol reduces obesity in high-fat diet-fed rats by modulation of gut microbiota. *Food Funct.* **2017**, *8*, 4644–4656. [CrossRef] [PubMed]

210. Hijona, E.; Aguirre, L.; Perez-Matute, P.; Villanueva-Millan, M.J.; Mosqueda-Solis, A.; Hasnaoui, M.; Nepveu, F.; Senard, J.M.; Bujanda, L.; Aldamiz-Echevarria, L.; et al. Limited beneficial effects of piceatannol supplementation on obesity complications in the obese Zucker rat: Gut microbiota, metabolic, endocrine, and cardiac aspects. *J. Physiol. Biochem.* **2016**, *72*, 567–582. [CrossRef] [PubMed]

211. Etxeberria, U.; Arias, N.; Boque, N.; Macarulla, M.T.; Portillo, M.P.; Martinez, J.A.; Milagro, F.I. Reshaping faecal gut microbiota composition by the intake of trans-resveratrol and quercetin in high-fat sucrose diet-fed rats. *J. Nutr. Biochem.* **2015**, *26*, 651–660. [CrossRef] [PubMed]

212. Tain, Y.L.; Lee, W.C.; Wu, K.L.H.; Leu, S.; Chan, J.Y.H. Resveratrol prevents the development of hypertension programmed by maternal plus post-weaning high-fructose consumption through modulation of oxidative stress, nutrient-sensing signals, and gut microbiota. *Mol. Nutr. Food Res.* **2018**. [CrossRef] [PubMed]

213. Most, J.; Penders, J.; Lucchesi, M.; Goossens, G.H.; Blaak, E.E. Gut microbiota composition in relation to the metabolic response to 12-week combined polyphenol supplementation in overweight men and women. *Eur. J. Clin. Nutr.* **2017**, *71*, 1040–1045. [CrossRef] [PubMed]

214. Samson, S.L.; Garber, A.J. Metabolic syndrome. *Endocrinol. Metab. Clin. N. Am.* **2014**, *43*, 1–23. [CrossRef] [PubMed]

215. Piotrowska, H.; Kucinska, M.; Murias, M. Biological activity of piceatannol: Leaving the shadow of resveratrol. *Mutat. Res.* **2012**, *750*, 60–82. [CrossRef] [PubMed]

216. Ryu, D.; Mouchiroud, L.; Andreux, P.A.; Katsyuba, E.; Moullan, N.; Nicolet-Dit-Félix, A.A.; Williams, E.G.; Jha, P.; Lo Sasso, G.; Huzard, D.; et al. Urolithin A induces mitophagy and prolongs lifespan in C. elegans and increases muscle function in rodents. *Nat. Med.* **2016**, *22*, 879–888. [CrossRef] [PubMed]

217. Li, J.; Riaz Rajoka, M.S.; Shao, D.; Jiang, C.; Jin, M.; Huang, Q.; Yang, H.; Shi, J. Strategies to increase the efficacy of using gut microbiota for the modulation of obesity. *Obes. Rev.* **2017**, *18*, 1260–1271. [CrossRef] [PubMed]

218. Nohr, M.K.; Kroager, T.P.; Sanggaard, K.W.; Knudsen, A.D.; Stensballe, A.; Enghild, J.J.; Olholm, J.; Richelsen, B.; Pedersen, S.B. SILAC-MS Based Characterization of LPS and Resveratrol Induced Changes in Adipocyte Proteomics-Resveratrol as Ameliorating Factor on LPS Induced Changes. *PLoS ONE* **2016**, *11*, e0159747. [CrossRef] [PubMed]

219. Etxeberria, U.; Castilla-Madrigal, R.; Lostao, M.P.; Martínez, J.A.; Milagro, F.I. Trans-resveratrol induces a potential anti-lipogenic effect in lipopolysaccharide-stimulated enterocytes. *Cell Mol. Biol.* **2015**, *61*, 9–16. [PubMed]

220. Elovaara, H.; Huusko, T.; Maksimow, M.; Elima, K.; Yegutkin, G.G.; Skurnik, M.; Dobrindt, U.; Siitonen, A.; McPherson, M.J.; Salmi, M.; et al. Primary Amine Oxidase of Escherichia coli Is a Metabolic Enzyme that Can Use a Human Leukocyte Molecule as a Substrate. *PLoS ONE* **2015**, *10*, e0142367. [CrossRef] [PubMed]

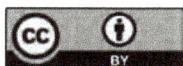

nutrients

MDPI

Article

Tissular Distribution and Metabolism of *trans*-ε-Viniferin after Intraperitoneal Injection in Rat

Arnaud Courtois [1,2], Claude Atgié [3], Axel Marchal [1], Ruth Hornedo-Ortega [1], Caroline Lapèze [1], Chrystel Faure [3], Tristan Richard [1] and Stéphanie Krisa [1,*]

[1] Unité de Recherche Œnologie, Molécules d'Intérêt Biologique, EA 4577, USC 1366 INRA,
Université de Bordeaux, Bordeaux INP, Institut des Sciences de la Vigne et du Vin, 210 Chemin de Leysottes,
33882 Villenave d'Ornon, France; arnaud.courtois@u-bordeaux.fr (A.C.); axel.marchal@u-bordeaux.fr (A.M.);
rhornedo@us.es (R.H.-O.); carolinelapeze@live.fr (C.L.); tristan.richard@u-bordeaux.fr (T.R.)
[2] Centre Antipoison et de Toxicovigilance de Nouvelle Aquitaine, Bâtiment UNDR, CHU de Bordeaux,
Place Amélie Raba Léon, 33076 Bordeaux, France
[3] Institut de Chimie et de Biologie des Membranes et des Nano-objets (CBMN), Equipe ClipIN (Colloïdes et
Lipides pour l'Industrie et la Nutrition) UMR 5248, CNRS, Université de Bordeaux, Bordeaux INP, Bât B14,
Allée Geoffroy Saint-Hilaire, 33600, Pessac, France; Claude.Atgie@enscbp.fr (C.A.);
chrystel.faure@enscbp.fr (C.F.)
* Correspondence: stephanie.krisa@u-bordeaux.fr; Tel.: +33-(0)5-57-57-59-53

Received: 11 October 2018; Accepted: 30 October 2018; Published: 4 November 2018

Abstract: Background: Recent studies showed that *trans*-ε-viniferin (ε-viniferin), a *trans*-resveratrol dehydrodimer, has anti-inflammatory and anti-obesity effects in rodents. The main purpose of this work was to assess the tissue distribution study of ε-viniferin and its metabolites after intraperitoneal (IP) administration in rat. Methods: After IP injection of 50 mg/kg, ε-viniferin and its metabolites were identified and quantified in plasma, liver, kidneys, adipose tissues, urine, and faeces by Liquid Chromatography-High Resolution Mass Spectrometry (LC-HRMS). Results: ε-Viniferin underwent a rapid hepatic metabolism mostly to glucuronides but also to a lesser extent to sulphate derivatives. The highest glucuronide concentrations were found in liver followed by plasma and kidneys whereas only traces amounts were found in adipose tissues. In contrast the highest ε-viniferin areas under concentration (AUC) and mean residence times (MRT) values were found in white adipose tissues. Finally, much lower levels of ε-viniferin or its metabolites were found in urine than in faeces, suggesting that biliary excretion is the main elimination pathway. Conclusion: A rapid and large metabolism of ε-viniferin and a high bioaccumulation in white adipose tissues were observed. Thus, these tissues could be a reservoir of the native form of ε-viniferin that could allow its slow release and a sustained presence within the organism.

Keywords: ε-viniferin; distribution; metabolism; adipose tissue

1. Introduction

Trans-ε-viniferin (ε-viniferin), a stilbene oligomer formed by two units of *trans*-resveratrol monomer (Figure 1), is found in various plant families such as Vitaceae, Gnetaceae, Cyperaceae, Fabaceae or Dipterocarpaceae [1–4]. ε-Viniferin is a major constituent of *Vitis* species [5]. In dietary terms, the principal source of ε-viniferin is wine and its amount ranging from 0.2 to 4.3 mg/L [6,7]. It is now considered nowadays as a potential bioactive molecule with promising antioxidant, anti-inflammatory, and cardioprotective activities [8–11].

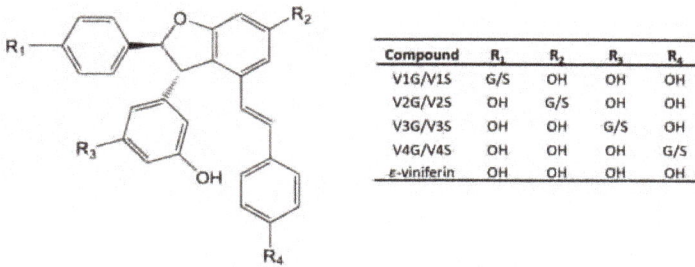

Figure 1. Structural representation of ε-viniferin and its glucuronide and sulphate metabolites. G: glucuronic acid, S: sulphate, OH: hydroxy group.

Recent studies have reported its strong potential anti-obesity effects and that it acts preventively against metabolic syndrome. In fact, ε-viniferin (50 µM) has been demonstrated to be able to inhibit adipogenesis in 3T3-L1 cells by decreasing lipid accumulation and expression of adipogenesis (PPARgamma) and anti-inflammatory (MCP-1) gene markers. In addition, the same authors showed in mice that administration over four weeks of a diet containing 0.2% of ε-viniferin significantly reduced subcutaneous, epididymal, and retroperitoneal adipose tissue weights and consequently the body weight. Moreover, a significantly decrease in inflammatory and obesity-related gene expression (tumor necrosis factor alpha, monocyte chemoattractant protein-1, and leptin) was observed in vitro and in vivo [12]. These results are in accordance with a study in which, ε-viniferin (2.5, 5, and 10 µM) decreased the size of lipid deposits in vitro. It also reduced the body weight and the weight ratio of mesenteric fat in mice (10 and 25 mg/kg/day, 5 weeks) [13]. These findings on the potential anti-obesity properties of ε-viniferin are opening a new and interesting line of research that has received little attention to date.

The persistent shadow of doubt when working with stilbene is its low bioavailability, which is often explained by low absorption and an extensive enteric and hepatic phase II metabolism. Generally, this metabolism results in conversion of the stilbene compound to conjugated metabolites that are rapidly excreted [14,15]. Recently, we described the in vitro metabolism of ε-viniferin using liver fractions. We found an intense metabolism in which more than 75% of the ε-viniferin was converted into glucuronide and sulphate metabolites in rat and human [16]. Mao and co-workers described the pharmacokinetic profile of δ-viniferin, another dehydrodimer of *trans*-resveratrol, in rats [17]. They found a total absorption of 31.5% for δ-viniferin and its glucuronide and sulphate metabolites and reported an absolute oral bioavailability of 2.3% for unchanged δ-viniferin, assuming a high metabolism [17]. Moreover, the apparent volume of distribution value in this study suggested that δ-viniferin and its metabolites could disseminate extensively into organs and tissues.

The biological activity of ε-viniferin may depend highly on its ability to be distributed in target tissues. To our knowledge, the only study that investigated the pharmacokinetic parameters of ε-viniferin was performed in mice [18]. The authors reported a low oral bioavailability of 0.771% and a high IP bioavailability of more than 85%. However, they did not study the metabolism and the tissue distribution of ε-viniferin.

Given the anti-obesity potential of ε-viniferin and that the onset and evolution of obesity depend on of the regional distribution of adipose tissue, it would be worth exploring the distribution of ε-viniferin and its metabolites in superficial and deep white adipose deposit [19,20]. Thus, the objective of our study was to describe the tissue distribution and excretion of ε-viniferin and its glucuronide and sulphate metabolites after IP injection in rat. A sensitive liquid chromatography-high resolution mass spectrometry (LC-HRMS) Orbitrap mass spectrometer was used to quantify ε-viniferin and its metabolites in plasma, liver, kidneys, adipose tissues, urine and faeces.

2. Materials and Methods

2.1. Material and Reagents

ε-Viniferin (purity ≥ 95%) was extracted and purified from grapevine shoot extract in our laboratory as described previously [21]. The chemical structure was confirmed by 1H NMR, and high-resolution mass spectrometry [22]. High pressure liquid chromatography (HPLC)-grade acetonitrile, methanol, ethanol, ethyl acetate and formic acid were purchased from Fisher Scientific (Illkirch, France). Ultrapure water used was obtained using a Purelab Ultra System (Elga Lab Water, High Wycombe, UK).

2.2. Pharmacokinetic Studies

The study was approved by the Bordeaux University Institutional Ethics Committee for Animal Research (IEC-AR/ MESR approval n°00289.0). All experiments were conducted in accordance with Directive 2010/63/EU on the protection of animals used for scientific purposes. The animals (male Wistar rats) were purchased from Janvier-LABS (Saint-Berthevin, France) (agreement n° A33063917, University of Bordeaux, France). Thirty-six male Wistar rats (250–300 g, 7 weeks old) were maintained in controlled conditions (12 h light/12 h dark cycle, humidity 50–60% and ambient temperature 24 ± 1 °C) and had free access to food and water. ε-Viniferin was dissolved in H_2O/ethanol (90/10) and administrated intraperitoneally at a dose of 50 mg/kg in a total volume of 1 mL/rat. For the distribution study, rats were sacrificed by a deep anesthesia with isoflurane followed by a rapid exsanguination in random groups of 6 rats at the following periods of time points: 15 and 30 min, and 1, 2, 4 h post-injection. Blood samples (500 μL) were collected in heparinised tubes and plasma was harvested by centrifugation at 4 °C and 10,000 g for 5 min. Rats were then perfused with saline prior to collecting and weighing liver, kidneys, interscapular brown adipose tissue (IBAT) and epididymal (EWAT) and retroperitoneal (RWAT) white adipose tissues. All biological samples were stored at −80 °C until analysis. For the excretion study, 6 rats were housed individually in metabolic cages fitted with urine/faeces separators. Urine and faeces (24 h) were collected after ε-viniferin intraperitoneal IP administration. Urine volumes were measured and faecal samples were weighed. All the samples were rapidly frozen at −80 °C until analysis.

2.3. Extraction of ε-Viniferin and its Metabolites from Plasma, Urine and Faeces

An aliquot of 100 μL of plasma was mixed with 300 μL of methanol. After vortex-mixing for 3 min and centrifugation at 12,000 g for 30 min at 4 °C, the supernatant was evaporated using a SpeedVac concentrator (Thermo Fisher Scientific, Waltham, MA USA). Four millilitres of urine were vortex-mixed with ethyl acetate (3 mL) for 1 min. After centrifugation at 12,000 g for 10 min at 4 °C, the supernatant was recovered and the residue was extracted again using ethyl acetate (3 mL). Both supernatants were combined and evaporated using a SpeedVac concentrator. Faeces were lyophilized, weighed and 100 mg of dried sample were mixed with 800 μL of methanol. The mixture was gently vortexed for 3 min and centrifuged at 12,000 g for 10 min at 4 °C. Finally, the supernatant was evaporated. The residue of plasma, urine and faeces extraction was reconstituted in 200 μL H_2O/methanol (90/10) and filtered through a 0.45 μm PTFE filter (Millex, Darmstadt, Germany) prior to LC-HRMS Orbitrap mass spectrometer analysis.

2.4. Extraction of ε-Viniferin and its Metabolites from Tissues

An aliquot of rat tissue (lower than 0.6 g) was homogenized in 3 mL of methanol/H_2O (80/20) using an Ultra-Turrax homogenizer (IKA, Staufen, Deutschland). Extraction was performed for 1 min in an ultrasonic bath, followed by vortex-mixing for 3 min. After centrifugation at 12,000 g for 20 min at 4 °C, the supernatant was recovered and the residue was extracted again using 3 mL of methanol/H_2O (80/20). Both supernatants were combined, evaporated, reconstituted in 1 mL H_2O/methanol (90/10) and filtered through a 0.45 μm PTFE filter. Some samples were diluted prior to LC-HRMS Orbitrap mass spectrometer analysis.

2.5. LC-HRMS Quantitation of ε-Viniferin and its Metabolites

The LC-HRMS platform consisted of an HTC PAL autosampler (CTC Analytics AG, Zwingen, Switzerland), an Accela U-HPLC system with quaternary pumps and an Exactive benchtop Orbitrap mass spectrometer equipped with a heated electrospray ionization (HESI) probe (both from Thermo Fisher Scientific, Bremen, Germany). For liquid chromatography separation, a C18 column was used as the stationary phase (BEH C18 2.1 mm × 100 mm, 1.7 μm particle size, Waters, Guyancourt, France). The mobile phases were (A) water and (B) acetonitrile both acidified with 0.1% formic acid. The flow rate was 450 μL/min and eluent B varied as follows: 0 min, 25%; 0.5 min, 25%; 3.6 min, 50%; 3.9 min, 50%; 4 min, 100%; 5.7 min, 100%; 5.8 min, 25%; 7 min, 25%. The injection volume was 5 μL. Data were acquired in negative Fourier transform mass spectrometry (FTMS) ionization mode at a unit resolution of 25,000 (m/Δm, full width at half maximum (FWHM) at 200 u). The sheath and auxiliary gas flows (both nitrogen) were optimized at 75 and 18 arbitrary units, respectively. The HESI probe and capillary temperatures were 320 °C and 350 °C, respectively. The electrospray voltage was set to −3 kV, the capillary voltage to −60 V, the tube lens voltage offset to −135 V and the skimmer voltage to −26 V. Mass spectra were recorded from 100 to 1800 Th, with an AGC value of 3×10^6. Before each series of analysis, the spectrometer was calibrated using Pierce® ESI Negative Ion Calibration solution (Thermo Fisher Scientific).

All data were processed using Qualbrowser and Quanbrowser applications from Xcalibur version 2.1 (Thermo Fisher Scientific, Waltham, MA USA). Peak areas were determined by automatic integration from the extracted ion chromatogram built for the deprotonated ion of ε-viniferin (m/z 453.1343 u), ε-viniferin glucuronide (m/z 629.1664 u) and ε-viniferin sulphate (m/z 533.0912 u) in a 5-ppm window. The ε-viniferin calibration curve was obtained by injections of standard solutions in a range of concentrations varying from 100 ng/L to 2 mg/L showing a good linearity ($R^2 = 0.9971$) with recovery ratio calculated between 89% and 104%. The quantification limit was set at 10 μg/L according to the methodology described by De Paepe et al. (2013) [23]. Injection of 5 replicates of calibration samples at 10 ug/L and 1 mg/L showed relative standard deviation (RDS) less than 7 and 5%, respectively. Metabolite concentrations were expressed as an equivalent of the ε-viniferin standard curve.

2.6. Data Analysis

Variables measured were expressed as mean ± SD of 6 rats for each timepoint. Maximum concentration (Cmax) and time to reach Cmax (Tmax) were recorded directly. Pharmacokinetic parameters such as area under concentration-time curve from time zero to the last point (AUC_{0-t}), area under concentration-time curve from time zero to infinity ($AUC_{0-\infty}$), elimination half-life (T1/2), and mean residence time (MRT) were analyzed by non-compartmental modelling using the PKSolver program [24].

3. Results

The plasma and tissue kinetic profiles of ε-viniferin and its metabolites (Figure 1) were assessed in rats. Animals were administered an IP bolus of 50 mg/kg ε-viniferin and were euthanized at different timepoints (15, 30 min, 1, 2 and 4 h) to obtain blood samples, and to collect the liver, kidneys, IBAT, EWAT and RWAT. ε-Viniferin and its metabolites were identified and quantified by LC-HRMS. The plasma and tissue concentrations of ε-viniferin and its metabolites are illustrated in Figure 2, and the relevant pharmacokinetic parameters are presented in Table 1.

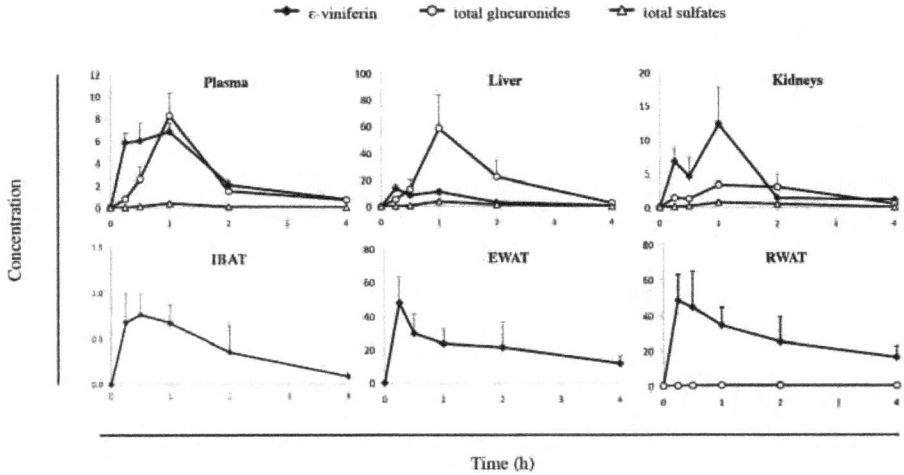

Figure 2. Kinetic profiles of ε-viniferin and its total glucuronide and total sulphate metabolites (*n* = 6). Concentrations were expressed in nmol/mL for plasma and nmol/g for the tissues. Interscapular brown adipose tissue (IBAT), epididymal white adipose tissue (EWAT), retroperitoneal white adipose tissue (RWAT).

Table 1. Pharmacokinetic parameters of ε-viniferin and metabolites in plasma and collected tissues.

Parameters	Plasma	Liver	Kidney	IBAT	EWAT	RWAT
ε-Viniferin						
Tmax	1.00	0.25	1.00	0.50	0.25	0.25
Cmax	6.80	13.41	12.30	0.76	47.78	48.32
T1/2	0.95	0.74	1.00	1.01	2.74	2.86
AUC_{0-t}	12.52	20.05	15.86	1.58	84.16	109.02
$AUC_{0-\infty}$	13.49	20.70	17.53	1.71	130.27	177.02
MRT	1.53	1.24	1.62	1.64	3.86	4.13
ε-Viniferin Glucuronides						
Tmax	1.00	1.00	1.00	nq	nq	1.00
Cmax	8.20	58.17	3.30	nq	nq	0.52
T1/2	0.90	0.65	1.08	nq	nq	5.79
AUC_{0-t}	10.14	85.01	8.42	nq	nq	1.61
$AUC_{0-\infty}$	11.00	87.31	9.27	nq	nq	4.67
MRT	1.66	1.52	2.03	nq	nq	8.81
ε-Viniferin Sulphates						
Tmax	1.00	1.00	1.00	nq	nq	nq
Cmax	0.38	3.82	0.74	nq	nq	nq
T1/2	0.49	0.35	0.72	nq	nq	nq
AUC_{0-t}	0.44	5.31	1.50	nq	nq	nq
$AUC_{0-\infty}$	0.44	5.31	1.55	nq	nq	nq
MRT	1.22	1.37	1.69	nq	nq	nq

Tmax, T1/2 and mean residence time (MRT) were expressed in h. Cmax were expressed in nmol/mL and AUC in nmol/mL×h for plasma, and nmol/g and nmol/g×h for the tissues. nq = non quantified. Interscapular brown adipose tissue (IBAT), epididymal white adipose tissue (EWAT), retroperitoneal white adipose tissue (RWAT).

Regarding ε-viniferin, we found a rapid and wide distribution of the native molecule in tissue within the time course examined (Figure 2). Plasma and tissue concentrations of ε-viniferin rapidly increased and reached a maximum concentration between 15 to 60 min after IP injection. The Tmax values for ε-viniferin were 15 min for EWAT and RWAT and liver, followed by IBAT (30 min) and by plasma and kidneys (1 h), as depicted in Table 1. Thereafter, ε-viniferin concentrations rapidly decreased within 4 h in plasma, liver, kidneys and IBAT. Interestingly, 4 h after injection, a high concentration of ε-viniferin still remained in both white adipose tissues (EWAT and RWAT) in which the MRT and T1/2 were the longest (3.86 and 4.13 h; 2.74 and 2.86 h, respectively). These values were more than 2-fold higher for white adipose tissue than for plasma, liver and kidneys (Table 1). Similarly, the highest AUC_{0-t} were found for EWAT and RWAT (84.16 and 109.02 nmol/g×h, respectively), which were from 4- to 8-fold higher than the values for plasma, liver and kidney (12.52, 20.05 and 15.86 nmol/g×h, respectively).

To obtain an accurate description of the pharmacokinetic profile of ε-viniferin in rat, its metabolism was studied. The mass spectra obtained from plasma and tissue analysis showed the presence of ε-viniferin phase-II metabolites: glucuronide and sulphate conjugates. These metabolites, previously characterized in our laboratory, were identified as being V1G, V2G, V3G and V4G for glucuronides and V1S, V2S, V3S, and V4S for sulphates (Figure 1) [16]. The plasma and tissue concentration-time profiles of total glucuronides and of total sulphates are shown in Figure 2.

Sulphate metabolite levels were lower than those of glucuronide metabolites in plasma and tissues. Glucuronides appeared rapidly in plasma, liver and kidneys and reached a maximum concentration after 60 min (Figure 2). Thereafter, they rapidly decreased both in plasma and liver, but slowly in kidneys. AUC_{0-t} values showed that glucuronides were mainly located in liver, followed by plasma and kidneys (85.01 nmol/mL×h, 10.14 and 8.42 nmol/g×h, respectively) (Table 1). Only traces of glucuronides were detectable in IBAT and EWAT while they were measurable in RWAT. In all tissues and plasma, the major metabolite was V2G, which represented more than 70% of the eight metabolites studied while total sulphates accounted for less than 10%. LC-HRMS chromatograms of ε-viniferin and its metabolites quantified in plasma, liver and kidney are presented in Figure 3.

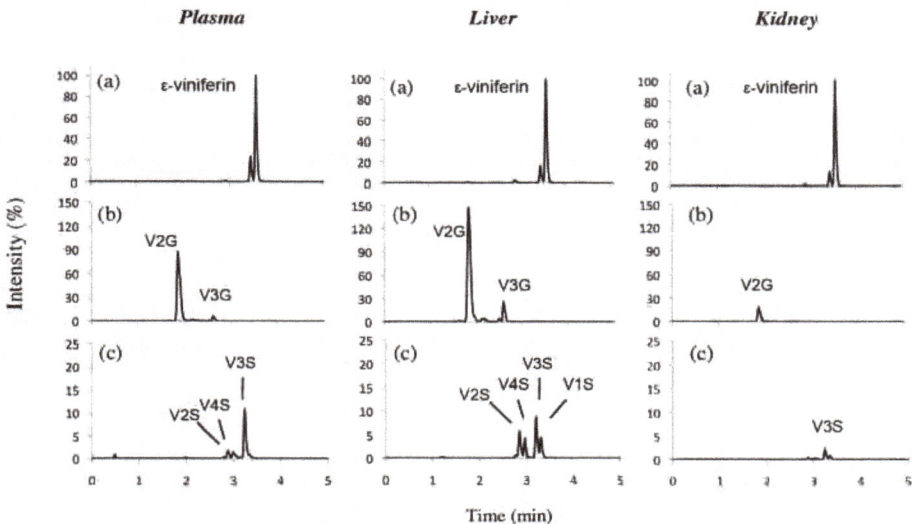

Figure 3. Liquid chromatography-high resolution mass spectrometry (LC-HRMS) extracted ions chromatograms of plasma, liver and kidney extracts from rat 1h after IP administration. (**a**) ε-viniferin (*m/z* 453.1343), (**b**) glucuronide metabolites (*m/z* 629.1664) and (**c**) sulphate metabolites (*m/z* 533.0912). For each tissue, the intensity was expressed relative to the ε-viniferin maximum (%).

The difference in tissue distribution is highlighted in Figure 4, which shows the 1 h time point (Tmax of ε-viniferin in plasma) for ε-viniferin and its glucurono- and sulpho-conjugates concentrations. Higher ε-viniferin concentrations were found in EWAT and RWAT (23.46 and 34.46 nmol/g, respectively) than in plasma, liver or kidneys (6.80, 11.02 and 12.30 nmol/g, respectively).

Regarding glucuronides, the highest concentrations were found in liver followed by plasma and kidneys, whereas only trace amounts were found in adipose tissues. Sulpho-conjugates were found only in very low levels in liver, kidney and plasma.

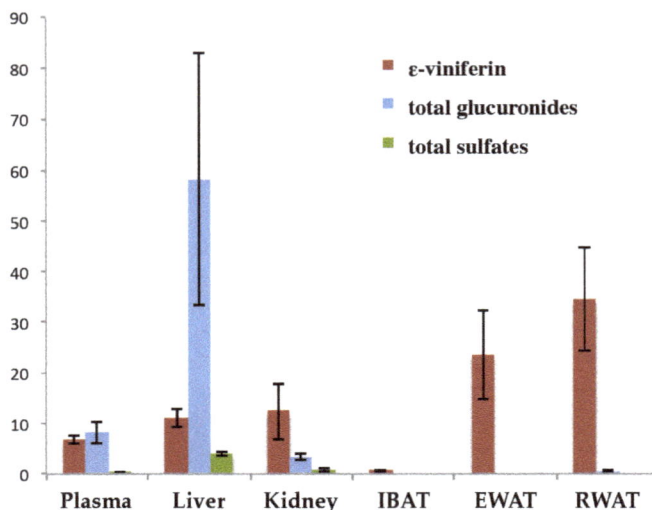

Figure 4. Concentrations ε-viniferin and its total glucuronide and total sulphate metabolites in plasma and organs 1 h after IP administration (*n* = 6). Concentrations were expressed in nmol/mL for plasma and nmol/g for the tissues.

Urine and faeces were collected 24 h after IP administration of 50 mg/kg ε-viniferin. In urine, ε-viniferin and its metabolites were detected but at less than 0.001% of the administered dose, while 9.7% of the administered dose was excreted in faeces. The major form of dehydrodimer in faeces was unchanged ε-viniferin, with 7.7 ± 1.2% of the initial dose. Glucuronides and sulphates were 0.6 ± 0.2% and 1.4 ± 0.4%, respectively.

4. Discussion

After IP injection, the appearance of the administered molecule requires a certain time to reach the systemic blood circulation. In this study, we observed that ε-viniferin was present in the plasma as early as 15 min after administration. Its concentration slowly increased during 1 h and then rapidly declined. This could be due to its rapid biotransformation in the liver (Tmax 15 min). Indeed, ε-viniferin glucuronides appeared as early as 15 min in liver and were present in much greater concentrations than ε-viniferin and the sulphate forms (Table 1). In plasma, kidneys and RWAT, glucuronides were also the main metabolites. Regarding another dehydrodimer of *trans*-resveratrol, δ-viniferin, Mao et al. (2016) showed in vivo that glucuronides were also much more present than sulphates in plasma after oral or intravenous administration. In a previous study using rat liver extracts, we showed that the in vitro metabolism of ε-viniferin produced four glucuronides (V1G, V2G, V3G and V4G) and four sulphates (V1S, V2S, V3S and V4S), with glucuronides being the major metabolites. V2G and V3G represented more than 90% of the total glucuronides, whereas sulphates metabolites were present in equal proportion [16]. We now confirm the same metabolic profile in vivo in rat liver both for glucuronides and sulphates, which is an important finding (Figure 3). Identification of the metabolic profile of ε-viniferin will allow us to perform additional studies into potential values of metabolites.

The AUC0–t for ε-viniferin glucuronides in liver were 8.4- and 10.1-fold higher than those measured in plasma and kidneys, respectively. Moreover, ε-viniferin glucuronides were present in faeces but not in the urine. Therefore, glucuronides were eliminated mainly by the hepato-biliary system, which could explain the low amount measured in plasma, kidneys and urine. Native ε-viniferin was also found in faeces (7.7% of the administered dose), which could be due to its biliary excretion or to the cleavage of glucuronide by glucuronidase in the intestinal lumen. The aglycone and glucuronide forms of *trans*-resveratrol are known to be eliminated mainly in faeces by the bile tract and not in the urine [25,26]. Interestingly, when the bile cannula from a bile-donor rat, which received an oral dose of *trans*-resveratrol, was diverted to the duodenum of a bile-recipient rat, *trans*-resveratrol and its glucuronide were found in the blood-stream of the latter. Therefore, *trans*-resveratrol could undergo an entero-hepatic re-circulation [25]. Moreover, Mao (2016) observed a double peak of δ-viniferin on the concentration-time curve in plasma after oral administration, suggesting the enterohepatic circulation of δ-viniferin [17]. It might thus be of interest to extend the time of exposure of the organism to ε-viniferin and lengthen its pharmacological activity. In urine, the amounts of ε-viniferin, its glucuronides and its sulphates were less than 0.001% of the initial dose, therefore strengthening the notion of an extremely weak urinary elimination. A recent study found that, after an oral dosage, δ-viniferin were eliminated in urine under unchanged, glucuronidated and sulphated forms at a low concentration (<0.05%) [17]. Therefore, urine does not seem to be a major route for eliminating these *trans*-resveratrol dehydrodimers.

In this study we collected two types of white adipose tissues: the epididymal (EWAT) and the retroperitoneal (RWAT), and one brown adipose tissue, the interscapular (IBAT). These two types do not have the same structures or functions. Brown adipose tissue is involved in thermogenesis whereas white adipose tissues regulates energy storage and metabolism through endocrine secretion of adipokines [27]. We report here that, ε-viniferin was found 15 min (Tmax 15 min) after injection in all adipose tissues, indicating a rapid uptake. In EWAT and RWAT, ε-viniferin Cmax were very high, even much higher than the concentration found in the other organs studied. Moreover, ε-viniferin was eliminated slowly, as attested by the high MRT values in EWAT and RWAT (3.83 and 4.13 h, respectively). Based on these results, we speculated that the large amount of the native ε-viniferin found in white adipose tissues could be due to its lipophilic characteristics, as confirmed by its poor aqueous solubility and a high octanol-water ratio partition coefficient (log *p* value 4.60) which promote rapid incorporation in unilocular lipid droplets of adipocytes. Surprisingly, the ε-viniferin concentration in IBAT was very low as compared to that in white adipose tissue. Indeed, brown adipocytes are multilocular with small lipid droplets, surrounded by many mitochondries with a high metabolic activity. This is not conducive to the accumulation of lipophilic compounds that occurs in white adipose tissue.

The very low levels of metabolites detected in each different adipose tissues studied could be due to one of the principal functions of the first pass metabolism, which enhance the hydrophilic characteristics of a compound in order to facilitate its elimination. The low level of glucuronidated and sulphated forms detected in these depots together with the high value of MRT of ε-viniferin suggests that ε-viniferin is not metabolized (or at a very low rate) and that its metabolites are not distributed in white adipose tissues.

Few studies have been conducted on the presence of polyphenols and their metabolites in adipose tissues after administration, and to our knowledge, no one concerning ε-viniferin. It was reported that after oral administration of a grape extract enriched in polyphenols, the unmodified flavanols were the major forms accumulated in mesenteric white adipose tissue. These authors suggested that white adipose tissue acts as a storage compartment for non-metabolized polyphenols [28,29]. To our knowledge, only two studies to date have quantified *trans*-resveratrol in adipose tissues. *Trans*-resveratrol was not present in the adipose tissue of rats, which received it in their diet (30 mg/kg/day) for 6 weeks, while several glucuronide and sulphate metabolites were detected [30]. On the other hand, *trans*-resveratrol and some of its metabolites were detected in pig 6 h after 6.25 mg/kg intragastric administration [31].

In other studies, ε-viniferin decreased the accumulation of lipids and inhibited of the enzyme HMG-CoA reductase, an enzyme involved in cholesterol synthesis, for a concentration range of 2.5 to 50 μM in 3T3-L1 adipocytes [12,13]. Thus, despite the weak adipose concentrations of ε-viniferin observed in our study as compared to those reported to exert an anti-adipogenic effect in vitro, we believe they are sufficient to induce an anti-adipogenic effect in vivo. Indeed, for a given compound, the effective in vitro concentrations are often far higher than the effective in vivo concentrations. Moreover, studies mentioned above also reported that an oral administration of ε-viniferin was found to limit weight gain in mice fed a hypercaloric diet without decreasing their food intake. The authors explained the weight loss by a decrease in the mass of mesenteric white adipose tissue [12,13]. This suggests that the rage of concentrations found in adipose tissue in our study may be responsible for the effect observed in studies in mice. Thus, white adipose tissue may be both a target organ for ε-viniferin and a reservoir of the native form, which might allow its slow release, thereby ensuring that the organism remains exposed to it. This is of interest because this phenomenon could lengthen its biological activity both in adipose tissue and in other organs.

5. Conclusions

This is the first demonstration that even if ε-viniferin is highly and rapidly metabolized, it is also bioaccumulated in its native form in white adipose tissues after IP injection in rats. These findings offer a new opportunity to develop innovative strategies to increase the bioavailability of ε-viniferin. Considering its potential in the fight against obesity, this bioaccumulation of ε-viniferin in adipose tissues warrants further investigations. If this lipid-lowering potential were to be confirmed, it would pave the way for new strategies aiming at the prevention or reduction of obesity and related metabolic disorders.

Author Contributions: Conceptualization, A.C., C.A. and S.K.; investigation and validation, A.C., C.A., C.L., A.M., R.H.-O., S.K. and T.R.; formal analysis, A.C., C.A., A.M., R.H.-O., C.F. and S.K.; writing-original draft preparation, A.C., C.A, A.M., R.H., C.F. and S.K.; funding acquisition, T.R.

Funding: This research received no external funding.

Acknowledgments: The authors would like to thank the Fundación Alfonso Martín Escudero for the postdoctoral fellowship of Ruth Hornedo-Ortega. The work was supported by the Bordeaux Metabolome Facility and MetaboHUB (ANR-11-INBS-0010 project).

Conflicts of Interest: The authors declare no conflict of interest.

References

1. Pawlus, A.D.; Waffo-Teguo, P.; Shaver, J.; Merillon, J.-M. Stilbenoid chemistry from wine and the genus Vitis, a review. *OENO One* **2012**, *46*, 57–111. [CrossRef]
2. Lin, M.; Yao, C.-S. Natural Oligostilbenes. In *Studies in Natural Products Chemistry*; Atta-ur-Rahman, Ed.; Elsevier: Amsterdam, The Netherlands, 2006; Volume 33, pp. 601–644.
3. Takaya, Y.; Yan, K.-X.; Terashima, K.; Ito, J.; Niwa, M. Chemical determination of the absolute structures of resveratrol dimers, ampelopsins A, B, D and F. *Tetrahedron* **2002**, *58*, 7259–7265. [CrossRef]
4. Mattivi, F.; Vrhovsek, U.; Malacarne, G.; Masuero, D.; Zulini, L.; Stefanini, M.; Moser, C.; Velasco, R.; Guella, G. Profiling of resveratrol oligomers, important stress metabolites, accumulating in the leaves of hybrid Vitis vinifera (merzling × teroldego) genotypes infected with Plasmopara viticola. *J. Agric. Food Chem.* **2011**, *59*, 5364–5375. [CrossRef] [PubMed]
5. Rivière, C.; Pawlus, A.D.; Mérillon, J.-M. Natural stilbenoids: Distribution in the plant kingdom and chemotaxonomic interest in Vitaceae. *Nat. Prod. Rep.* **2012**, *29*, 1317–1333. [CrossRef] [PubMed]
6. El Khawand, T.; Courtois, A.; Valls, J.; Richard, T.; Krisa, S. A review of dietary stilbenes: Sources and bioavailability. *Phytochem. Rev.* **2018**. [CrossRef]
7. Vitrac, X.; Bornet, A.; Vanderlinde, R.; Valls, J.; Richard, T.; Delaunay, J.-C.; Mérillon, J.-M.; Teissédre, P.-L. Determination of stilbenes (δ-viniferin, trans-astringin, trans-piceid, cis- and trans-resveratrol, ε-viniferin) in Brazilian wines. *J. Agric. Food Chem.* **2005**, *53*, 5664–5669. [CrossRef] [PubMed]

8. Privat, C.; Telo, J.P.; Bernardes-Genisson, V.; Vieira, A.; Souchard, J.-P.; Nepveu, F. Antioxidant properties of trans-epsilon-viniferin as compared to stilbene derivatives in aqueous and nonaqueous media. *J. Agric. Food Chem.* **2002**, *50*, 1213–1217. [CrossRef] [PubMed]

9. Zghonda, N.; Yoshida, S.; Ezaki, S.; Otake, Y.; Murakami, C.; Mliki, A.; Ghorbel, A.; Miyazaki, H. ε-Viniferin is more effective than its monomer resveratrol in improving the functions of vascular endothelial cells and the heart. *Biosci. Biotechnol. Biochem.* **2012**, *76*, 954–960. [CrossRef] [PubMed]

10. Zghonda, N.; Yoshida, S.; Araki, M.; Kusunoki, M.; Mliki, A.; Ghorbel, A.; Miyazaki, H. Greater effectiveness of ε-viniferin in red wine than its monomer resveratrol for inhibiting vascular smooth muscle cell proliferation and migration. *Biosci. Biotechnol. Biochem.* **2011**, *75*, 1259–1267. [CrossRef] [PubMed]

11. Nassra, M.; Krisa, S.; Papastamoulis, Y.; Kapche, G.D.; Bisson, J.; André, C.; Konsman, J.-P.; Schmitter, J.-M.; Mérillon, J.-M.; Waffo-Téguo, P. Inhibitory activity of plant stilbenoids against nitric oxide production by lipopolysaccharide-activated microglia. *Planta Med.* **2013**, *79*, 966–970. [CrossRef] [PubMed]

12. Ohara, K.; Kusano, K.; Kitao, S.; Yanai, T.; Takata, R.; Kanauchi, O. ε-Viniferin, a resveratrol dimer, prevents diet-induced obesity in mice. *Biochem. Biophys. Res. Commun.* **2015**, *468*, 877–882. [CrossRef] [PubMed]

13. Lu, Y.-L.; Lin, S.-Y.; Fang, S.-U.; Hsieh, Y.-Y.; Chen, C.-R.; Wen, C.-L.; Chang, C.-I.; Hou, W.-C. Hot-water extracts from roots of *Vitis thunbergii* var. taiwaniana and identified ε-viniferin improve obesity in high-fat diet-induced mice. *J. Agric. Food Chem.* **2017**, *65*, 2521–2529. [CrossRef] [PubMed]

14. Gambini, J.; Inglés, M.; Olaso, G.; Lopez-Grueso, R.; Bonet-Costa, V.; Gimeno-Mallench, L.; Mas-Bargues, C.; Abdelaziz, K.M.; Gomez-Cabrera, M.C.; Vina, J.; et al. Properties of resveratrol: In vitro and in vivo studies about metabolism, bioavailability, and biological effects in animal models and humans. *Oxid. Med. Cell. Longev.* **2015**, *2015*, 837042. [CrossRef] [PubMed]

15. Wenzel, E.; Soldo, T.; Erbersdobler, H.; Somoza, V. Bioactivity and metabolism of trans-resveratrol orally administered to Wistar rats. *Mol. Nutr. Food Res.* **2005**, *49*, 482–494. [CrossRef] [PubMed]

16. Courtois, A.; Jourdes, M.; Dupin, A.; Lapèze, C.; Renouf, E.; Biais, B.; Teissedre, P.-L.; Mérillon, J.-M.; Richard, T.; Krisa, S. In vitro glucuronidation and sulfation of ε-viniferin, a resveratrol dimer, in humans and rats. *Molecules* **2017**, *22*, 733. [CrossRef] [PubMed]

17. Mao, P.; Lei, Y.; Zhang, T.; Ma, C.; Jin, B.; Li, T. Pharmacokinetics, bioavailability, metabolism and excretion of δ-viniferin in rats. *Acta Pharm. Sin. B* **2016**, *6*, 243–252. [CrossRef] [PubMed]

18. Kim, J.; Min, J.S.; Kim, D.; Zheng, Y.F.; Mailar, K.; Choi, W.J.; Lee, C.; Bae, S.K. A simple and sensitive liquid chromatography-tandem mass spectrometry method for trans-ε-viniferin quantification in mouse plasma and its application to a pharmacokinetic study in mice. *J. Pharm. Biomed. Anal.* **2017**, *134*, 116–121. [CrossRef] [PubMed]

19. Gómez-Hernández, A.; Beneit, N.; Díaz-Castroverde, S.; Escribano, Ó. Differential role of adipose tissues in obesity and related metabolic and vascular complications. *Int. J. Endocrinol.* **2016**, *2016*, 1216783. [CrossRef] [PubMed]

20. Wajchenberg, B.L. Subcutaneous and visceral adipose tissue: Their relation to the metabolic syndrome. *Endocr. Rev.* **2000**, *21*, 697–738. [CrossRef] [PubMed]

21. Biais, B.; Krisa, S.; Cluzet, S.; Da Costa, G.; Waffo-Teguo, P.; Mérillon, J.-M.; Richard, T. Antioxidant and cytoprotective activities of grapevine stilbenes. *J. Agric. Food Chem.* **2017**, *65*, 4952–4960. [CrossRef] [PubMed]

22. ISVV—Polyphenols Reference Database. Available online: https://mib-polyphenol.eu/ (accessed on 4 September 2018).

23. De Paepe, D.; Servaes, K.; Noten, B.; Diels, L.; De Loose, M.; Van Droogenbroeck, B.; Voorspoels, S. An improved mass spectrometric method for identification and quantification of phenolic compounds in apple fruits. *Food Chem.* **2013**, *136*, 368–375. [CrossRef] [PubMed]

24. Zhang, Y.; Huo, M.; Zhou, J.; Xie, S. PKSolver: An add-in program for pharmacokinetic and pharmacodynamic data analysis in Microsoft Excel. *Comput. Methods Programs Biomed.* **2010**, *99*, 306–314. [CrossRef] [PubMed]

25. Marier, J.-F.; Vachon, P.; Gritsas, A.; Zhang, J.; Moreau, J.-P.; Ducharme, M.P. Metabolism and disposition of resveratrol in rats: Extent of absorption, glucuronidation, and enterohepatic recirculation evidenced by a linked-rat model. *J. Pharmacol. Exp. Ther.* **2002**, *302*, 369–373. [CrossRef] [PubMed]

26. Maier-Salamon, A.; Hagenauer, B.; Reznicek, G.; Szekeres, T.; Thalhammer, T.; Jäger, W. Metabolism and disposition of resveratrol in the isolated perfused rat liver: Role of Mrp2 in the biliary excretion of glucuronides. *J. Pharm. Sci.* **2008**, *97*, 1615–1628. [CrossRef] [PubMed]

27. Landrier, J.-F.; Marcotorchino, J.; Tourniaire, F. Lipophilic micronutrients and adipose tissue biology. *Nutrients* **2012**, *4*, 1622–1649. [CrossRef] [PubMed]
28. Arola-Arnal, A.; Oms-Oliu, G.; Crescenti, A.; del Bas, J.M.; Ras, M.R.; Arola, L.; Caimari, A. Distribution of grape seed flavanols and their metabolites in pregnant rats and their fetuses. *Mol. Nutr. Food Res.* **2013**, *57*, 1741–1752. [CrossRef] [PubMed]
29. Margalef, M.; Pons, Z.; Iglesias-Carres, L.; Arola, L.; Muguerza, B.; Arola-Arnal, A. Gender-related similarities and differences in the body distribution of grape seed flavanols in rats. *Mol. Nutr. Food Res.* **2016**, *60*, 760–772. [CrossRef] [PubMed]
30. Alberdi, G.; Rodríguez, V.M.; Miranda, J.; Macarulla, M.T.; Arias, N.; Andrés-Lacueva, C.; Portillo, M.P. Changes in white adipose tissue metabolism induced by resveratrol in rats. *Nutr. Metab.* **2011**, *8*, 29. [CrossRef] [PubMed]
31. Azorín-Ortuño, M.; Yáñez-Gascón, M.J.; Vallejo, F.; Pallarés, F.J.; Larrosa, M.; Lucas, R.; Morales, J.C.; Tomás-Barberán, F.A.; García-Conesa, M.T.; Espín, J.C. Metabolites and tissue distribution of resveratrol in the pig. *Mol. Nutr. Food Res.* **2011**, *55*, 1154–1168. [CrossRef] [PubMed]

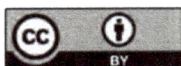

Article

Effects of Resveratrol on the Renin-Angiotensin System in the Aging Kidney

In-Ae Jang [1], Eun Nim Kim [2], Ji Hee Lim [2], Min Young Kim [2], Tae Hyun Ban [1,3], Hye Eun Yoon [1,4], Cheol Whee Park [1,3], Yoon Sik Chang [1,5] and Bum Soon Choi [1,6,*]

[1] Department of Internal medicine, College of Medicine, The Catholic University of Korea, Seoul 06591, Korea; inae623@hanmail.net (I.-A.J.); deux0123@catholic.ac.kr (T.H.B.); berrynana@catholic.ac.kr (H.E.Y.); cheolwhee@catholic.ac.kr (C.W.P.); ysc543@unitel.co.kr (Y.S.C.)

[2] Division of Medical Cell Biology, Department of Biomedical Science, College of Medicine, The Catholic University of Korea, Seoul 06591, Korea; kun0512@hanmail.net (E.N.K.); didsuai@hanmail.net (J.H.L.); sweetshow@naver.com (M.Y.K.)

[3] Division of Nephrology, Department of Internal Medicine, Seoul St. Mary's Hospital, Seoul 06591, Korea

[4] Division of Nephrology, Department of Internal Medicine, Incheon St. Mary's Hospital, Incheon 21431, Korea

[5] Division of Nephrology, Department of Internal Medicine, Yeouido St. Mary's Hospital, Seoul 07345, Korea

[6] Division of Nephrology, Department of Internal Medicine, St. Paul's Hospital, Seoul 02559, Korea

* Correspondence: sooncb@catholic.ac.kr; Tel.: +82-2-2558-6040

Received: 8 October 2018; Accepted: 9 November 2018; Published: 12 November 2018

Abstract: The renin-angiotensin system (RAS), especially the angiotensin II (Ang II)/angiotensin II type 1 receptor (AT1R) axis, plays an important role in the aging process of the kidney, through increased tissue reactive oxygen species production and progressively increased oxidative stress. In contrast, the angiotensin 1-7 (Ang 1-7)/Mas receptor (MasR) axis, which counteracts the effects of Ang II, is protective for end-organ damage. To evaluate the ability of resveratrol (RSV) to modulate the RAS in aging kidneys, eighteen-month-old male C57BL/6 mice were divided into two groups that received either normal mouse chow or chow containing resveratrol, for six months. Renal expressions of RAS components, as well as pro- and antioxidant enzymes, were measured and mouse kidneys were isolated for histopathology. Resveratrol-treated mice demonstrated better renal function and reduced albuminuria, with improved renal histologic findings. Resveratrol suppressed the Ang II/AT1R axis and enhanced the AT2R/Ang 1-7/MasR axis. Additionally, the expression of nicotinamide adenine dinucleotide phosphate oxidase 4, 8-hydroxy-2′-deoxyguanosine, 3-nitrotyrosine, collagen IV, and fibronectin was decreased, while the expression of endothelial nitric oxide synthase and superoxide dismutase 2 was increased by resveratrol treatment. These findings demonstrate that resveratrol exerts protective effects on aging kidneys by reducing oxidative stress, inflammation, and fibrosis, through Ang II suppression and MasR activation.

Keywords: renin-angiotensin system; angiotensin converting enzyme 2; kidney; resveratrol; aging

---

1. Introduction

Aging causes progressive deterioration of organs, leading to impaired tissue function, increased vulnerability to stress, and death [1,2]. The kidney is one of the most susceptible target organs of age-associated tissue damage [3], and the high incidence of chronic kidney disease, in the elderly, is a health problem, worldwide [4,5].

Various processes are involved in the deterioration seen in aging kidneys, including oxidative stress, mitochondrial dysfunction, inflammation, altered calcium regulation, and activation of the renin-angiotensin system (RAS) [6,7]. The RAS modulates cell growth and senescence by activating the classic RAS axis—angiotensin converting enzyme (ACE)/Ang II/AT1R. This axis suppresses pro-survival genes and enhances reactive oxygen species (ROS) and pro-inflammatory cytokines production, resulting in chronic inflammation and cell senescence [8,9]. In contrast, the ACE2/Ang 1-7/MasR axis acts as a counter-regulator of classic Ang II-mediated effects [10–12].

Resveratrol is a polyphenolic phytoalexin that exists naturally in various plant parts and products, such as grapes, red wine, berries, and peanut skins, and has numerous beneficial health effects [13,14]. It acts as an activator of silent information regulator 1 (SIRT1) [15,16], exerting anti-senescent effects, as well as antioxidant and anti-inflammatory activities [17,18]. We previously reported that resveratrol exerts renal protective effect by activating Nrf2 and SIRT1 signaling pathways [19]. In this study, we hypothesized that resveratrol would attenuate the aging process in the kidney of mice by modulating RAS components, especially by the activation of the ACE2/Ang 1-7/MasR axis, and furthermore, we examined pro-inflammatory and antioxidant molecular changes in kidneys of aging mice.

2. Materials and Methods

2.1. Study Design and Animals

Eighteen-month-aged male C57BL/6 mice were purchased from the Korea Research Institute of Bioscience and Biotechnology (Chungcheongbuk-do, Korea). The Animal Care Committee of the Catholic University of Korea approved the experimental protocol and the experiments were performed in accordance with our institutional animal care guidelines. Mice were housed in a controlled temperature and controlled light environment with 12:12-h light-dark cycles and had free access to water. The aged male C57BL/6 mice were divided into two groups: The control group ($n = 7$) received normal mice chow (PicoLab Rodent Diet 20 5053, Labdiet, St. Louis, MO, USA) and the resveratrol-treated group ($n = 7$) received normal mice chow mixed with resveratrol (40 mg/kg, Sigma, St. Louis, MO, USA). The food was changed every 24 h and a calculated regular amount of food was fed daily, for a six month period. The experimental conditions were set with reference to the article of Baur et al. [20]. The mice were sacrificed at the age of twenty-four month.

2.2. Evaluation of the Renal Function

Mice were placed in individual mouse metabolic cages (Tecniplast, Gazzada, Italy) with access to water and food for 24 h. Urine collection was done every four weeks and data from month 18 and 24 was used in this experiment. Albuminuria (Albuwell M, Exocell, Philadelphia, PA, USA) and urine creatinine concentration (The Creatinine Companion, Exocell, Philadelphia, PA, USA) were measured using ELISA kits. Serum creatinine concentrations and Blood urea nitrogen were measured using i-STAT system Cartridges (CHEM8+, Abbott Point of Care, Abbott Park, IL, USA). Creatinine clearance was calculated using a standard formula (urine creatinine (mg/dL) × urine volume (mL/24 h)/serum creatinine (mg/dL) × 1440 (min/24 h)).

2.3. Histological Assessment of the Renal Tissue

Kidney tissue samples were fixed in 10% formalin. The tissues were embedded in low-temperature melting paraffin, and 4 microns, thick sections were processed and stained with a periodic acid–Schiff (PAS), and Masson's trichrome. The glomerular volume and mesangial matrix were quantified for kidney tissue cross-sections, using PAS staining. The relative mesangial area was expressed as mesangial/glomerular surface area. A finding of tubulointerstitial fibrosis was defined as a matrix-rich expansion of the interstitium in Masson's trichrome. Ten randomly selected fields, per section, were assessed. All of these sections were examined in a blinded manner, using a color-image analyzer (TDI Scope Eye, Version 3.5 for Windows, Olympus, Tokyo, Japan) and quantified using image J (Wayne Rasband national institutes of health, Bethesda, MD, USA).

2.4. Immunohistochemistry

Immunohistochemistry was performed to determine changes of Ang II, angiotensin target receptors (AT1R, AT2R and MasR) and oxidative stress using 8-hydroxy-deoxyguanosine (8-OHdG) and 3-nitrotyrosine. Paraffin sections were deparaffinized in xylene and hydrated in ethanol, before staining, and treated with an antigen-unmasking solution, consisting of 10 mM sodium citrate, pH 6.0 and then washed with phosphate-buffered saline. Sections were incubated with 3% H_2O_2, in methanol, to block the endogenous peroxidase activity. Nonspecific binding was blocked with 10% normal horse serum. After incubating with the primary antibody to Ang II, AT2R and MasR (Novus Biologicals, Littleton, CO, USA), AT1R and 3-nitrotyrosine (Santa Cruz Biotechnology, Dallas, TX, USA), and 8-OHdG (Japan Institute for the Control of Aging, Shizuoka, Japan), at 4 °C, overnight, antibodies were visualized with a peroxidase conjugated secondary antibody, using the Vector Impress kit (Vector Laboratories, Burlingame, CA, USA). Sections were then dehydrated in ethanol, cleared in xylene and mounted without counterstaining. All sections were assessed using a color-image analyzer (TDI Scope Eye, Version 3.5 for Windows, Olympus, Tokyo, Japan).

2.5. Western Blot Analysis

Total protein was extracted from the kidney tissues, using Pro-Prep Protein Extraction Solution (Intron Biotechnology, Gyeonggi-Do, Korea), according to the manufacturer's instructions. Extracted protein was subjected to SDS-polyacrylamide gel electrophoresis and transferred onto a Nitrocellulose membrane (Amersham Biosciences, Amersham, UK). Membranes blocked with 3% nonfat milk in Tris-buffered saline (TBS), containing 0.1% Tween-20 for 1 h, at room temperature. Then membranes were incubated overnight, at 4 °C, with primary antibodies in 3% nonfat milk or 3% BSA in Tris-buffered saline (TBS), containing 0.1%. After that, the membranes were washed in TBS containing 0.1% Tween-20 and were then incubated with peroxidase-conjugated secondary antibody, for 2 h, at room temperature. Immunoreactive bands were detected using Amersham ECL Prime Western Blotting Detection Reagent (Amersham Biosciences, Amersham, UK). Western blot analysis was performed using the following antibodies—transforming growth factor-β (TGF-β, R&D Systems, Minneapolis, MN, USA), collagen IV (Abcam, Cambridge, UK), fibronectin (Proteintech Group Inc, Chicago, IL, USA), ACE (Santa Cruz Biotechnology, Dallas, TX, USA), ACE2 (R&D Systems, Minneapolis, MN, USA), AT1R (Santa Cruz Biotechnology, Dallas, TX, USA), AT2R (Novus Biologicals, Littleton, CO, USA), prorenin receptor (PRR, Sigma life science, St. Louis, MO, USA), MasR (Novus Biologicals, Littleton, CO, USA), endothelial nitric oxide synthase (eNOS, Cell Signaling Technology Inc., Beverly, MA, USA), phosphorylated (phospho)-Ser1177 eNOS (Cell Signaling Technology Inc., Beverly, MA, USA), Nicotinamide adenine dinucleotide phosphate oxidase 2 (NOX2, BD Biosciences, Mountain View, MD, USA), Nicotinamide adenine dinucleotide phosphate oxidase 4 (NOX4, Santa Cruz Biotechnology, Dallas, TX, USA), superoxide dismutase 1 (SOD1, Enzo Life Sciences, Farmingdale, NY, USA), superoxide dismutase 2 (SOD2, Abcam, Cambridge, UK), and β-actin (Sigma Life Science, St. Louis, MO, USA).

2.6. Enzyme Immunoassay

Levels of Ang II and Ang 1-7 in Serum and renal tissue homogenates were measured using competitive enzyme immunoassay (Cusabio Biotech Co., Wuhan, China), according to the manufacturer's protocols.

2.7. Statistical Analysis

Data are expressed as means ± standard deviation (SD). Differences between the groups were examined for statistical significance, using ANOVA and unpaired *t*-test (SPSS v. 19.0, IBM, Armonk, NY, USA). *p* values of less than 0.05 were considered significant.

3. Results

3.1. Effects of Resveratrol on Renal Function in Aging Mice

Changes in renal function of aging mice were measured, before and after resveratrol treatment, and the results were compared with control mice. Serum creatinine was decreased in resveratrol-treated mice, compared with the control group mice (control 0.53 ± 0.05 vs. resveratrol 0.25 ± 0.02 mg/dL, Figure 1a). Creatinine clearance was significantly greater in the resveratrol-treated group than the control group (control 0.10 ± 0.01 vs. resveratrol 0.27 ± 0.03 mL/min, Figure 1b). Twenty-four hour albuminuria was significantly decreased in the resveratrol-treated group, compared with the control group (control 47.60 ± 1.97 vs. resveratrol 29.47 ± 5.85 µg/24 h, Figure 1c). These results show that resveratrol reduces albuminuria and, thus, improves kidney function in aging mice.

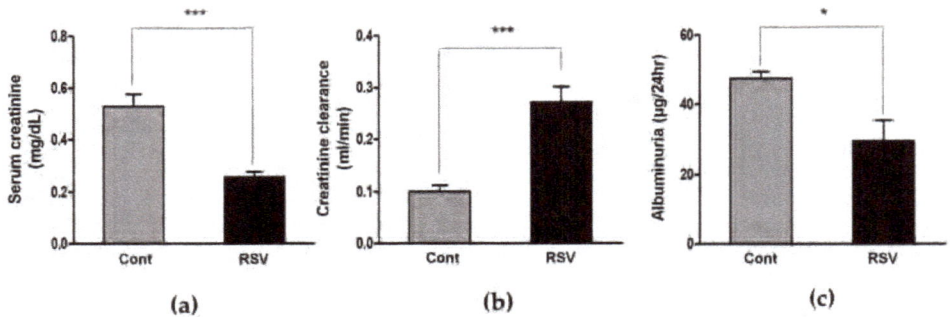

Figure 1. Effects of resveratrol on renal function of eighteen-month-old male C57BL/6 mice. Compared to the control group, resveratrol group showed (**a**) lower serum creatinine, (**b**) increased creatinine clearance, and (**c**) reduced 24 h albuminuria (* $p < 0.05$, *** $p < 0.001$).

3.2. Effects of Resveratrol on the Renal Histological Changes in Aging Mice

Histological examination demonstrated that the fractional mesangial area was reduced in the resveratrol-treated group, as compared to the control group (control 52.75 ± 2.18 vs. resveratrol $41.03 \pm 0.92\%$, Figure 2a,c). Additionally, tubulointerstitial fibrosis was substantially less in the resveratrol-treated group than in the control group (control 14.68 ± 2.69 vs. resveratrol $4.89 \pm 1.11\%$, Figure 2b,d). Thus, renal histological deterioration induced by aging was improved by resveratrol treatment.

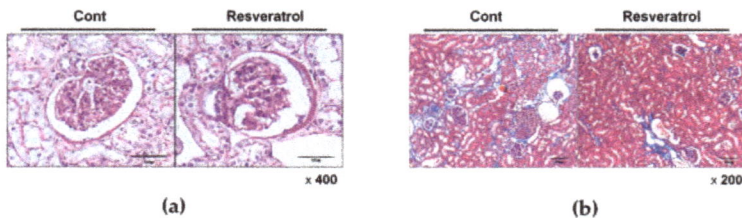

Figure 2. *Cont.*

(c)

(d)

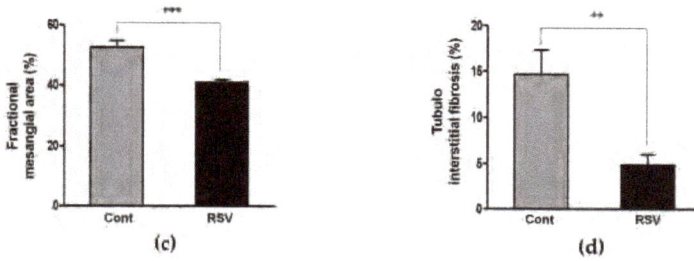

Figure 2. Effects of resveratrol on aging-related histological renal injury. (**a**) Representative photomicrographs of the periodic acid–Schiff-(PAS)-stained kidney showed less expansion of the mesangial area in the RSV group (original magnification 400×). (**b**) Representative sections of the Masson's trichrome-stained kidney showed significantly less tubulointerstitial fibrosis in the RSV group (original magnification 200×). (**c**) Quantitative assessments of the areas of extracellular matrix in the glomerulus. (**d**) Quantitative assessment of the areas of tubulointerstitial fibrosis in the control and RSV groups (** $p < 0.01$, *** $p < 0.001$).

3.3. Resveratrol Inhibits the Ang II/AT1R Axis in Aging Mice

The RAS plays an important role in the aging process of kidneys, through increased tissue ROS production and progressively increased oxidative stress. Expression of the PRR, ACE, and Ang II was measured by western blot analyses. Expression of the PRR decreased significantly in the resveratrol-treated group, compared with the control group (control 1.00 ± 0.02 vs. resveratrol 0.49 ± 0.02-fold, Figure 3).

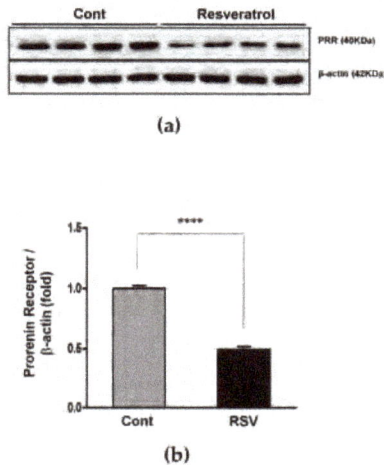

(a)

(b)

Figure 3. Effects of resveratrol on the expression of prorenin receptors. (**a**) Representative western blot analysis of prorenin receptors expression. (**b**) Prorenin receptors levels were decreased in the RSV group. Quantitative analysis of the results is shown (**** $p < 0.0001$).

The expression of ACE, which converts Ang I to Ang II, was decreased significantly in the resveratrol-treated group, compared to the control group (control 1.00 ± 0.01 vs. resveratrol 0.62 ± 0.02-fold, Figure 4a,b).

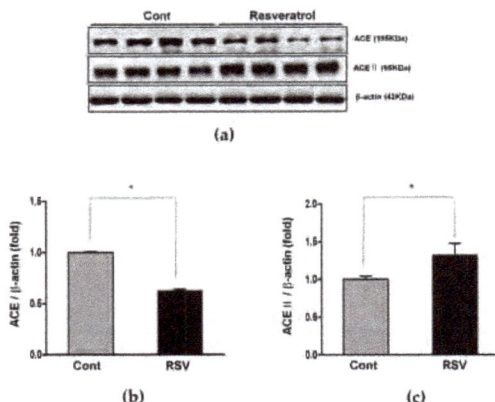

Figure 4. Effects of resveratrol on the angiotensin converting enzyme (ACE) and ACEII protein expressions. (**a**) Representative western blots of ACE and ACEII protein levels. (**b**) The protein levels of ACE were lower in the RSV group than in the control (Cont.) group. (**c**) The protein levels of ACEII were higher in the RSV group than in the control group. Quantitative analysis of the results is shown (* $p < 0.05$).

Consequently, Ang II was also decreased in the resveratrol-treated group, compared with the control group; immunohistochemistry for Ang II showed decreased Ang II-positive areas (control 1.18 ± 0.49 vs. resveratrol $0.17 \pm 0.08\%$, Figure 5a,c). enzyme immunoassay demonstrated significantly reduced renal Ang II levels (control 40.09 ± 3.76 vs. resveratrol 29.06 ± 2.85 pg/mL, Figure 5b) as well as decreased serum levels of Ang II (control 40.67 ± 1.16 vs. resveratrol 20.00 ± 2.43 pg/mL, Figure 5d).

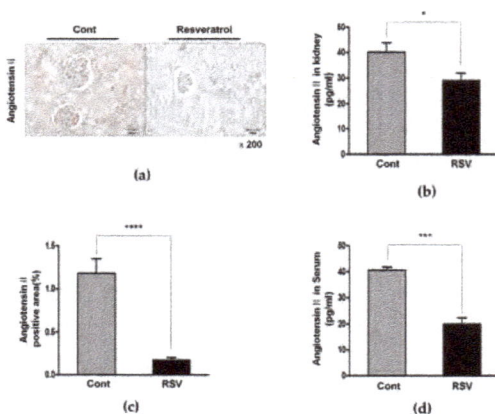

Figure 5. Effects of resveratrol on the Ang II. (**a**) Representative images of immunohistochemical staining with Ang II in aging kidney glomerulus (original magnification 200×). (**b**) The expression of Ang II in kidney was significantly decreased in the RSV group. (**c**) Ang II-positive area in kidney were observed to be significantly smaller in the RSV group; (**d**) The expression of Ang II in serum was also significantly decreased in the RSV group (* $p < 0.05$, *** $p < 0.001$, **** $p < 0.0001$).

Furthermore, the expression of AT1R was decreased significantly (control 1.00 ± 0.06 vs. resveratrol 0.76 ± 0.05-fold, Figure 6a,b), as well as AT1R-positive areas, by immunohistochemistry (control 7.02 ± 2.88 vs. resveratrol $0.84 \pm 1.19\%$, Figure 6d,e).

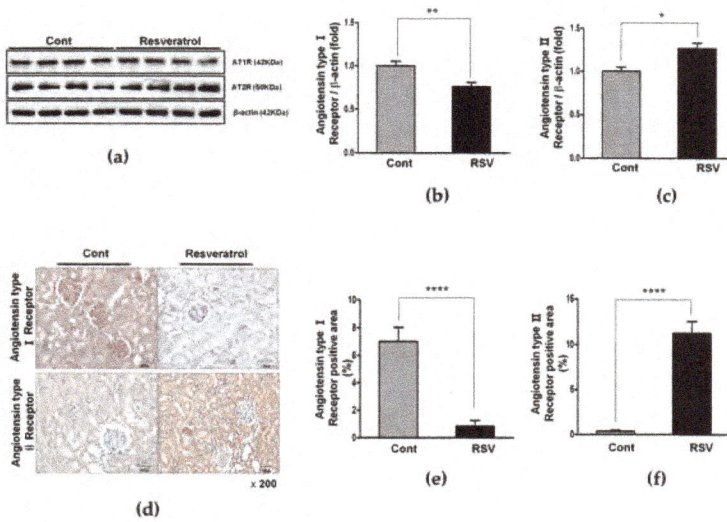

Figure 6. Effects of resveratrol on the AT1R and AT2R. (**a**) Representative western blots of AT1R and AT2R. (**b**) The expression of AT1R was significantly decreased in the RSV group. (**c**) The expression of AT2R was significantly increased in the RSV group. (**d**) Representative images of immunohistochemistry for AT1R and AT2R, in the aging kidney glomerulus (original magnification × 200). (**e**) The expression of AT1R-positive area in the kidney was markedly decreased in the RSV group. (**f**) The expression of AT2R-positive area in the kidney was markedly increased in the RSV group (* $p < 0.05$, ** $p < 0.01$, **** $p < 0.0001$).

3.4. Resveratrol Stimulates Angiotensin II Type 2 Receptors (AT2R) and Mas Receptor in Aging Mice

The RAS has another pathway comprised of ACE2, Ang 1-7, and MasRs that exerts a counter-regulatory function to Ang II activity. The expression of ACE2, which converts Ang II to Ang 1-7, was significantly increased in the resveratrol-treated group, compared to the control group (control 1.00 ± 0.04 vs. resveratrol 1.32 ± 0.16-fold, Figure 4a,c). Renal and serum levels of Ang 1-7 were analyzed by an enzyme immunoassay. Both the renal and serum levels of Ang 1-7 were significantly increased in the resveratrol-treated group, compared to the control group (control 618 ± 6 vs. resveratrol 632 ± 10 pg/mL, Figure 7a; and control 15.09 ± 0.91 vs. resveratrol 19.16 ± 2.18 pg/mL, Figure 7b; respectively).

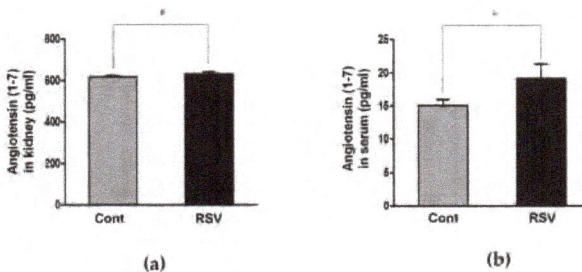

Figure 7. ELISA for serum and kidney levels of Ang 1-7. (**a**) Renal levels of Ang 1-7 significantly increased in the RSV group, compared to Cont. groups. (**b**) Serum levels of Ang 1-7 significantly increased in the RSV group, compared to Cont. groups. Quantitative analysis of the results is shown (* $p < 0.05$).

Accordingly, MasR, the effecter of Ang 1-7, was also significantly increased (control 1.00 ± 0.02 vs. resveratrol 1.19 ± 0.01-fold, Figure 8b,d).

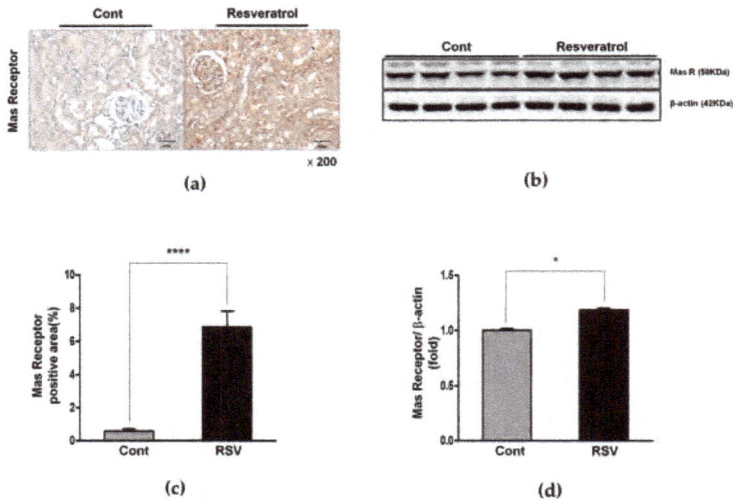

(a)

(b)

(c)

(d)

Figure 8. Effects of resveratrol on MasR. (**a**) Representative images of immunohistochemical staining of MasR in the aging kidney glomerulus (original magnification 200×). (**b**) Representative western blots of MasR. (**c**) MasR-positive area in the kidney was significantly increased in the RSV group. (**d**) The expression of MasR was significantly increased in the RSV group (* $p < 0.05$, **** $p < 0.0001$).

The expression of AT2R, the negative regulator of AT1R, was increased significantly in the resveratrol-treated group, compared with the control group (control 1.00 ± 0.05 vs. resveratrol 1.27 ± 0.06-fold, Figure 6a,c). Immunohistochemistry for AT2R and MasR was performed and the results reinforced these findings. AT2R- and MasR-positive areas increased in the resveratrol-treated group (control 0.37 ± 0.27 vs. resveratrol $11.28 \pm 1.28\%$, $p < 0.001$, Figure 6d,f; and control 0.57 ± 0.39 vs. resveratrol $6.86 \pm 2.72\%$, $p < 0.001$, Figure 8a,c, respectively). These results showed that resveratrol inhibited the ACE/AT1R axis and that the ACEII/AT2R/MasR axis was activated.

3.5. Effects of the Resveratrol on the Oxidative Stress Marker

Previous reports show that oxidative stress and chronic exposure to ROS are key steps to age-related kidney changes [7,21,22]. Using western blot analyses, we examined the changes of the ROS generators NOX2 and NOX4. The expression of NOX2 tended to decrease without any statistical significance, while NOX4 was decreased significantly, in the resveratrol-treated group (control 1.00 ± 0.07 vs. resveratrol 0.64 ± 0.20-fold, Figure 9).

To evaluate changes in oxidative stress markers, immunohistochemical analyses of 8-OHdG and 3-nitrotyrosine were performed. The positive area of 8-OHdG (control 4.93 ± 1.41 vs. resveratrol $1.10 \pm 0.55\%$, Figure 10a) and 3-nitrotyrosine (control 4.13 ± 1.22 vs. resveratrol 0.39 ± 0.17, Figure 10b) were significantly decreased in the resveratrol—treated group, compared with the control group. These findings indicated that resveratrol diminished the renal oxidative stress in the aging mice.

(a)

(b)　　　　　　　　　　　　　　　　(c)

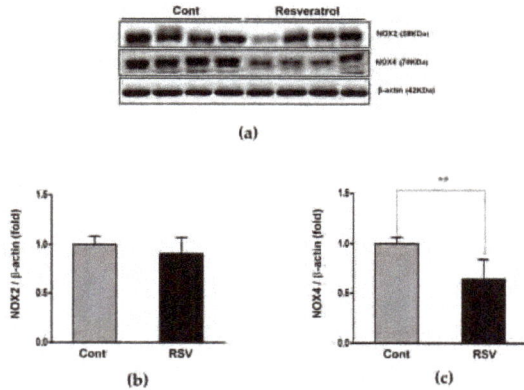

Figure 9. Effects of resveratrol on NOX2 and NOX4. (**a**) Representative western blots of NOX2 and NOX4 levels. (**b**) The expression of NOX2 showed a tendency of decrease in the RSV group, compared with the Cont. group, but it was not statistically significant. (**c**) The expression of Nox4 was significantly decreased in the RSV group. Quantitative analysis of the results is shown (** $p < 0.01$).

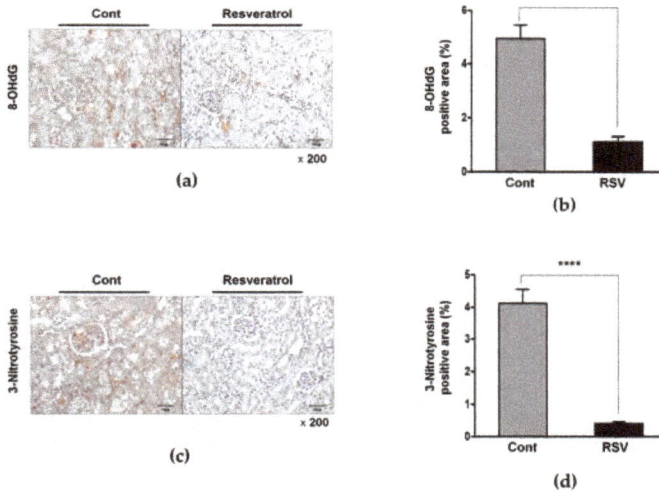

(a)　　　　　　　　　　　　　　　　(b)

(c)　　　　　　　　　　　　　　　　(d)

Figure 10. Effects of resveratrol on renal oxidative stress. (**a**) Representative images of immunohistochemistry for 8-OHdG in aging kidney glomerulus (original magnification 200×). (**b**) The positive area expression of 8-OHdG in the renal tissue was decreased in the RSV group, compared to that in the Cont. group. (**c**) Representative images of immunohistochemistry for 3-Nitrotyrosine in the aging kidney glomerulus (original magnification 200×). (**d**) The positive area expression of 3-Nitrotyrosine in the renal tissue was also decreased in the RSV group (**** $p < 0.0001$).

3.6. Effects of Resveratrol on the Antioxidant Enzyme

The influence of resveratrol on eNOS and the antioxidant enzymes SOD1 and SOD2 was examined by western blot analyses. The ratio of phospho-Ser1177 eNOS to the total eNOS was increased in the resveratrol-treated mice (control 1.00 ± 0.07 vs. resveratrol 1.27 ± 0.19-fold, Figure 11).

(a)

(b)

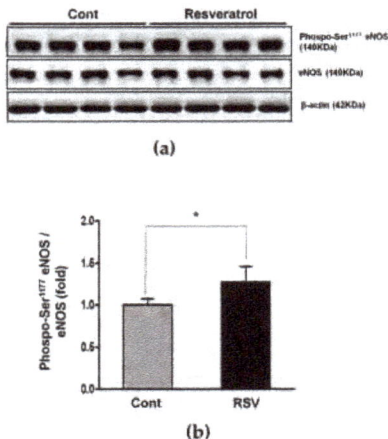

Figure 11. Effects of resveratrol on phospho-Ser1177eNOS/eNOS. (a) Representative western blots of phospho-Ser1177eNOS/eNOS levels. (b) The expression of phospho-Ser1177eNOS/eNOS was significantly increased in the RSV group. Quantitative analysis of the results is shown (* $p < 0.05$).

SOD2 protein levels were increased in the resveratrol-treated mice (control 1.00 ± 0.02 vs. resveratrol 1.23 ± 0.06-fold, Figure 12).

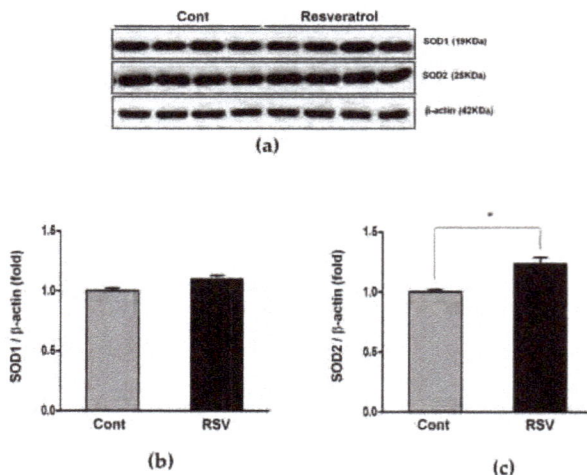

(a)

(b)   (c)

Figure 12. Effects of resveratrol on SOD1 and SOD2. (a) Representative western blots of SOD1 and SOD2 levels. (b) The expression of SOD1 showed a tendency of increase in the RSV group, compared with the Cont. group, but it was not statistically significant. (c) The expression of SOD2 was significantly increased in the RSV group. Quantitative analysis of the results is shown (* $p < 0.05$).

3.7. Anti-Inflammatory Effects of Resveratrol

To evaluate the anti-inflammatory effects of resveratrol, we examined the expression of TGF-β, collagen IV, and fibronectin in kidneys, using a western blot analyses. TGF-β expression was decreased non-significantly in the resveratrol-treated group. The expression of collagen IV (control 1.00 ± 0.08 vs. resveratrol 0.66 ± 0.08-fold) and fibronectin (control 1.00 ± 0.19 vs. resveratrol 0.64 ± 0.21-fold) were decreased significantly by the resveratrol (Figure 13).

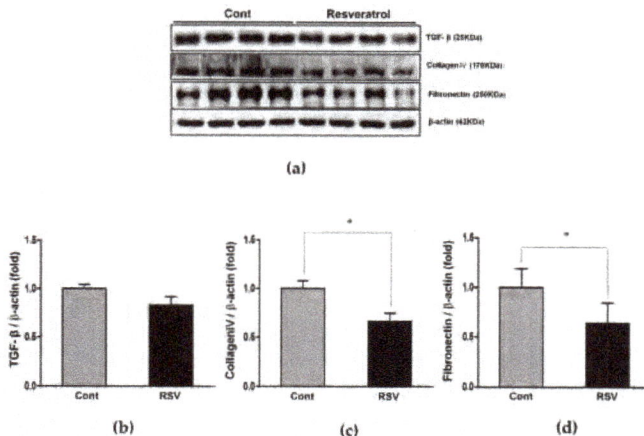

Figure 13. Effects of resveratrol on the TGF-β, collagen IV and fibronectin. (**a**) Representative western blots of TGF-β, collagen IV and fibronectin levels. (**b**) The expression of TGF-β showed a tendency of decrease in the RSV group, compared with the Cont. group, but it was not statistically significant. (**c,d**) The expression of collagen IV and fibronectin was significantly decreased in the RSV group. Quantitative analysis of the results is shown (* $p < 0.05$).

4. Discussion

In this study, we investigated the beneficial effects of resveratrol on the kidneys of aging mice. A six-month treatment with resveratrol resulted in a reduced albuminuria, better renal function, and improved renal histological changes, including diminished tubulointerstitial fibrosis, glomerulosclerosis, and inflammatory cell infiltration. Positive changes of the RAS were also observed in the resveratrol-treated aging mice. Specifically, the expression of ACE, Ang II, and AT1R was suppressed, while the expression of ACE2, Ang 1-7, AT2R, and particularly, MAS was stimulated. Furthermore, the expression of oxidative stress markers (NOX4, 8-OhdG, 3-nitrotyrosine) and inflammation markers (collagen IV, fibronectin) was improved in the resveratrol-treated mice. The novel finding of the present study is that resveratrol not only inhibits ACE, Ang II, and AT1R, the well-known classic axis, but also stimulates the ACE2/Ang 1-7/MasR axis in the aging kidneys. The altered expression of RAS components was confirmed by the western blot, as well as immunohistochemical assays.

Aging is a complex, multifactorial process, characterized by gradual deterioration of function and progressive structural changes [6,7]. Various possible mechanisms for aging and consequent anti-aging therapies have been studied including the free radical theory, immunological theory and mitochondrial theory, but the exact mechanism is still obscure [2,23–25]. Among potential mechanisms of aging, changes in the RAS, especially activation of the Ang II axis and inhibition of the MasR axis, are particularly important [26,27]. Previous reports have shown that chronic RAS activation promotes end-organ damage associated with aging [9,28] and the RAS blockade protects against renal aging caused by increasing the tissue and mitochondrial oxidative stress [29,30].

Recently, multiple lines of evidence suggested an association between an increased ACE2 signaling and improvements in the aging-related tissue injury. First, activation of ACE2 improved metabolic profiles during aging [31]. Second, endothelial dysfunction with aging was augmented in the ACE2-deficient mice [32]. Third, administration of an Ang 1-7 analogue was associated with improved aging-related neuroinflammation [33].

Numerous studies have reported that aging induces changes in the RAS [26,27]. For example, the baseline plasma renin level decreases and plasma renin activity is reduced with aging, which is associated with a reduction in both renin synthesis and release in the juxtaglomerular apparatuses [34,35]. This suppression of the systemic RAS leads to an impaired response to RAS stimuli, as well as to RAS inhibition [36]. Despite the decline in RAS activity, local secretion of Ang II, in the aging kidney, is markedly increased [37] and responsiveness to Ang II is enhanced [38]. In contrast, the ACE2/Ang 1-7/MasR axis is reduced with aging. Decreased expression of ACE2 and MasR is observed in the aortas of aging mice [39] and lower Ang 1-7 levels, in the mouse brains, are noted during aging [31]. Together, these events lead to age-associated functional and structural changes in the kidney. Many studies searching for anti-senescence antioxidants have been conducted. Resveratrol, a polyphenolic compound that occurs in many plants and plant products with potent antioxidant and anti-inflammatory activities, is among the numerous agents tested [13,40,41]. Resveratrol is a known activator of the AMP-activated protein kinase and SIRT1, which downregulate the expression of AT1R [42–45]. Previously, Miyasaki et al. reported that, in rat vascular smooth muscle cells, resveratrol downregulated the expression of AT1R via the activation of SIRT1 [46]. While Kim et al. revealed that inflammation, fibrosis, and oxidative stress in the aging aorta were attenuated by a resveratrol treatment, through regulation of the systemic and tissue-specific RAS [47]. Similarly, the results of the present study showed that resveratrol treatment attenuated oxidative stress, inflammation and fibrosis in the aging kidney, and modulated age-associated changes in the RAS components, by suppressing the PRR/ACE/Ang II axis and activating the ACE2/Ang 1–7/AT2R/MasR axis, in the mouse kidney.

Many of the molecular and cellular effects of Ang II are mediated by stimulating the production of ROS. Of the many types of ROS generated, NOX is considered as the prime producer [48,49]. To date, seven isoforms of NOX have been identified (NOX1–5, dual oxidase 1 and 2). NOX1, NOX2, and NOX4 are found in the kidney. NOX4 is the predominant renal form, whereas NOX1 and NOX2 have less functional importance [50,51]. Ang II is a potent stimulator of NOX. It activates the enzyme, increases expression of NOX subunits, and stimulates superoxide production [52–54]. Increased NOX activity and overproduction of mitochondrial ROS underlie the oxidative stress associated with aging and promote inflammation and tissue damage [55–57]. To date, numerous studies have been conducted about the organ-protective effect of the ACE2/Ang 1-7/MasR axis, through NOX suppression. Lo et al. reported that an infusion of the recombinant ACE2, lowered plasma Ang II, and increased the plasma Ang 1-7 levels, resulting in a significantly reduced NOX4, along with a lowered blood pressure [58]. In addition, Tanno et al. found that AT1R blockade enhanced the ACE2/Ang 1-7/MasR axis and suppressed the NOX4 expression, resulting in improved cardiac hypertrophy [59]. Our results congruently noted that a suppressed NOX4 expression, after the resveratrol treatment, was accompanied by an activation of the ACE2/Ang 1-7/MasR axis.

5. Conclusions

Our results demonstrated that the resveratrol treatment improves kidney function, albuminuria, glomerulosclerosis, tubular interstitial fibrosis, inflammation, and oxidative stress of age-related renal injury. These changes occur through decreases in the PRR/ACE/Ang II/AT1R axis and increases in the ACE2/Ang 1-7/MasR axis. A therapeutic strategy targeting the ACE2/Ang 1-7/MasR axis with resveratrol may postpone age-related renal structural and functional deterioration, through its antioxidant and antifibrotic effects. However, additional clinical investigations of the safety and anti-aging efficacy of resveratrol, are necessary.

Author Contributions: H.E.Y. and B.S.C. conceived and designed the experiments. I.-A.J., E.N.K. and M.Y.K performed the experiments E.N.K., M.Y.K., and J.H.L. analyzed the experimental data. T.H.B. contributed to discussions. I.-A.J. wrote this paper. C.W.P., Y.S.C. and B.S.C. critically revised the manuscript. All authors have read and approved the final manuscript.

Funding: This research was supported by the Basic Science Research Program through the National Research Foundation of Korea (NRF) funded by the Ministry of Education, Science and Technology (NRF-2016R1A6A3A11930177 and NRF-2016R1D1A1A09919985).

Conflicts of Interest: The authors declare no conflict of interest.

References

1. López-Otín, C.; Blasco, M.A.; Partridge, L.; Serrano, M.; Kroemer, G. The hallmarks of aging. *Cell* **2013**, *153*, 1194–1217. [CrossRef] [PubMed]
2. Tosato, M.; Zamboni, V.; Ferrini, A.; Cesari, M. The aging process and potential interventions to extend life expectancy. *Clin. Interv. Aging* **2007**, *2*, 401–412. [PubMed]
3. Denic, A.; Glassock, R.J.; Rule, A.D. Structural and functional changes with the aging kidney. *Adv. Chronic Kidney Dis.* **2016**, *23*, 19–28. [CrossRef] [PubMed]
4. Ozieh, M.N.; Bishu, K.G.; Dismuke, C.E.; Egede, L.E. Trends in healthcare expenditure in united states adults with chronic kidney disease: 2002–2011. *BMC Health Serv. Res.* **2017**, *17*, 368. [CrossRef] [PubMed]
5. Lee, R.; Mason, A. Cost of aging. *Financ. Dev.* **2017**, *54*, 7–9.
6. Kovacic, J.C.; Moreno, P.; Nabel, E.G.; Hachinski, V.; Fuster, V. Cellular senescence, vascular disease, and aging: Part 2 of a 2-part review: Clinical vascular disease in the elderly. *Circulation* **2011**, *123*, 1900–1910. [CrossRef] [PubMed]
7. O'Sullivan, E.D.; Hughes, J.; Ferenbach, D.A. Renal aging: Causes and consequences. *J. Am. Soc. Nephrol.* **2017**, *28*, 407–420. [CrossRef] [PubMed]
8. Capettini, L.S.; Montecucco, F.; Mach, F.; Stergiopulos, N.; Santos, R.A.; da Silva, R.F. Role of renin-angiotensin system in inflammation, immunity and aging. *Curr. Pharm. Des.* **2012**, *18*, 963–970. [CrossRef] [PubMed]
9. Conti, S.; Cassis, P.; Benigni, A. Aging and the renin-angiotensin system. *Hypertension* **2012**, *60*, 878–883. [CrossRef] [PubMed]
10. Santos, R.A.; Ferreira, A.J.; Verano-Braga, T.; Bader, M. Angiotensin-converting enzyme 2, angiotensin-(1-7) and mas: New players of the renin-angiotensin system. *J. Endocrinol.* **2013**, *216*, R1–R17. [CrossRef] [PubMed]
11. Shi, Y.; Lo, C.S.; Padda, R.; Abdo, S.; Chenier, I.; Filep, J.G.; Ingelfinger, J.R.; Zhang, S.L.; Chan, J.S. Angiotensin-(1-7) prevents systemic hypertension, attenuates oxidative stress and tubulointerstitial fibrosis, and normalizes renal angiotensin-converting enzyme 2 and mas receptor expression in diabetic mice. *Clin. Sci.* **2015**, *128*, 649–663. [CrossRef] [PubMed]
12. Chappell, M.C. Emerging evidence for a functional angiotensin-converting enzyme 2-angiotensin-(1-7)-mas receptor axis: More than regulation of blood pressure? *Hypertension* **2007**, *50*, 596–599. [CrossRef] [PubMed]
13. Baur, J.A.; Pearson, K.J.; Price, N.L.; Jamieson, H.A.; Lerin, C.; Kalra, A.; Prabhu, V.V.; Allard, J.S.; Lopez-Lluch, G.; Lewis, K.; et al. Resveratrol improves health and survival of mice on a high-calorie diet. *Nature* **2006**, *444*, 337–342. [CrossRef] [PubMed]
14. Wahab, A.; Gao, K.; Jia, C.; Zhang, F.; Tian, G.; Murtaza, G.; Chen, J. Significance of resveratrol in clinical management of chronic diseases. *Molecules* **2017**, *22*, 1329. [CrossRef] [PubMed]
15. Kitada, M.; Koya, D. Renal protective effects of resveratrol. *Oxid. Med. Cell. Longev.* **2013**, *2013*, 568093. [CrossRef] [PubMed]
16. Wen, D.; Huang, X.; Zhang, M.; Zhang, L.; Chen, J.; Gu, Y.; Hao, C.M. Resveratrol attenuates diabetic nephropathy via modulating angiogenesis. *PLoS ONE* **2013**, *8*, e82336. [CrossRef] [PubMed]
17. Albertoni, G.; Schor, N. Resveratrol plays important role in protective mechanisms in renal disease-mini-review. *Braz. J. Nephrol.* **2015**, *37*, 106–114. [CrossRef] [PubMed]
18. Cho, S.; Namkoong, K.; Shin, M.; Park, J.; Yang, E.; Ihm, J.; Thu, V.T.; Kim, H.K.; Han, J. Cardiovascular protective effects and clinical applications of resveratrol. *J. Med. Food* **2017**, *20*, 323–334. [CrossRef] [PubMed]
19. Kim, E.N.; Lim, J.H.; Kim, M.Y.; Ban, T.H.; Jang, I.-A.; Yoon, H.E.; Park, C.W.; Chang, Y.S.; Choi, B.S. Resveratrol, an Nrf2 activator, ameliorates aging-related progressive renal injury. *Aging* **2018**, *10*, 83–99. [CrossRef] [PubMed]
20. Baur, J.A.; Ungvari, Z.; Minor, R.K.; Le Couteur, D.G.; De Cabo, R. Are sirtuins viable targets for improving healthspan and lifespan? *Nat. Rev. Drug Discov.* **2012**, *11*, 443–461. [CrossRef] [PubMed]
21. Ozbek, E. Induction of oxidative stress in kidney. *Int. J. Nephrol.* **2012**, *2012*, 465897. [CrossRef] [PubMed]
22. Rhee, H.; Han, M.; Kim, S.S.; Kim, I.Y.; Lee, H.W.; Bae, S.S.; Ha, H.K.; Jung, E.S.; Lee, M.Y.; Seong, E.Y. The expression of two isoforms of matrix metalloproteinase-2 in aged mouse models of diabetes mellitus and chronic kidney disease. *Kidney Res. Clin. Pract.* **2018**, *37*, 222–229. [CrossRef] [PubMed]
23. Jin, K. Modern biological theories of aging. *Aging Dis.* **2010**, *1*, 72–74. [PubMed]
24. Sergiev, P.; Dontsova, O.; Berezkin, G. Theories of aging: An ever-evolving field. *Acta Nat.* **2015**, *7*, 9–18.

25. Davalli, P.; Mitic, T.; Caporali, A.; Lauriola, A.; D'Arca, D. ROS, cell senescence, and novel molecular mechanisms in aging and age-related diseases. *Oxid. Med. Cell. Longev.* **2016**, *2016*, 3565127. [CrossRef] [PubMed]

26. Yoon, H.E.; Choi, B.S. The renin-angiotensin system and aging in the kidney. *Korean J. Intern. Med.* **2014**, *29*, 291–295. [CrossRef] [PubMed]

27. Musso, C.G.; Jauregui, J.R. Renin-angiotensin-aldosterone system and the aging kidney. *Expert Rev. Endocrinol. Metab.* **2014**, *9*, 543–546. [CrossRef]

28. Benigni, A.; Cassis, P.; Remuzzi, G. Angiotensin ii revisited: New roles in inflammation, immunology and aging. *EMBO Mol. Med.* **2010**, *2*, 247–257. [CrossRef] [PubMed]

29. Diz, D.I.; Lewis, K. Dahl memorial lecture: The renin-angiotensin system and aging. *Hypertension* **2008**, *52*, 37–43. [CrossRef] [PubMed]

30. Gilliam-Davis, S.; Payne, V.S.; Kasper, S.O.; Tommasi, E.N.; Robbins, M.E.; Diz, D.I. Long-term at1 receptor blockade improves metabolic function and provides renoprotection in fischer-344 rats. *Am. J. Physiol.-Heart Circ. Physiol.* **2007**, *293*, H1327–H1333. [CrossRef] [PubMed]

31. Jiang, T.; Xue, L.-J.; Yang, Y.; Wang, Q.-G.; Xue, X.; Ou, Z.; Gao, Q.; Shi, J.-Q.; Wu, L.; Zhang, Y.-D. Ave0991, a nonpeptide analogue of ang-(1-7), attenuates aging-related neuroinflammation. *Aging* **2018**, *10*, 645. [CrossRef] [PubMed]

32. Pena Silva, R.A.; Chu, Y.; Miller, J.D.; Mitchell, I.J.; Penninger, J.M.; Faraci, F.M.; Heistad, D.D. Impact of ace2 deficiency and oxidative stress on cerebrovascular function with aging. *Stroke* **2012**, *43*, 3358–3363. [CrossRef] [PubMed]

33. Bruce, E.B.; Sakarya, Y.; Kirichenko, N.; Toklu, H.Z.; Sumners, C.; Morgan, D.; Tumer, N.; Scarpace, P.J.; Carter, C.S. Ace2 activator diminazene aceturate reduces adiposity but preserves lean mass in young and old rats. *Exp. Gerontol.* **2018**, *111*, 133–140. [CrossRef] [PubMed]

34. Weidmann, P.; De Myttenaere-Bursztein, S.; Maxwell, M.H.; de Lima, J. Effect of aging on plasma renin and aldosterone in normal man. *Kidney Int.* **1975**, *8*, 325–333. [CrossRef] [PubMed]

35. Jung, F.F.; Kennefick, T.M.; Ingelfinger, J.R.; Vora, J.P.; Anderson, S. Down-regulation of the intrarenal renin-angiotensin system in the aging rat. *J. Am. Soc. Nephrol.* **1995**, *5*, 1573–1580. [PubMed]

36. Tank, J.E.; Vora, J.P.; Houghton, D.C.; Anderson, S. Altered renal vascular responses in the aging rat kidney. *Am. J. Physiol.-Ren. Physiol.* **1994**, *266*, F942–F948. [CrossRef] [PubMed]

37. Musso, C.G.; Oreopoulos, D.G. Aging and physiological changes of the kidneys including changes in glomerular filtration rate. *Nephron Physiol.* **2011**, *119* (Suppl. 1), p1–p5. [CrossRef]

38. Dinh, Q.N.; Drummond, G.R.; Kemp-Harper, B.K.; Diep, H.; Silva, T.M.D.; Kim, H.A.; Vinh, A.; Robertson, A.A.B.; Cooper, M.A.; Mansell, A.; et al. Pressor response to angiotensin ii is enhanced in aged mice and associated with inflammation, vasoconstriction and oxidative stress. *Aging* **2017**, *9*, 1595–1605. [CrossRef] [PubMed]

39. Yoon, H.E.; Kim, E.N.; Kim, M.Y.; Lim, J.H.; Jang, I.A.; Ban, T.H.; Shin, S.J.; Park, C.W.; Chang, Y.S.; Choi, B.S. Age-associated changes in the vascular renin-angiotensin system in mice. *Oxid. Med. Cell. Longev.* **2016**, *2016*, 6731093. [CrossRef] [PubMed]

40. Labinskyy, N.; Csiszar, A.; Veress, G.; Stef, G.; Pacher, P.; Oroszi, G.; Wu, J.; Ungvari, Z. Vascular dysfunction in aging: Potential effects of resveratrol, an anti-inflammatory phytoestrogen. *Curr. Med. Chem.* **2006**, *13*, 989–996. [CrossRef] [PubMed]

41. Ichiki, T.; Miyazaki, R.; Kamiharaguchi, A.; Hashimoto, T.; Matsuura, H.; Kitamoto, S.; Tokunou, T.; Sunagawa, K. Resveratrol attenuates angiotensin ii-induced senescence of vascular smooth muscle cells. *Regul. Pept.* **2012**, *177*, 35–39. [CrossRef] [PubMed]

42. D'Onofrio, N.; Vitiello, M.; Casale, R.; Servillo, L.; Giovane, A.; Balestrieri, M.L. Sirtuins in vascular diseases: Emerging roles and therapeutic potential. *Biochim. Biophys. Acta BBA-Mol. Basis Dis.* **2015**, *1852*, 1311–1322. [CrossRef] [PubMed]

43. Kitada, M.; Kume, S.; Takeda-Watanabe, A.; Kanasaki, K.; Koya, D. Sirtuins and renal diseases: Relationship with aging and diabetic nephropathy. *Clin. Sci.* **2013**, *124*, 153–164. [CrossRef] [PubMed]

44. Hamza, S.M.; Dyck, J.R. Systemic and renal oxidative stress in the pathogenesis of hypertension: Modulation of long-term control of arterial blood pressure by resveratrol. *Front. Physiol.* **2014**, *5*, 292. [CrossRef] [PubMed]

45. Kim, Y.; Park, C.W. Adenosine monophosphate–activated protein kinase in diabetic nephropathy. *Kidney Res. Clin. Pract.* **2016**, *35*, 69–77. [CrossRef] [PubMed]

46. Miyazaki, R.; Ichiki, T.; Hashimoto, T.; Inanaga, K.; Imayama, I.; Sadoshima, J.; Sunagawa, K. Sirt1, a longevity gene, downregulates angiotensin ii type 1 receptor expression in vascular smooth muscle cells. *Arterioscler. Thromb. Vasc. Biol.* **2008**, *28*, 1263–1269. [CrossRef] [PubMed]

47. Kim, E.N.; Kim, M.Y.; Lim, J.H.; Kim, Y.; Shin, S.J.; Park, C.W.; Kim, Y.S.; Chang, Y.S.; Yoon, H.E.; Choi, B.S. The protective effect of resveratrol on vascular aging by modulation of the renin-angiotensin system. *Atherosclerosis* **2018**, *270*, 123–131. [CrossRef] [PubMed]

48. Sachse, A.; Wolf, G. Angiotensin ii–induced reactive oxygen species and the kidney. *J. Am. Soc. Nephrol.* **2007**, *18*, 2439–2446. [CrossRef] [PubMed]

49. Montezano, A.C.; Nguyen Dinh Cat, A.; Rios, F.J.; Touyz, R.M. Angiotensin ii and vascular injury. *Curr. Hypertens. Rep.* **2014**, *16*, 431. [CrossRef] [PubMed]

50. Sedeek, M.; Nasrallah, R.; Touyz, R.M.; Hebert, R.L. Nadph oxidases, reactive oxygen species, and the kidney: Friend and foe. *J. Am. Soc. Nephrol.* **2013**, *24*, 1512–1518. [CrossRef] [PubMed]

51. Gill, P.S.; Wilcox, C.S. Nadph oxidases in the kidney. *Antioxid. Redox Signal.* **2006**, *8*, 1597–1607. [CrossRef] [PubMed]

52. Oudot, A.; Vergely, C.; Ecarnot-Laubriet, A.; Rochette, L. Angiotensin ii activates nadph oxidase in isolated rat hearts subjected to ischaemia–reperfusion. *Eur. J. Pharmacol.* **2003**, *462*, 145–154. [CrossRef]

53. Garrido, A.M.; Griendling, K.K. Nadph oxidases and angiotensin ii receptor signaling. *Mol. Cell. Endocrinol.* **2009**, *302*, 148–158. [CrossRef] [PubMed]

54. Fazeli, G.; Stopper, H.; Schinzel, R.; Ni, C.W.; Jo, H.; Schupp, N. Angiotensin ii induces DNA damage via at1 receptor and nadph oxidase isoform nox4. *Mutagenesis* **2012**, *27*, 673–681. [CrossRef] [PubMed]

55. Oudot, A.; Martin, C.; Busseuil, D.; Vergely, C.; Demaison, L.; Rochette, L. Nadph oxidases are in part responsible for increased cardiovascular superoxide production during aging. *Free Radic. Biol. Med.* **2006**, *40*, 2214–2222. [CrossRef] [PubMed]

56. Nguyen Dinh Cat, A.; Montezano, A.C.; Burger, D.; Touyz, R.M. Angiotensin ii, nadph oxidase, and redox signaling in the vasculature. *Antioxid. Redox Signal.* **2013**, *19*, 1110–1120. [CrossRef] [PubMed]

57. Munzel, T.; Camici, G.G.; Maack, C.; Bonetti, N.R.; Fuster, V.; Kovacic, J.C. Impact of oxidative stress on the heart and vasculature: Part 2 of a 3-part series. *J. Am. Coll. Cardiol.* **2017**, *70*, 212–229. [CrossRef] [PubMed]

58. Lo, J.; Patel, V.B.; Wang, Z.; Levasseur, J.; Kaufman, S.; Penninger, J.M.; Oudit, G.Y. Angiotensin-converting enzyme 2 antagonizes angiotensin ii-induced pressor response and nadph oxidase activation in wistar-kyoto rats and spontaneously hypertensive rats. *Exp. Physiol.* **2013**, *98*, 109–122. [CrossRef] [PubMed]

59. Tanno, T.; Tomita, H.; Narita, I.; Kinjo, T.; Nishizaki, K.; Ichikawa, H.; Kimura, Y.; Tanaka, M.; Osanai, T.; Okumura, K. Olmesartan inhibits cardiac hypertrophy in mice overexpressing renin independently of blood pressure: Its beneficial effects on ace2/ang (1–7)/mas axis and nadph oxidase expression. *J. Cardiovasc. Pharmacol.* **2016**, *67*, 503–509. [CrossRef] [PubMed]

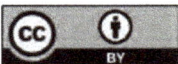

nutrients

MDPI

Article

Potential Involvement of Peripheral Leptin/STAT3 Signaling in the Effects of Resveratrol and Its Metabolites on Reducing Body Fat Accumulation

Andrea Ardid-Ruiz [1], Maria Ibars [1], Pedro Mena [2], Daniele Del Rio [3,4,5], Begoña Muguerza [1,6], Cinta Bladé [1], Lluís Arola [1,6], Gerard Aragonès [1,*] and Manuel Suárez [1]

[1] Department of Biochemistry and Biotechnology, Nutrigenomics Research Group, Universitat Rovira i Virgili, 43007 Tarragona, Spain; andrea.ardid@urv.cat (A.A.-R.); maria.ibars@urv.cat (M.I.); begona.muguerza@urv.cat (B.M.); mariacinta.blade@urv.cat (C.B.); lluis.arola@urv.cat (L.A.); manuel.suarez@urv.cat (M.S.)

[2] Department of Food and Drugs, Human Nutrition Unit, University of Parma, 43125 Parma, Italy; pedromiguel.menaparreno@unipr.it

[3] Department of Veterinary Medicine, University of Parma, 43125 Parma, Italy; daniele.delrio@unipr.it

[4] School for Advanced Studies on Food and Nutrition, University of Parma, 43125 Parma, Italy

[5] Microbiome Research Hub, University of Parma, 43125 Parma, Italy

[6] Eurecat, Centre Tecnològic de Catalunya, Unit of Nutrition and Health, 43204 Reus, Spain

* Correspondence: gerard.aragones@urv.cat; Tel.: +34-977-558-188

Received: 30 October 2018; Accepted: 12 November 2018; Published: 14 November 2018

Abstract: Bioactive compounds such as polyphenols have increased in importance in recent years, and among them, resveratrol (3,5,4′-trihydroxy-trans-stilbene) has generated great interest as an anti-obesity agent. Recent investigations have highlighted the importance of leptin signaling in lipid metabolism in peripheral organs. The aims of this study were (1) to investigate whether resveratrol can reduce fat accumulation in peripheral tissues by increasing their leptin sensitivity and (2) to identify which resveratrol-derived circulating metabolites are potentially involved in these metabolic effects. Serum leptin levels and the leptin signaling pathway were assessed in diet-induced obese rats. Moreover, serum metabolites of resveratrol were studied by ultra-high performance liquid chromatography–mass spectrometry (UHPLC-MS^n). The daily consumption of 200 mg/kg of resveratrol, but not doses of 50 and 100 mg/kg, reduced body weight and fat accumulation in obese rats and restored leptin sensitivity in the periphery. These effects were due to increases in sirtuin 1 activity in the liver, leptin receptors in muscle and protection against endoplasmic reticulum (ER)-stress in adipose tissue. In general, the resveratrol metabolites associated with these beneficial effects were derived from both phase II and microbiota metabolism, although only those derived from microbiota increased proportionally with the administered dose of resveratrol. In conclusion, resveratrol reversed leptin resistance caused by diet-induced obesity in peripheral organs using tissue-specific mechanisms.

Keywords: cafeteria diet; leptin resistance; metabolites; microbiota; obesity; sirtuin

1. Introduction

Obesity, defined by the World Health Organization (WHO) as excessive fat accumulation, has been increasing in recent decades and is now reaching epidemic proportions [1]. The increased consumption of energy-dense foods and the significant reduction of physical activity in our daily lives have led to the dysregulation of the homeostatic control of energy balance and, consequently, body weight [2]. The current options for body weight management are energy restriction and physical activity [3]. However, compliance with these treatments is frequently poor, especially in the long term, and thus they are less successful than expected [4]. In this context, the scientific community is interested in naturally occurring bioactive compounds such as polyphenols that may be useful in body weight management [5]. Among these molecules, resveratrol (3,5,4′-trihydroxy-trans-stilbene, RSV), a 14-carbon skeleton stilbene consisting of two aromatic rings with hydroxyl groups in position 3, 5, and 4′, joined by a double styrene bond, has been found to provide a wide range of benefits for many metabolic diseases, including cardiovascular and neurological protective, thermogenic, antioxidant, anti-inflammatory, antiviral and anticancer activities [6–11]. Over recent years, these properties have been widely studied in animal and human models, both in vitro and in vivo. Additionally, in most studies in rodent models of diet-induced obesity, RSV alleviated the effects of this dietary pattern [12–14]. In addition, RSV is a well-described activator of NAD^+-dependent deacetylase sirtuin 1 (SIRT1) [15] and adenosine monophosphate-(AMP)-activated protein kinase (AMPK) [16], both of which are considered metabolic sensors that act on gene expression according to the metabolic state of the cell and are closely linked with the benefits of caloric restriction [17].

Leptin, a hormone secreted mainly from white adipose tissue, is the main messenger that carries information about peripheral energy stores to the hypothalamus [18]. The interaction of leptin with its longest receptor isoform (ObRb) promotes the phosphorylation of signal transducer and activator of transcription-3 (STAT3). Subsequently, STAT3 dimerizes and translocates from the cytoplasm into the nucleus, stimulating anorexigenic factors and reducing body weight [19]. For this reason, the role of leptin in controlling energy homeostasis has thus far focused on hypothalamic receptors and neuroendocrine signaling pathways [20,21]. However, accumulating evidence indicates that leptin's effects on energy balance are also mediated by direct peripheral actions on key metabolic organs such as the liver, skeletal muscle, and adipose tissue [22]. In fact, several studies have recently indicated that peripheral leptin signaling regulates cellular lipid balance to stimulate lipolysis and fatty acid oxidation in white adipose tissues [22–24] and skeletal muscle [22,25], decrease triglyceride content and secretion rates in liver [22,26], and even suppress insulin expression and secretion in pancreatic β-cells [22]. However, leptin is unable to exert its effect during diet-induced obesity, and several molecular alterations have been associated with attenuated leptin/STAT3 signaling. These include enhanced endoplasmic reticulum stress (ER-stress) and inflammation, impaired SIRT1 activity and the overexpression of inhibitory factors such as suppressor of cytokine signaling 3 (SOCS3) and protein-tyrosine phosphatase (PTP1B) [19,27].

In this context, we previously showed that a polyphenol-rich extract from grape seeds could improve peripheral and central leptin signaling by increasing SIRT1 functionality and protecting against neuroinflammation [28]. However, to the best of our knowledge, RSV has not been previously studied for its impact on leptin signaling in these organs. Therefore, the aim of the present study was to examine whether RSV exerts part of its anti-obesity effect by modulating leptin sensitivity in the liver, skeletal muscle and adipose tissue. Thus, both serum leptin concentrations and the leptin/STAT3 signaling pathway were evaluated in diet-induced obese animals to investigate the effects of this compound in hyperleptinemic animals with impaired leptin signaling. In addition, as RSV is quickly metabolized by both phase II enzymes and gut microbiota, it was necessary to simultaneously analyze its derived circulating metabolites to obtain a better understanding of the mechanism of action of this compound.

2. Materials and Methods

2.1. Animal Handling

The study was conducted in accordance with the Declaration of Helsinki and was approved by the Ethics Review Committee for Animal Experimentation of the Universitat Rovira i Virgili (reference number 4249 by Generalitat de Catalunya). Male Wistar rats ($n = 30$; 200 ± 50 g body weight) were purchased from Charles River Laboratories (Barcelona, Spain). The animals were housed in pairs under a 12 h light-dark cycle at 22 °C, fed a standard chow diet (Panlab A04, Barcelona, Spain) ad libitum, and were provided access to tap water during the adaptation week. Then, the animals were distributed into equal groups composed of 6 rats. One group was fed a standard chow diet (STD group) with a calorie breakdown of 14% protein, 8% fat and 73% carbohydrates, while the others were fed an STD plus cafeteria diet (CAF group). The CAF diet was composed of 14% protein, 35% fat and 51% carbohydrates and consisted of bacon, carrots, cookies, foie gras, cupcakes, cheese and sugary milk. Nine weeks later, an oral treatment with RSV (Fagron Iberica, Barcelona, Spain) was administered together with the CAF diet for 22 days. The treatment groups were supplemented daily with 50, 100 or 200 mg/kg body weight of RSV dissolved in low-fat sugary milk diluted 1:1 in water. The STD and CAF diet groups were supplemented with the same quantity of vehicle (750 µL) (Figure S1, Supplemental Data). Before supplementation, all rats were trained to voluntarily lick the milk to avoid oral gavage. On the day of sacrifice, the rats received vehicle or RSV and then were fasted for 3 h before sacrifice by decapitation. Blood was collected, and the serum was obtained by centrifugation (1500× g, 4 °C and 15 min) and stored at −80 °C. Metabolic tissues such as the liver, calf skeletal muscle and epididymal and retroperitoneal white adipose tissues (eWAT and rWAT, respectively) were excised, weighed, immediately frozen in liquid nitrogen and stored at −80 °C until further analysis.

2.2. Body Weight and Composition Analysis

Body weight was monitored weekly until the end of the experiment. In addition, the day before sacrifice, total body composition in live animals was assessed by nuclear magnetic resonance (NMR) using an EchoMRI-700 system (Echo Medical Systems, Houston, TX, USA). Direct measurements of fat mass were obtained in triplicate for each animal, and the results were expressed as a percentage of total body weight.

2.3. Hormonal and Metabolic Serum Parameters

Serum glucose (Ref. #998282), total cholesterol (TC) (Ref. #995280) and triacylglycerol (TAG) (Ref. #992320) were measured by enzymatic colorimetric kits (QCA, Barcelona, Spain). Serum leptin (Ref. #EZRL-83K) and insulin (Ref. #EZRMI-13K) concentrations were measured using ELISA kits (Millipore, Madrid, Spain) according to the manufacturer's instructions.

2.4. Tissue Lipid Analysis

The total lipid content in liver, calf skeletal muscle and eWAT was extracted using the Folch method [29]. Briefly, 0.5 g of either liver or eWAT or 0.1 g of calf skeletal muscle was homogenized with 0.45% NaCl in chloroform:methanol (2:1) in an orbital shaker at 4 °C overnight. Then, the homogenate was filtered and washed with 0.45% NaCl solution and 0.9% NaCl solution. An aliquot of each extract was subjected to gravimetric analysis to measure the total lipid concentration. The remainder was allowed to evaporate under nitrogen flow, dissolved in isopropanol and stored at −80 °C until further analysis. The TAG and TC concentrations from the extracts were also measured using QCA enzymatic colorimetric kits (QCA).

2.5. Leptin Signaling Analysis

Leptin signaling in the liver, calf skeletal muscle and eWAT was assessed by calculating the activation of STAT3 using an ELISA kit (Abcam, Cambridge, UK)with a phospho-specific antibody for STAT3 phosphorylation (pSTAT3) at tyrosine 705. Briefly, 100 µL of the positive control or sample homogenate was added to wells in duplicate and incubated at room temperature for 2.5 h on an orbital microtiter plate shaker. After washing, 100 µL of the anti-pSTAT3 antibody was applied, and the plate was sealed and incubated for 1 h with shaking. After washing, 100 µL of horseradish peroxidase (HRP)-conjugated anti-rabbit IgG against rabbit anti-pSTAT3 was applied, and the plate was sealed and incubated for 1 h with shaking. Then, the wells were washed, and the 3,3′,5,5′-tetramethylbenzidine (TMB) one-step substrate reagent was incubated for 30 min in the dark. Finally, 50 µL of the stop solution was added, and the plates were immediately read at 450 nm on an microplate automatic plate reader (BioTek, Winooski, VT, USA).

2.6. Leptin Sensitivity Index

As cellular pSTAT3 levels are mainly attributable to leptin action in peripheral tissues, leptin sensitivity in the liver, calf skeletal muscle and eWAT was objectively estimated as the ratio of pSTAT3 levels in each tissue to the leptin concentration in serum.

2.7. qRT-PCR Analysis

Total RNA was extracted from the liver, calf skeletal muscle and eWAT using TRIzol LS Reagent (Thermo Fisher, Madrid, Spain) and RNeasy Mini Kit (Qiagen, Madrid, Spain) according to the manufacturers' protocols. The quantity and purity of RNA were measured using a NanoDrop 1000 Spectrophotometer (Thermo Scientific, Madrid, Spain). Only samples with an adequate RNA concentration (A260/A280 $\geq$ 1.8) and purity (A230/A260 $\geq$ 2.0) were selected for reverse transcription. Complementary DNA (cDNA) was generated using the High-Capacity cDNA Reverse Transcription Kit (Thermo Fisher), and 10 ng was subjected to quantitative PCR (qPCR) with iTaq Universal SYBR Green Supermix (Bio-Rad, Barcelona, Spain) using the 7900HT Real-Time PCR system (Applied Biosystems, Foster City, CA, USA). The thermal profile settings were 50 °C for 2 min, 95 °C for 2 min, and then 40 cycles at 95 °C for 15 s and 60 °C for 2 min. The forward (FW) and reverse (RV) primers used in this study were obtained from Biomers.net (Ulm, Germany) and can be found in Table S1 in the Supplemental Data. A cycle threshold (Ct) value was generated by setting the threshold during the geometric phase of the cDNA sample amplification. The relative expression of each gene was calculated by referring to cyclophilin peptidylprolyl isomerase A (*Ppia*) mRNA levels and normalized to the STD group. The ΔΔCt method was used and corrected for primer efficiency [30]. Only samples with a quantification cycle lower than 35 were used for fold change calculation.

2.8. Western Blot Analysis

Protein levels of the ObRb leptin receptor isoform in the liver, calf skeletal muscle and eWAT were determined by western blot analysis. Tissues were homogenized at 4 °C in 800–1000 µL of radio-immunoprecipitation assay (RIPA) lysis buffer (100 mM Tris-HCl and 300 mM NaCl pH 7.4, 10% Tween, 10% Na-Deox) containing protease and phosphatase inhibitor cocktails using a TissueLyser LT (Qiagen, Madrid, Spain). The homogenate was incubated for 30 min at 4 °C and then centrifuged at $12,000 \times g$ for 20 min at 4 °C. The supernatant was placed in fresh tubes and used to determine total protein and for immunoblotting analyses. The total protein content of the supernatant was measured using the Pierce bicinchoninic acid assay (BCA) protein assay kit (Thermo Scientific, Madrid, Spain). Samples were denatured by mixing with loading buffer solution (Tris-HCl 0.5 M pH 6.8, glycerol, sodium dodecyl sulfate (SDS), β-mercaptoethanol and Bromophenol Blue) and then heated at 99 °C for 5 min in a thermocycler (Multigen Labnet, Barcelona, Spain). Acrylamide gels were prepared using TGX Fast Cast Acrylamide Kit(Bio-Rad, Barcelona, Spain), and 25 µg of protein was subjected to SDS-polyacrylamide gel electrophoresis (PAGE) in electrophoresis buffer (glycine 192 mM, Tris base 25 mM and 1% SDS). Proteins were electrotransferred onto supported polyvinylidene difluoride (PVDF) membranes (Trans-Blot Turbo Mini PVDF Transfer Packs, Bio-Rad). After blocking with 5% non-fat dried milk, the membranes were incubated with gentle agitation overnight at 4 °C with a specific antibody for ObRb (ab177469, Abcam, Cambridge, UK) diluted 1:1000. For β-actin analysis as a loading control, membranes were incubated with a rabbit anti-actin primary antibody (A2066, Sigma-Aldrich, Madrid, Spain) diluted 1:1000. Finally, membranes were incubated with anti-rabbit horseradish peroxidase secondary antibody (NA9344, GE Healthcare, Barcelona, Spain) diluted 1:10,000. Protein levels were detected with the chemiluminescent detection reagent ECL Select (GE Healthcare, Barcelona, Spain) and GeneSys image acquisition software (G:Box series, Syngene, Barcelona, Spain). The protein bands were quantitated by densitometry using ImageJ software (W.S Rasband, Bethesda, MD, USA), and each band was normalized by the corresponding β-actin band, and finally, the treatment groups were normalized by the STD group.

2.9. SIRT1 Activity Assay

The SIRT1 activity in liver, calf skeletal muscles and eWAT was determined using a SIRT1 direct fluorescent screening assay kit (Cayman, Ann Arbor, MI, USA) as previously described [31]. Briefly, a total of 25 µL of assay buffer (50 mM Tris-HCl, pH 8.0, containing 137 mM NaCl, 2.7 mM KCl, and 1 mM MgCl$_2$), 5 µL of tissue extract (1.5 mg/mL), and 15 µL of substrate (Arg-His-Lys-Lys(ε-acetyl)–7-amino-4-methylcoumarin) solution were added to all wells. The fluorescence intensity was monitored every 2 min for 1 h using a BertholdTech TriStar2S fluorescence plate reader (Berthold Technologies, Bad Wildbad, Germany) at an excitation wavelength of 355 nm and an emission wavelength of 460 nm. The results were expressed as the rate of reaction for the first 30 min, when there was a linear relationship between fluorescence and time.

2.10. Resveratrol Metabolite Extraction from Serum Samples

Serum samples were extracted as previously reported by Savi et al. [32] with minor modifications. Briefly, 300 µL of serum was diluted with 1 mL of acidified acetonitrile (2% formic acid, Sigma-Aldrich, Madrid, Spain). The samples were vortexed vigorously, ultrasonicated for 10 min, and centrifuged at 12,000 rpm for 5 min. Then, the supernatant was dried under vacuum by rotary evaporation, and the pellet was suspended in 100 µL of methanol 50% (*v*/*v*) acidified with formic acid 0.1% (*v*/*v*) and centrifuged at 12,000 rpm for 5 min prior to analysis by ultra-high performance liquid chromatography–mass spectrometry (UHPLC-MS).

2.11. UHPLC-MS^n Analysis

Samples were analyzed by an Accela UHPLC 1250 coupled to a linear ion trap-mass spectrometer (LTQ XL, Thermo Fisher Scientific Inc., San Jose, CA, USA) fitted with a heated-electrospray ionization source (H-ESI-II; Thermo Fisher Scientific Inc., Madrid, Spain). The chromatographic and ionization parameters for the analysis of the samples were set as previously described [33]. Metabolite identification was performed by comparing the retention time with authentic standards and/or MS^n fragmentation patterns in negative ionization mode (Table S2 in Supplemental Data). The glucuronide forms of RSV and dihydroresveratrol (DRSV) were fragmented using a collision-induced dissociation (CID) value of 16 (arbitrary units), whereas aglycones and sulfate conjugates required CID values of 34 and 23, respectively. Pure helium gas was used for CID. Data processing was performed using Xcalibur software from Thermo Scientific (Madrid, Spain). Quantification was performed using specific MS2 full scans and calibration curves of pure standards in the case of RSV, resveratrol-3-sulfate (R3S), resveratrol-4′-sulfate (R4S), resveratrol-3-glucuronide (R3G) and DRSV. Calibration curves were prepared, in the range of expected concentrations, by supplementation with known concentrations of available standards. When a standard was not available, the conjugated metabolites were quantified based on the most structurally similar compound and expressed as their equivalents. All of them were quantified using a nine-point calibration curve which ranged from 0.1 to 100 µM. Spiked samples were extracted and subsequently analysed by using the same procedure as the serum samples. The calibration curves were finally generated for each standard by plotting the peak abundance versus the concentration and fitting to a linear regression. Quality parameters were determined to validate and evaluate the suitability of the developed quantitative method as was done previously [33].

2.12. Statistical Analysis

The data are expressed as the means ± standard errors of the means (SEM). Groups were compared by Student's *t*-test or two-way ANOVA and Bonferroni's test. Outliers were determined by Grubbs' test. MetaboAnalyst (Xia Lab, McGill University, Montréal, Quebec, Canada) was used to perform multivariate statistical analyses. Correlation analysis was performed using the nonparametric Spearman test. Statistical analyses were performed using XLSTAT 2017 (Addinsoft, Paris, France). Graphics were prepared using GraphPad Prism 6 (GraphPad Software, San Diego, CA, USA). $p < 0.05$ was considered statistically significant, and $p < 0.1$ was considered to indicate a tendency.

3. Results

3.1. RSV Attenuates Diet-Induced Body Fat Increase, Hypertriglyceridemia and Hyperleptinemia

The CAF diet for 12 weeks consistently resulted in obesity, as indicated by the significantly higher body weight gain (50.1% higher) and total body fat mass (124.3% higher, assessed by NMR scanning) compared to the STD group. Notably, the body weight gain was 17% lower in animals supplemented with RSV at 200 mg/kg daily compared to the CAF group (Figure 1A), and this reduction was associated with a significant decrease in total body fat mass (Figure 1B). Notably, at this dose, no differences were found among groups in food intake (data not shown). Importantly, the consumption of 200 mg/kg of RSV partially reversed the hyperleptinemia induced by CAF diet (40.1% lower) (Figure 1C), reinforcing the robust metabolic correlation between leptin levels and total body fat mass in our experimental model ($\rho = 0.93$, $p < 0.05$). In addition, at this dose, RSV was also effective in normalizing serum concentrations of TAG, glucose and insulin in a fasting state (Figure 1D–F), indicating that RSV has an insulin-sensitizing effect in diet-induced obesity. By contrast, the daily consumption of 50 and 100 mg/kg of RSV for 22 days did not exert any beneficial effects with respect to body weight, total body fat accumulation and hormonal and metabolic serum parameters.

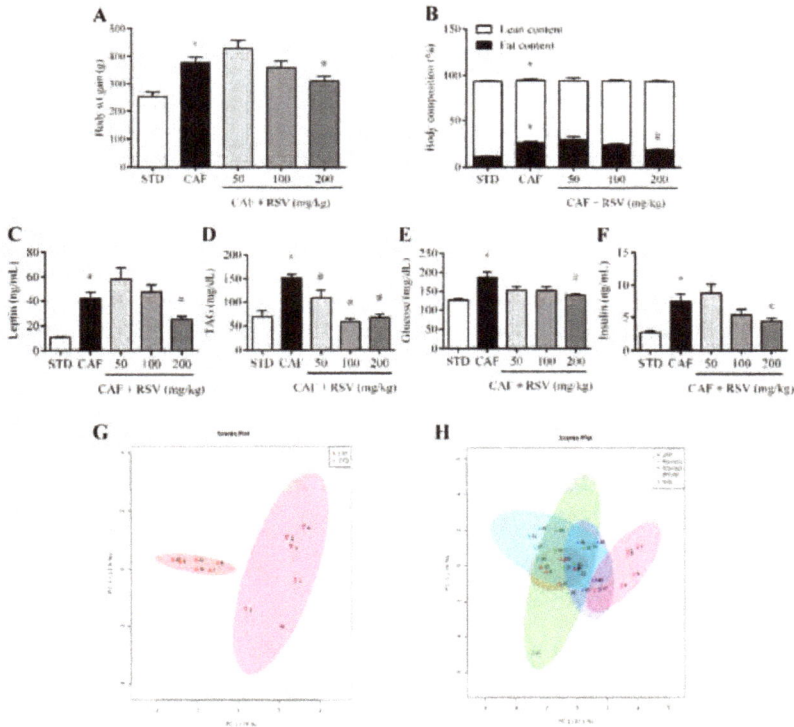

Figure 1. Metabolic parameters. The rats were fed the STD or CAF diet for 9 weeks. Then, the rats in the STD and CAF groups were treated orally with RSV (50, 100 or 200 mg per kg of body weight) or vehicle for 3 weeks. (**A**) Body weight gain (g) from the first day of the experiment until the last day; (**B**) Body composition (%) assessed by NMR, including fat and lean content; Serological levels of (**C**) leptin, (**D**) TAG, (**E**) glucose and (**F**) insulin. (**G**) and (**H**) are PCAs representing the clusters between the different groups according to the studied biometric parameters. Data are expressed as the mean ± SEM, $n = 6$. * denotes $p < 0.05$, Student's *t*-test comparing the CAF group to the STD group. # denotes $p < 0.05$ and $^\varepsilon$ $p < 0.1$, Student's *t*-test comparing the RSV group to the CAF group. CAF: cafeteria diet; NMR: nuclear magnetic resonance; RSV: resveratrol; STD: standard chow diet; TAG: triacylglycerol.

3.2. Multivariate Analysis Shows That RSV Partially Reverses the Metabolic Alterations Induced by the Cafeteria Diet

To further evaluate the effect of RSV from a multivariate point of view, principal component analysis (PCA) was performed to analyze globally the distribution of animals among all anthropometric, metabolic and biochemical variables. Accordingly, the PCA score plot for the STD and CAF groups accounted for 91.6% of the variance of the original matrix, and each animal was clearly clustered according to their diet (Figure 1G). In addition, when the multivariate analysis was used to evaluate the effect of RSV consumption on diet-induced obesity, we observed that animals treated at doses of 50 and 100 mg/kg could not be clustered separately with respect to CAF animals, and only animals daily supplemented at a dose of 200 mg/kg were clustered in an intermediate position between the CAF and STD groups, indicating that RSV at this dose could exert a tendency to reverse the metabolic alterations induced by an obesogenic diet and a return to the basal situation (Figure 1H).

3.3. RSV Decreases Diet-Induced Lipid Content in Liver, Skeletal Muscle and Adipose Tissues

To assess the contribution of visceral fat accumulation to the decrease in total body fat mass, we next evaluated the effect of RSV on fat deposition in three important metabolic peripheral tissues: visceral white adipose tissue, liver and skeletal muscle. Again, the CAF diet for 12 weeks resulted in a significant increase in two different visceral WAT depots compared to the STD group, including eWAT (18.6 ± 1.4 vs. 8.9 ± 0.9 g, respectively) and retroperitoneal WAT (rWAT, 8.4 ± 0.9 vs. 3.6 ± 0.1 g, respectively). Notably, at a dose of 200 mg/kg, RSV elicited a significant decrease in the weights of these depots compared with CAF animals, and this effect was more evident in eWAT (14.6 ± 1.4 g, 21% lower) than in rWAT (7.1 ± 0.7 g, 16% lower). In addition, RSV also tended to reduce the total fat content in eWAT (Figure 2A) and significantly in the liver (Figure 2B), but above all in the skeletal muscle, although not in a dose-dependent manner (Figure 2C). Interestingly, this decrease in fat depots in peripheral organs was directly associated with significant reductions of both cholesterol and TAG content (Table S3, Supplemental Data), and in turn, it was positively and significantly related to serum leptin levels in the liver ($\rho = 0.54$, $p < 0.05$) and eWAT ($\rho = 0.43$, $p < 0.05$ in eWAT), implicating leptin in the regulation of lipid metabolism in peripheral tissues.

3.4. RSV Directly Down-Regulates Leptin Transcription in Adipose Tissues

To further examine the mechanism by which RSV regulates lipid accumulation in peripheral tissues, we assessed the gene expression of lipid-regulating enzymes by RT-qPCR in the liver, skeletal muscle and eWAT. Completely contrary to our expectations, we found that the expression levels of genes involved in lipogenesis but not fatty acid oxidation, such as *Acc*, *Scd1* and *Fas*, were significantly increased in the liver of animals supplemented with 50 and 100 mg/kg of RSV (Figure 2D). By contrast, no significant changes were observed in the expression of genes encoding enzymes for lipogenesis, whereas RSV down-regulated fatty acid oxidation in eWAT (Figure 2E). Moreover, we did not observe any significant changes in thermogenesis, mitochondrial biogenesis and fatty acid oxidation in skeletal muscle (Figure 2F). Importantly, in eWAT and rWAT, at a dose of 200 mg/kg, RSV consumption tended to down-regulate leptin mRNA levels compared with CAF animals (Figure 2G,H), indicating that animals undergoing RSV treatment more efficiently regulated leptin production and secretion in these tissues than those in the CAF group.

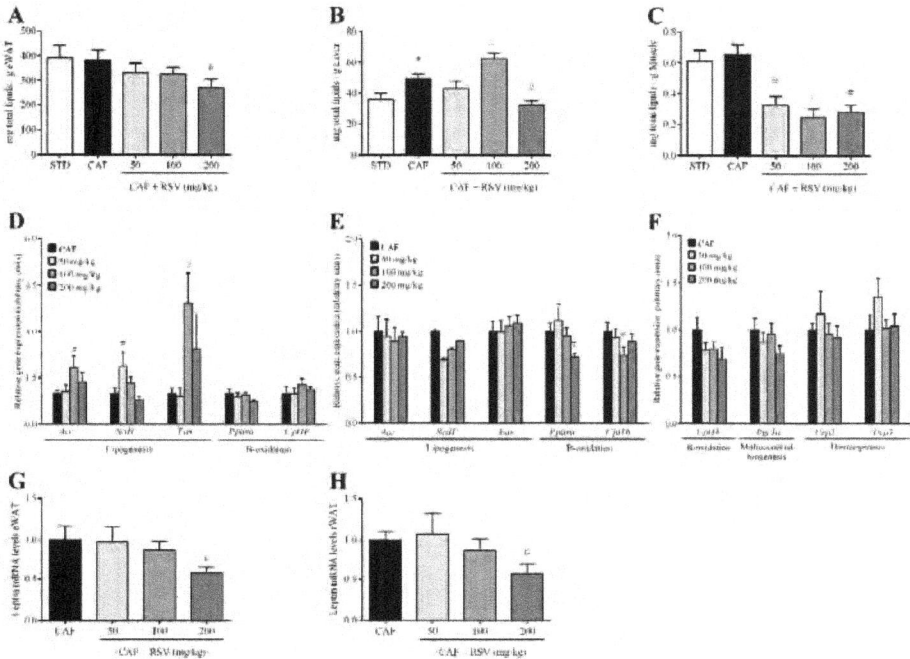

Figure 2. Lipid profile. The rats were fed the STD or CAF diet for 9 weeks. Then, the rats in the STD and CAF groups were treated orally with RSV (50, 100 or 200 mg per kg of body weight) for 3 weeks. Total lipids in (**A**) eWAT, (**B**) liver and (**C**) calf skeletal muscle in mg for each g of tissue. (**D**) Expression in the liver of genes related to lipogenesis (*Acc*, *Scd1* and *Fas*) and β-oxidation (*Ppara* and *Cpt1b*). (**E**) Expression in eWAT of genes related to lipogenesis (*Acc*, *Scd1* and *Fas*) and β-oxidation (*Ppara* and *Cpt1b*). (**F**) Expression in calf skeletal muscle of genes related to β-oxidation (*Cpt1b*), mitochondrial biogenesis (*Pgc1a*) and thermogenesis (*Ucp2* and *Ucp3*). Leptin gene expression in (**G**) eWAT and (**H**) rWAT. Data are expressed as the mean ± SEM, n = 6. * denotes p < 0.05, Student's t-test comparing the CAF group to the STD group. # indicates p < 0.05 and ε p < 0.1, Student's t-test comparing the RSV group to the CAF group. CAF: cafeteria diet; eWAT: epididymal white adipose tissue; RSV: resveratrol; rWAT: retroperitoneal white adipose tissue; STD: standard chow diet. *Acc* (acetyl-CoA carboxylase); *Cpt1b* (carnitine palmitoyltransferase 1b); *Fas* (fatty acid synthase); *Pgc1a* (peroxisome proliferator-activated receptor gamma coactivator 1-alpha), *Ppara* (peroxisome proliferator activated receptor alpha); *Scd1* (stearoyl-CoA desaturase 1); *Ucp2* (mitochondrial uncoupling protein 2); *Ucp3* (mitochondrial uncoupling protein 3).

3.5. RSV Potentiates Leptin Sensitivity in Liver, Skeletal Muscle and Adipose Tissue

To determine if the observed decreases in leptin production and circulating levels could indicate that RSV directly affects leptin signaling in peripheral tissues, we assessed leptin sensitivity in liver, skeletal muscle and eWAT by detecting STAT3 activation (pSTAT3). Because pSTAT3 levels are mainly attributable to leptin action in theses tissues, we assessed the ratio of tissue-specific levels of pSTAT3 to the circulating leptin concentration to estimate the degree of sensitivity of each tissue to this hormone. In this context, the leptin sensitivity of CAF animals was significantly reduced compared to the STD group in all three tissues studied, and importantly, when RSV was administered at dose of 200 mg/kg, the leptin sensitivity significantly increased to basal levels, indicating partial reversion of the situation observed in CAF animals (Figure 3A). By contrast, no significant effects on leptin sensitivity were observed at lower doses in any of the tissues assessed.

135

Next, we studied the gene expression levels of Socs3 and Ptp1b, negative feedback regulatory molecules involved in leptin signaling, by qRT-PCR. However, *Socs3* and *Ptp1b* mRNA levels were not significantly altered by RSV consumption (Figure S2, Supplemental Data). Finally, we also investigated the impact of RSV on two metabolic processes closely associated with leptin signaling disruption: local inflammation and ER stress. However, *iNos* mRNA expression levels were not significantly regulated in any tissue (Figure S3, Supplemental Data). In a similar manner, in liver and muscle, transcripts related to ER stress were not modulated in any group of animals undergoing RSV supplementation (Figure S4, Supplemental Data). Interestingly, a significant decrease in ER-stress markers was observed in eWAT in animals under the highest dose of RSV (Figure 3B).

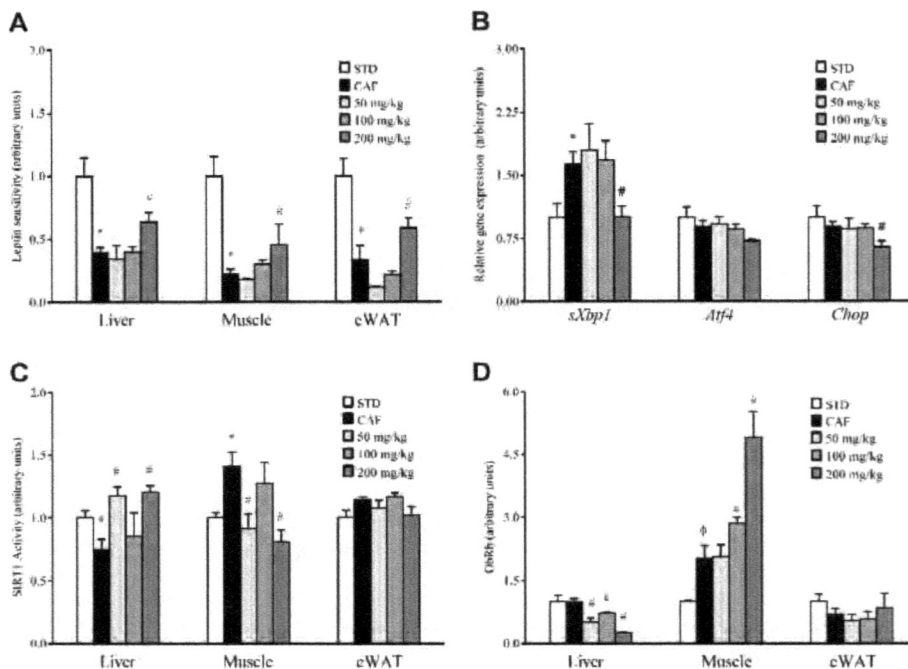

Figure 3. Leptin sensitivity and signaling. The rats were fed the STD or CAF diet for 9 weeks. Then, the STD and CAF rats were treated orally with RSV (50, 100 or 200 mg per kg of body wt) or vehicle for 3 weeks. (**A**) The leptin sensitivity index. (**B**) Gene expression of ER-stress markers in eWAT. (**C**) SIRT1 activity. (**D**) WB results for ObRb. Data are expressed as the mean ± SEM, $n = 6$. * $p < 0.05$ and $^\varphi$ $p < 0.1$, Student's *t*-test comparing the CAF group with the STD group. # $p < 0.05$ and $^\varepsilon$ $p < 0.1$, Student's *t*-test comparing the RSV group with the CAF group. CAF: cafeteria diet; ER: endoplasmic reticulum; eWAT: epididymal white adipose tissue; LSI: leptin sensitivity index; ObRb: leptin receptor isoform b; RSV: resveratrol; SIRT1: NAD$^+$-dependent deacetylase sirtuin-1; STD: standard chow diet; VH: vehicle; WB: western blot; wt: weight. *Atf4* (activating transcription factor 4), *Chop* (DNA damage inducible transcript 3), s*Xbp1* (spliced x-box binding protein 1).

3.6. RSV Distinctively Modulates Sirtuin-1 (SIRT1) Activity and Leptin Receptor (ObRb) Protein Expression in Peripheral Tissues

To elucidate the molecular mechanisms by which RSV potentially rescues leptin sensitivity in these tissues, we next evaluated whether RSV consumption could result in enhanced SIRT1 functionality, which could be an additional mechanism involved in the regulation of leptin signal transduction in the periphery. Thus, we analyzed the deacetylase activity of SIRT1 in liver, skeletal muscle and eWAT

(Figure 3C). Notably, robust activation of SIRT1 was observed in the liver of animals supplemented with 50 and 200 mg/kg of RSV, indicating that a relatively low dose of RSV (50 mg/kg) is sufficient to efficiently activate this enzyme in the liver. By contrast, at these same doses, SIRT1 activity was notably decreased in skeletal muscle and was not significantly affected in eWAT, suggesting that if RSV is a true leptin sensitizer, this activity is not mediated by an increase in SIRT1 functionality in skeletal muscle and eWAT. Therefore, we also investigated by immunoblotting whether the modulation of leptin sensitivity in these tissues could also be directly mediated by increasing the cell content of the long leptin receptor isoform ObRb (Figure 3D). Interestingly, the consumption of RSV resulted in a dose-dependent significant increase in ObRb protein levels in skeletal muscle, although statistically significant differences were only observed at a dose of 200 mg/kg. Importantly, in contrast to skeletal muscle, ObRb protein levels in liver were decreased significantly in animals under RSV at doses of 50 and 200 mg/kg, whereas in eWAT, ObRb protein levels were not significantly affected at any dose. These results indicate that RSV can modulate different cellular processes in a tissue-specific manner.

3.7. Different RSV Metabolites, Including Microbial and Phase II Conjugates, Could Explain the Body Fat-Lowering Effects of RSV Consumption

Since the efficacy of orally administered RSV depends on its absorption and metabolism, we next investigated whether RSV and its metabolites found in the bloodstream can account for the observed anti-obesity effects after the daily consumption of RSV for 22 days. Table 1 details the serum concentrations of each metabolite of RSV. The administration of RSV at 50, 100 and 200 mg/kg led to high serum concentrations of some metabolites, in the range of μM. Interestingly, 10 different RSV-derived metabolites, but not the parent compound, were detected in serum 3 h after the last RSV treatment. These metabolites included seven phase II metabolites of RSV (R3G, R4G, RDG, R3S, R4S, RDS and RSG) and three gut microbiota-derived metabolites, including the glucuronide and sulfate conjugates of DRSV (DRG, DRS and DRGS). When the serum distribution of these two types of metabolites was analyzed, phase II RSV metabolites were found to be predominant over DRSV metabolites derived from microbiota by more than two fold (Figure 4A). Interestingly, the concentration of microbial DRSV metabolites significantly increased at a dose of 200 mg/kg, whereas the opposite occurred for phase II RSV metabolites. Thus, the largest circulating levels of microbial metabolites were found at the highest dose of 200 mg/kg. In addition, total glucuronide metabolites (R3G, R4G, RDG and DRG) were also detected in higher levels than total sulfate conjugates (R3S, R4S, RDS and DRS) at all doses (Figure 4B). However, the concentration of glucuronide conjugates tended to decrease when the RSV dosage was increased, whereas sulfate metabolites significantly increased at doses of 100 and 200 mg/kg.

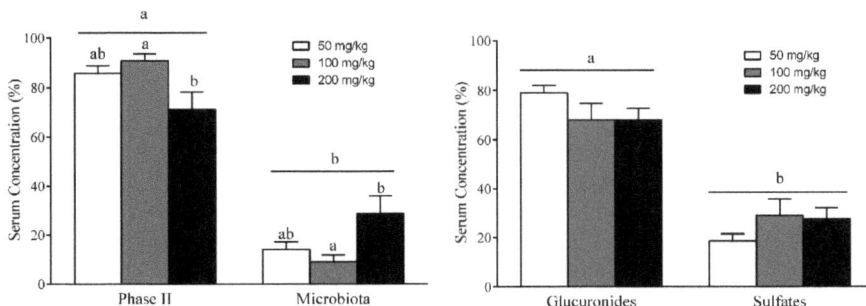

Figure 4. Serum resveratrol metabolites. The rats were fed the STD or CAF diet for 9 weeks. Then, the STD and CAF rats were treated orally with RSV (50, 100 or 200 mg per kg of body wt) or vehicle for 3 weeks. The metabolites present in serum were classified as (**A**) phase II RSV metabolites or microbial metabolites and as (**B**) glucuronide or sulfate metabolites. Data are expressed as the mean ± SEM, *n* = 6. [a,b] denote significant differences between groups ($p < 0.05$; two-way ANOVA and Bonferroni's test).

Table 1. The results obtained for each metabolite (μM) present in serum respect each group of rats treated with RSV.

RSV Metabolites (μM)		50 mg/Kg	100 mg/Kg	200 mg/Kg
Phase II	R4G	18.52 ± 4.54	15.45 ± 1.69	20.53 ± 7.73
	R3G	12.44 ± 4.85	8.43 ± 3.79	1.84 ± 0.61 *
	RDG	0.19 ± 0.04	0.29 ± 0.09	0.23 ± 0.04
	R4S	0.12 ± 0.02	0.16 ± 0.05	0.27 ± 0.09
	R3S	7.06 ± 2.66	5.69 ± 1.21	5.59 ± 2.04
	RDS	0.80 ± 0.31	1.39 ± 0.31	0.66 ± 0.09
	RSG	0.83 ± 0.15	1.00 ± 0.14	0.83 ± 0.21
Microbiota	DRG	3.95 ± 0.60	2.72 ± 0.66	9.43 ± 2.28 *
	DRS	1.15 ± 0.46	1.24 ± 0.63	3.92 ± 1.30
	DRSG	0.11 ± 0.02	0.15 ± 0.04	0.21 ± 0.06

Abbreviations: R4G: resveratrol-4′-glucuronide; R3G: resveratrol-3-glucuronide; R3S: resveratrol-3-sulfate; R4S: resveratrol-4′-sulfate; RDS: resveratrol-disulfate; RDG: resveratrol-diglucoronide; RSG: resveratrol-sulfate-glucuronide; DRG: dihydroresveratrol-glucuronide; DRS: dihydroresveratrol-sulfate; DRSG: dihydroresveratrol-sulfate-glucuronide. * $p < 0.05$.

Finally, to determine which blood RSV metabolites could potentially be involved in the anti-obesity effects of RSV, we used the Spearman's correlation test to evaluate the relationship of RSV metabolites with body and fat mass as well as with leptin sensitivity in each peripheral tissue (Table S4, Supplemental Data). R4G and R3S were the only phase II RSV metabolites that showed significant and negative correlations with total body fat mass ($\rho = -0.67$ and -0.76, $p = 0.033$ and 0.011, respectively) and circulating leptin levels ($\rho = -0.66$ and -0.60, $p = 0.038$ and 0.067, respectively). In addition, R4G was also positively associated with leptin sensitivity in liver ($\rho = 0.72$, $p = 0.03$), skeletal muscle ($\rho = 0.69$, $p = 0.05$) and adipose tissue ($\rho = 0.79$, $p = 0.021$), whereas R4S was positively associated with leptin sensitivity in skeletal muscle ($\rho = 0.81$, $p = 0.015$) and adipose tissue ($\rho = 0.79$, $p = 0.021$). When the correlation coefficients were analyzed for the microbial DRSV metabolites, only DRSG presented a negative and significant correlation with diet-induced body weight increase ($\rho = 0.66$, $p = 0.038$). In addition, DRSG was related to leptin sensitivity in skeletal muscle ($\rho = 0.81$, $p = 0.015$) and adipose tissue ($\rho = 0.71$, $p = 0.047$), whereas DRS was related to leptin sensitivity in skeletal muscle ($\varrho = 0.69$, $p = 0.05$).

4. Discussion

Previous studies by our group indicated that chronic consumption of grape-seed proanthocyanidins for three weeks by diet-induced obese rats significantly decreased both hepatic fat content and circulating plasmatic leptin levels, presumably by restoring SIRT1 functionality and leptin signaling in both the hypothalamus and liver [28,31]. Nonetheless, studies of other compounds with complementary or more powerful effects are necessary to combat metabolic diseases associated with leptin dysfunction, such as obesity. Accordingly, in the present study, we demonstrated that RSV, a dietary non-flavonoid polyphenol found in grapes and red wine, decreased body fat mass and leptinemia by restoring leptin sensitivity in the liver, skeletal muscle and adipose tissue.

Leptin is a pleiotropic hormone with a variety of functions within the organism and activity in different tissues. Liver and skeletal muscle are the tissues with greatest metabolic activity and, together with adipose tissue, constitute important targets for the leptin regulation of lipid metabolism [34,35]. However, pathological states such as obesity have been related to peripheral leptin resistance development, and dietary components have been proposed to modulate leptin actions in these peripheral tissues, suggesting that leptin resistance may also result from specific nutrient intake [36,37]. In this sense, our CAF-induced obesity rat model exhibited body weight/fat increase, hyperleptinemia and peripheral leptin resistance as indicated by the impairment of leptin-induced STAT3 phosphorylation in these tissues. pSTAT3 levels are widely studied to evaluate leptin sensitivity as STAT3 is proportionally activated by leptin concentrations in these tissues [38].

Remarkably, our results showed an ability of RSV at 200 mg/kg to normalize tissue fat content and leptin expression and secretion as well as to enhance peripheral leptin sensitivity, highlighting the overall beneficial effect of RSV in the modulation of diet-induced obesity at this dose. Conversely, RSV did not regulate the gene expression of enzymes directly involved in peripheral lipid metabolism, such as *Acc*, *Fas*, *Cpt1b* and *Scd1*. Nevertheless, other possibilities cannot be discarded, such as that RSV could regulate the proteins involved in fatty acid oxidation by post-transcriptional mechanisms that are not detectable by qRT-PCR analysis, or that RSV could induce lipid oxidation in tissues other than those examined in this study. Alternatively, RSV could also induce the catabolism of fatty acids to ketone bodies as previously suggested in $Csb^{m/m}$ mice fed a standard diet supplemented with 100 mg/kg$_{chow}$ RSV ad libitum [39]. In addition, RSV did not down-regulate the gene expression of relevant enzymes involved in leptin signaling, such as Socs3 and Ptp1b. Contradictory results have been published about the effect of RSV on these markers of leptin signaling in different tissues [40–42], indicating that the duration of the treatment and the grade of obesity achieved can directly influence the effect of RSV in these tissues.

The daily consumption of 50 and 100 mg/kg of RSV for 22 days in combination with the CAF diet did not change any metabolic parameter or leptin sensitivity in our experimental model. Some contradictory results have been published about the effectiveness of RSV on metabolic alterations in rodents. Andrade et al. reported that the consumption of 30 mg/kg of RSV by FVN/N mice for 60 days in combination with a CAF-rich diet exerted beneficial effects on body fat and weight [43]. By contrast, supplementation of diet-induced obese C57BL/6J mice with 22.5 and 45 mg/kg of RSV for 12 weeks [44] or 200 mg/kg for 20 weeks [45] did not cause any significant change in body weight, indicating that the effect of RSV in rodents might depend on the treatment length, RSV dosage and the percentage of fat present in the diet. In our study, the impact of the CAF diet was too robust, as the lowest doses of RSV administered could not counteract the diet-induced dysregulation of lipid metabolism and leptin signaling.

Other mechanisms have been proposed to explain the effects of phenolic compounds on body weight in mammals, including their inhibitory effects on food intake and fat absorption as well as on intestinal permeability and gut microbiota. However, as we did not evaluate the effect of RSV on all of these mechanisms, we cannot be completely sure that the consumption of this compound exclusively prevents fat accumulation through the leptin signaling activation in peripheral tissues. Thus, more studies are needed that elucidate the molecular mechanisms involved in this beneficial effect.

The induction of peripheral leptin resistance in diet-induced models has been primarily attributed to the induction of pro-inflammatory signaling and ER stress [27]. However, in this study, we did not find significant differences in inflammatory status in any of the three tissues studied as indicated by the *iNos* gene expression levels, but important anti-inflammatory effects of RSV in these animals cannot be excluded. In this sense, in contrast to our results, Kimbrough et al. observed the down-regulation of *iNos* by RSV in hepatocytes in an inflammatory experimental model [46], as did Centeno-Baez et al. in muscle and WAT in lipopolysaccharide (LPS)-treated C57BL6 mice [47]. Conversely, our results showed a significant reduction of *sXBP1* gene expression in adipose tissue, suggesting that this local decrease in ER stress in adipocytes is one of the mechanisms by which RSV re-establishes appropriate leptin sensitivity in this tissue. In addition, SIRT1 functionality and ObRb levels have been highlighted as mediators of leptin action in peripheral organs. Thus, both the overexpression of *Sirt1* in the liver and the enhanced *ObRb* protein content in skeletal muscle induced by RSV could be mechanisms by which this compound increases leptin signaling in these tissues. In fact, this beneficial effect of RSV on SIRT1 activity in the liver is in accordance with a previous report [48]. However, the different responses of the liver, muscle and adipose to RSV suggest different functions of SIRT1 and ObRb in peripheral tissues, and thus further studies are required to clarify the molecular mechanism by which RSV regulates leptin signaling in each tissue under obesogenic conditions.

The efficacy of orally administered RSV depends on its absorption and metabolism. RSV is quickly absorbed in the intestine via simple intestinal transepithelial transport and by ATP-dependent binding cassette transporters, but most RSV undergoes rapid and extensive phase II metabolism in enterocytes before entering the blood and further into the liver [49,50]. Accordingly, RSV is mainly converted into glucuronide and sulfate metabolites. Interestingly, in the present study, we detected RSV metabolites but not RSV. Our results are in line with some previously published findings of RSV metabolites but not free RSV in different peripheral tissues when rats were supplemented with 300 [51] or 60 mg/kg [52]. In addition, total glucuronide RSV metabolites (R3G, R4G and RDG) were also detected in higher levels than total sulfate RSV conjugates (R3S, R4S and RDS) at all doses. Similarly, in a previous study using male Sprague–Dawley rats, Marier et al. observed 46 times more glucuronidated forms in plasma than other metabolites 4 h after oral administration of 50 mg/kg of RSV [53]. However, other researchers have reported that the sulfate forms were prevalent over glucuronides in male Wistar rats orally supplemented with 300 mg/kg of RSV for 8 weeks, whereas no RSV conjugates were detected in the group with a dose of 50 mg/kg [51].

Notably, in our study, the concentration of glucuronide RSV conjugates tended to decrease as the RSV dosage increased, whereas the sulfate RSV metabolites increased at the highest doses. Similarly, Andres-Lacueva et al. observed that as the dose of RSV in rats increased (6, 30 and 60 mg/kg/day for 6 weeks), there was an increase in the sulfate forms compared with the glucuronides [52]. These results may suggest that glucuronidation but not sulfation could be a saturable metabolic pathway, at least in the range of doses used in the present study. Nevertheless, the potential degradation of glucuronide metabolites cannot be discarded. Consequently, further studies are needed to better elucidate this issue.

Only a few studies have considered the determination of RSV-derived microbial metabolites after RSV consumption. Consequently, we also assessed DRSV concentrations in serum in free form or as glucuronide and sulfate conjugates. Notably, in our study, the largest circulating levels of microbial metabolites were found at the highest dose of 200 mg/kg. These data could provide a clue to explain the protective effects on body fat accumulation and leptin sensitivity observed only at this dose of RSV. In fact, our results showed negative correlations of levels of DRSG metabolites from microbiota with body fat mass, circulating leptin levels and body weight gain. However, the levels of most of these DRSV metabolites detected in serum were low in comparison to RSV metabolites, and thus it is difficult to understand how they contributed to the effects observed. In addition, some studies also showed that, in 3T3-L1 cells, R3S, R3G and R4G decreased both mRNA and leptin secretion [54], increased the expression of Atgl, Cpt1, Sirt1 and Pgc1a, and decreased the expression of Fas [55]. Consequently, more studies are needed to explain the in vivo effects induced by this polyphenol after long-term treatment.

5. Conclusions

In summary, we can conclude that RSV can reverse the disruption of metabolic parameters and the lipid profile in a diet-induced obese rat model. This beneficial effect could be explained by the restoration of leptin sensitivity in the three peripheral organs described as more metabolically active. In the liver, RSV could act via a SIRT1-dependent manner, whereas in muscle and adipose tissue, its action was mediated by increasing ObRb content and protecting against ER stress, respectively. However, further studies are required to clarify the molecular mechanisms by which RSV regulates leptin signaling in obesity. Finally, the metabolites derived from the gut microbiota may partially explain the contribution of the highest dose of RSV to reducing the metabolic alteration caused by obesity.

Supplementary Materials: The following are available online at http://www.mdpi.com/2072-6643/10/11/1757/s1, Table S1: A summary of the rat-specific primer sequences used for qRT-PCR analysis, Table S2: Chromatographic and fragmentation characteristics of RSV metabolites identified by UHPLC-MSn in serum samples, Table S3: Different biochemical parameters of liver, calf skeletal muscle and eWAT, Table S4. Correlation analysis of the most relevant biochemical parameters and the metabolites concentrations of RSV present in the serum of rats treated with 50, 100 or 200 mg/kg RSV, Figure S1: A scheme of the distribution of animals in the study, Figure S2: Inhibitors of the leptin signaling, Figure S3: iNos gene expression, Figure S4: Gene expression analysis of ER-stress markers.

Author Contributions: Conceptualization, C.B., L.A., M.S. and G.A.; methodology, A.A.-R. and M.I., formal analysis, A.A.-R., M.S., P.M. and G.A.; writing—original draft preparation, A.A.-R.; writing—review and editing, P.M., D.D.R., M.S. and G.A.; funding acquisition, C.B., B.M. and L.A.

Funding: This research was funded by the Ministerio de Economía, Industria y Competitividad (AGL2013-40707-R, AGL2016-77105-R and FPU14/01202). G.A. is a Serra Húnter fellow.

Acknowledgments: We gratefully acknowledge the aid of Niurka Dariela Llópiz and Rosa Pastor, the laboratory technicians. Authors also thank Luca Calani for his valuable support in metabolite identification.

Conflicts of Interest: The authors declare no conflict of interest.

References

1. WHO. *Overweight and Obesity*; WHO: Geneva, Switzerland, 2016.
2. WHO. *Fact Sheet, N° 311*; WHO: Geneva, Switzerland, 2016.
3. Wadden, T.A.; Webb, V.L.; Moran, C.H.; Bailer, B.A. Lifestyle modification for obesity: New developments in diet, physical activity, and behavior therapy. *Circulation* **2012**, *125*, 1157–1170. [CrossRef] [PubMed]
4. Weinsier, R.L.; Hunter, G.R.; Heini, A.F.; Goran, M.I.; Sell, S.M. The etiology of obesity: Relative contribution of metabolic factors, diet, and physical activity. *Am. J. Med.* **1998**, *105*, 145–150. [CrossRef]
5. Riccardi, G.; Capaldo, B.; Vaccaro, O. Functional foods in the management of obesity and type 2 diabetes. *Curr. Opin. Clin. Nutr. Metab. Care* **2005**, *8*, 630–635. [CrossRef] [PubMed]
6. Bremer, A.A. Resveratrol use in metabolic syndrome. *Metab. Syndr. Relat. Disord.* **2014**, *12*, 493–495. [CrossRef] [PubMed]
7. Baur, J.A.; Sinclair, D.A. Therapeutic potential of resveratrol: The in vivo evidence. *Nat. Rev. Drug Discov.* **2006**, *5*, 493–506. [CrossRef] [PubMed]
8. Lopez, M.S.; Dempsey, R.J.; Vemuganti, R. Resveratrol neuroprotection in stroke and traumatic CNS injury. *Neurochem. Int.* **2015**, *89*, 75–82. [CrossRef] [PubMed]
9. Lançon, A.; Frazzi, R.; Latruffe, N. Anti-Oxidant, anti-Inflammatory and anti-Angiogenic properties of resveratrol in ocular diseases. *Molecules* **2016**, *21*, 304. [CrossRef] [PubMed]
10. Annunziata, G.; Maisto, M.; Schisano, C.; Ciampaglia, R.; Narciso, V.; Tenore, G.C.; Novellino, E. Resveratrol as a Novel Anti-Herpes Simplex Virus Nutraceutical Agent: An Overview. *Viruses* **2018**, *10*, 473. [CrossRef] [PubMed]
11. Serrano, A.; Asnani-Kishnani, M.; Rodríguez, A.M.; Palou, A.; Ribot, J.; Bonet, M.L. Programming of the beige phenotype in white adipose tissue of adult mice by mild resveratrol and nicotinamide riboside supplementations in early postnatal life. *Mol. Nutr. Food Res.* **2018**, *62*, e1800463. [CrossRef] [PubMed]
12. Aguirre, L.; Fernández-Quintela, A.; Arias, N.; Portillo, M.P. Resveratrol: Anti-obesity mechanisms of action. *Molecules* **2014**, *19*, 18632–18655. [CrossRef] [PubMed]
13. Sheen, J.M.; Yu, H.R.; Tain, Y.L.; Tsai, W.L.; Tiao, M.M.; Lin, I.C.; Tsai, C.C.; Lin, Y.J.; Huang, L.T. Combined maternal and postnatal high-fat diet leads to metabolic syndrome and is effectively reversed by resveratrol: A multiple-organ study. *Sci. Rep.* **2018**, *8*, 5607. [CrossRef] [PubMed]
14. Fernández-Quintela, A.; Milton-Laskibar, I.; González, M.; Portillo, M.P. Antiobesity effects of resveratrol: Which tissues are involved? *Ann. N. Y. Acad. Sci.* **2017**, *1403*, 118–131. [CrossRef] [PubMed]
15. Howitz, K.T.; Bitterman, K.J.; Cohen, H.Y.; Lamming, D.W.; Lavu, S.; Wood, J.G.; Zipkin, R.E.; Chung, P.; Kisielewski, A.; Zhang, L.L.; et al. Small molecule activators of sirtuins extend Saccharomyces cerevisiae lifespan. *Nature* **2003**, *425*, 191–196. [CrossRef] [PubMed]
16. Trepiana, J.; Milton-Laskibar, I.; Gómez-Zorita, S.; Eseberri, I.; González, M.; Fernández-Quintela, A.; Portillo, M.P. Involvement of 5′-Activated Protein Kinase (AMPK) in the Effects of Resveratrol on Liver Steatosis. *Int. J. Mol. Sci.* **2018**, *19*, 3473. [CrossRef] [PubMed]
17. Cantó, C.; Gerhart-Hines, Z.; Feige, J.N.; Lagouge, M.; Noriega, L.; Milne, J.C.; Elliott, P.J.; Puigserver, P.; Auwerx, J. AMPK regulates energy expenditure by modulating NAD$^+$ metabolism and SIRT1 activity. *Nature* **2009**, *458*, 1056–1060. [CrossRef] [PubMed]
18. Bjørbaek, C.; Kahn, B.B. Leptin signaling in the central nervous system and the periphery. *Recent Prog. Horm. Res.* **2004**, *59*, 305–331. [CrossRef] [PubMed]
19. Aragonès, G.; Ardid-Ruiz, A.; Ibars, M.; Suárez, M.; Bladé, C. Modulation of leptin resistance by food compounds. *Mol. Nutr. Food Res.* **2016**, *60*, 1789–1803. [CrossRef] [PubMed]

20. Pan, W.W.; Myers, M.G., Jr. Leptin and the maintenance of elevated body weight. *Nat. Rev. Neurosci.* **2018**, *19*, 95–105. [CrossRef] [PubMed]

21. Flak, J.N.; Myers, M.G., Jr. Minireview: CNS Mechanisms of Leptin Action. *Mol. Endocrinol.* **2016**, *30*, 3–12. [CrossRef] [PubMed]

22. Margetic, S.; Gazzola, C.; Pegg, G.G.; Hill, R.A. Leptin: A review of its peripheral actions and interactions. *Int. J. Obes. Relat. Metab. Disord.* **2002**, *26*, 1407–1433. [CrossRef] [PubMed]

23. Zeng, W.; Pirzgalska, R.M.; Pereira, M.M.A.; Martins, G.G.; Barateiro, A.; Seixas, E.; Lu, Y.H.; Kozlova, A.; Voss, H.; Martins, G.G.; et al. Sympathetic Neuro-adipose Connections Mediate Leptin-Driven Lipolysis. *Cell* **2015**, *163*, 84–94. [CrossRef] [PubMed]

24. Buettner, C.; Muse, E.D.; Cheng, A.; Chen, L.; Scherer, T.; Pocai, A.; Su, K.; Cheng, B.; Li, X.; Harvey-White, J.; et al. Leptin controls adipose tissue lipogenesis via central, STAT3-independent mechanisms. *Nat. Med.* **2008**, *14*, 667–675. [CrossRef] [PubMed]

25. Ceddia, R.B.; William, W.N., Jr.; Curi, R. The response of skeletal muscle to leptin. *Front. Biosci.* **2001**, *6*, D90–D97. [CrossRef] [PubMed]

26. Huang, W.; Dedousis, N.; Bandi, A.; Lopaschuk, G.D.; O'Doherty, R.M. Liver triglyceride secretion and lipid oxidative metabolism are rapidly altered by leptin in vivo. *Endocrinology* **2006**, *147*, 1480–1487. [CrossRef] [PubMed]

27. Ye, Z.; Liu, G.; Guo, J.; Su, Z. Hypothalamic endoplasmic reticulum stress as a key mediator of obesity-induced leptin resistance. *Obes. Rev.* **2018**, *19*, 770–785. [CrossRef] [PubMed]

28. Ibars, M.; Ardid-Ruiz, A.; Suárez, M.; Muguerza, B.; Bladé, C.; Aragonès, G. Proanthocyanidins potentiate hypothalamic leptin/STAT3 signalling and Pomc gene expression in rats with diet-induced obesity. *Int. J. Obes. (Lond.)* **2017**, *41*, 129–136. [CrossRef] [PubMed]

29. Folch, J.; Lees, M.; Sloane Stanley, G.H. A simple method for the isolation and purification of total lipids from animal tissues. *J. Biol. Chem.* **1957**, *226*, 497–509. [PubMed]

30. Plut, C.; Ribière, C.; Giudicelli, Y.; Dausse, J.P. Hypothalamic leptin receptor and signaling molecule expressions in cafeteria diet-fed rats. *J. Pharmacol. Exp. Ther.* **2003**, *307*, 544–549. [CrossRef] [PubMed]

31. Aragonès, G.; Suárez, M.; Ardid-Ruiz, A.; Vinaixa, M.; Rodríguez, M.A.; Correig, X.; Arola, L.; Bladé, C. Dietary proanthocyanidins boost hepatic NAD(+) metabolism and SIRT1 expression and activity in a dose-dependent manner in healthy rats. *Sci. Rep.* **2016**, *6*, 24977. [CrossRef] [PubMed]

32. Savi, M.; Bocchi, L.; Mena, P.; Dall'Asta, M.; Crozier, A.; Brighenti, F.; Stilli, D.; Del Rio, D. In vivo administration of urolithin A and B prevents the occurrence of cardiac dysfunction in streptozotocin-induced diabetic rats. *Cardiovasc. Diabetol.* **2017**, *16*, 80. [CrossRef] [PubMed]

33. Bresciani, L.; Calani, L.; Bocchi, L.; Delucchi, F.; Savi, M.; Ray, S.; Brighenti, F.; Stilli, D.; Del Rio, D. Bioaccumulation of resveratrol metabolites in myocardial tissue is dose-time dependent and related to cardiac hemodynamics in diabetic rats. *Nutr. Metab. Cardiovasc. Dis.* **2014**, *24*, 408–415. [CrossRef] [PubMed]

34. Houseknecht, K.L.; Spurlock, M.E. Leptin regulation of lipid homeostasis: Dietary and metabolic implications. *Nutr. Res. Rev.* **2003**, *16*, 83–96. [CrossRef] [PubMed]

35. Muoio, D.M.; Lynis Dohm, G. Peripheral metabolic actions of leptin. *Best Pract. Res. Clin. Endocrinol. Metab.* **2002**, *16*, 653–666. [CrossRef] [PubMed]

36. Vasselli, J.R.; Scarpace, P.J.; Harris, R.B.; Banks, W.A. Dietary components in the development of leptin resistance. *Adv. Nutr.* **2013**, *4*, 164–175. [CrossRef] [PubMed]

37. Sáinz, N.; Barrenetxe, J.; Moreno-Aliaga, M.J.; Martínez, J.A. Leptin resistance and diet-induced obesity: Central and peripheral actions of leptin. *Metabolism* **2015**, *64*, 35–46. [CrossRef] [PubMed]

38. Robertson, S.A.; Leinningerm, G.M.; Myersm, M.G., Jr. Molecular and neural mediators of leptin action. *Physiol. Behav.* **2008**, *94*, 637–642. [CrossRef] [PubMed]

39. Scheibye-Knudsen, M.; Mitchell, S.J.; Fang, E.F.; Iyama, T.; Ward, T.; Wang, J.; Dunn, C.A.; Singh, N.; Veith, S.; Hasan-Olive, M.M.; et al. A high-fat diet and NAD(+) activate Sirt1 to rescue premature aging in cockayne syndrome. *Cell Metab.* **2014**, *20*, 840–855. [CrossRef] [PubMed]

40. Sun, C.; Zhang, F.; Ge, X.; Yan, T.; Chen, X.; Shi, X.; Zhai, Q. SIRT1 improves insulin sensitivity under insulin-resistant conditions by repressing PTP1B. *Cell Metab.* **2007**, *6*, 307–319. [CrossRef] [PubMed]

41. Franco, J.G.; Lisboa, P.C.; Lima, N.S.; Amaral, T.A.; Peixoto-Silva, N.; Resende, A.C.; Oliveira, E.; Passos, M.C.; Moura, E.G. Resveratrol attenuates oxidative stress and prevents steatosis and hypertension in obese rats programmed by early weaning. *J. Nutr. Biochem.* **2013**, *24*, 960–966. [CrossRef] [PubMed]

42. Pan, Q.R.; Ren, Y.L.; Liu, W.X.; Hu, Y.J.; Zheng, J.S.; Xu, Y.; Wang, G. Resveratrol prevents hepatic steatosis and endoplasmic reticulum stress and regulates the expression of genes involved in lipid metabolism, insulin resistance, and inflammation in rats. *Nutr. Res.* **2015**, *35*, 576–584. [CrossRef] [PubMed]

43. Andrade, J.M.; Paraíso, A.F.; de Oliveira, M.V.; Martins, A.M.; Neto, J.F.; Guimarães, A.L.; de Paula, A.M.; Qureshi, M.; Santos, S.H. Resveratrol attenuates hepatic steatosis in high-fat fed mice by decreasing lipogenesis and inflammation. *Nutrition* **2014**, *30*, 915–919. [CrossRef] [PubMed]

44. Jiang, M.; Li, X.; Yu, X.; Liu, X.; Xu, X.; He, J.; Gu, H.; Liu, L. Oral Administration of Resveratrol Alleviates Osteoarthritis Pathology in C57BL/6J Mice Model Induced by a High-Fat Diet. *Mediat. Inflamm.* **2017**, *2017*, 7659023. [CrossRef] [PubMed]

45. Jeon, B.T.; Jeong, E.A.; Shin, H.J.; Lee, Y.; Lee, D.H.; Kim, H.J.; Kang, S.S.; Cho, G.J.; Choi, W.S.; Roh, G.S. Resveratrol attenuates obesity-associated peripheral and central inflammation and improves memory deficit in mice fed a high-fat diet. *Diabetes* **2012**, *61*, 1444–1454. [CrossRef] [PubMed]

46. Kimbrough, C.W.; Lakshmanan, J.; Matheson, P.J.; Woeste, M.; Gentile, A.; Benns, M.V.; Zhang, B.; Smith, J.; Harbrecht, B.G. Resveratrol decreases nitric oxide production by hepatocytes during inflammation. *Surgery* **2015**, *158*, 1095–1101. [CrossRef] [PubMed]

47. Centeno-Baez, C.; Dallaire, P.; Marette, A. Resveratrol inhibition of inducible nitric oxide synthase in skeletal muscle involves AMPK but not SIRT1. *Am. J. Physiol. Endocrinol. Metab.* **2011**, *301*, E922–E930. [CrossRef] [PubMed]

48. Vetterli, L.; Maechler, P. Resveratrol-activated SIRT1 in liver and pancreatic β-cells: A Janus head looking to the same direction of metabolic homeostasis. *Aging (Albany NY)* **2011**, *3*, 444–449. [CrossRef] [PubMed]

49. Gambini, J.; Inglés, M.; Olaso, G.; Lopez-Grueso, R.; Bonet-Costa, V.; Gimeno-Mallench, L.; Mas-Bargues, C.; Abdelaziz, K.M.; Gomez-Cabrera, M.C.; Vina, J.; et al. Properties of Resveratrol: In Vitro and In Vivo Studies about Metabolism, Bioavailability, and Biological Effects in Animal Models and Humans. *Oxid. Med. Cell. Longev.* **2015**, *2015*, 837042. [CrossRef] [PubMed]

50. Wenzel, E.; Somoza, V. Metabolism and bioavailability of trans-resveratrol. *Mol. Nutr. Food Res.* **2005**, *49*, 472–481. [CrossRef] [PubMed]

51. Wenzel, E.; Soldo, T.; Erbersdobler, H.; Somoza, V. Bioactivity and metabolism of trans-resveratrol orally administered to Wistar rats. *Mol. Nutr. Food Res.* **2005**, *49*, 482–494. [CrossRef] [PubMed]

52. Andres-Lacueva, C.; Macarulla, M.T.; Rotches-Ribalta, M.; Boto-Ordóñez, M.; Urpi-Sarda, M.; Rodríguez, V.M.; Portillo, M.P. Distribution of resveratrol metabolites in liver, adipose tissue, and skeletal muscle in rats fed different doses of this polyphenol. *J. Agric. Food Chem.* **2012**, *60*, 4833–4840. [CrossRef] [PubMed]

53. Marier, J.F.; Vachon, P.; Gritsas, A.; Zhang, J.; Moreau, J.P.; Ducharme, M.P. Metabolism and disposition of resveratrol in rats: Extent of absorption, glucuronidation, and enterohepatic recirculation evidenced by a linked-rat model. *J. Pharmacol. Exp. Ther.* **2002**, *302*, 369–373. [CrossRef] [PubMed]

54. Eseberri, I.; Lasa, A.; Churruca, I.; Portillo, M.P. Resveratrol metabolites modify adipokine expression and secretion in 3T3-L1 pre-adipocytes and mature adipocytes. *PLoS ONE* **2013**, *8*, e63918. [CrossRef] [PubMed]

55. Lasa, A.; Churruca, I.; Eseberri, I.; Andrés-Lacueva, C.; Portillo, M.P. Delipidating effect of resveratrol metabolites in 3T3-L1 adipocytes. *Mol. Nutr. Food Res.* **2012**, *56*, 1559–1568. [CrossRef] [PubMed]

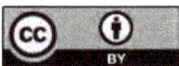

nutrients

MDPI

Article

In Vitro Anticancer Properties of Table Grape Powder Extract (GPE) in Prostate Cancer

Avinash Kumar [1], Melinee D'silva [1], Kshiti Dholakia [1] and Anait S. Levenson [2,*]

[1] Arnold & Marie Schwartz College of Pharmacy and Health Sciences, Long Island University, Brooklyn, NY 11201, USA; avinash.kumar@liu.edu (A.K.); melinee.dsilva@my.liu.edu (M.D.); kshiti.dholakia@my.liu.edu (K.D.)
[2] College of Veterinary Medicine, Long Island University, Brookville, NY 11548, USA
* Correspondence: anait.levenson@liu.edu; Tel.: +1-516-299-3692 or +1-718-246-6323

Received: 1 November 2018; Accepted: 15 November 2018; Published: 20 November 2018

Abstract: Although the link between diet and cancer is complex, epidemiological data confirm that diet is a risk factor for prostate cancer and indicate a reduced prostate cancer incidence associated with a diet rich in vegetables and fruits. Because of the known protective effect of grape seed extract (GSE) against prostate cancer, we evaluated the effects of grape powder extract (GPE) on cell viability, proliferation, and metastatic capability. Importantly, we explored the possible novel mechanism of GPE through metastasis-associated protein 1 (MTA1) downregulation in prostate cancer, since our previous studies indicated resveratrol (Res)- and pterostilbene (Pter)-induced MTA1-mediated anticancer activities in prostate cancer. We found that GPE inhibited the cell viability and growth of prostate cancer cells only at high 100 µg/mL concentrations. However, at low 1.5–15 µg/mL concentrations, GPE significantly reduced the colony formation and wound healing capabilities of both DU145 and PC3M cells. Moreover, we found that GPE inhibited MTA1 in a dose-dependent manner in these cells, albeit with considerably less potency than Res and Pter. These results indicate that stilbenes such as Res and Pter specifically and potently inhibit MTA1 and MTA1-associated proteins compared to GPE, which contains low concentrations of Res and mainly consists of other flavonoids and anthocyanidins. Our findings support continued interest in GPE as a chemopreventive and anti-cancer agent against prostate cancer but also emphasize the unique and specific properties of stilbenes on MTA1-mediated anticancer effects on prostate cancer.

Keywords: grape powder extract; prostate cancer; MTA1

1. Introduction

Despite progresses in understanding the molecular mechanisms of prostate cancer (PCa), it is still the most frequently diagnosed cancer in men in the United States, specifically in recent years, in which life expectancy has increased. Most men acquire PCa during their lifetime because of risk factors such as age and diet. Dietary bioactive polyphenols with anti-inflammatory, antioxidant, and anticancer properties have been of intense interest for use as chemopreventive agents against PCa. Particularly, stilbenes such as resveratrol (*trans*-3,5,4'-trihydroxystilbene, Res) and its natural analogs including pterostilbene (*trans*-3,5-dimethoxystilbene, Pter), found in grapes and berries [1,2], have attracted attention as potential pharmacological approaches for primary and clinical chemoprevention of PCa [3–16].

However, only limited studies support separate polyphenol(s) use in human chemoprevention due to their low bioavailability and rapid metabolism [17–19]. Therefore, grape extract, which contains a mix of various polyphenols including stilbenes, might present improved pharmacokinetics and superior pharmacological potency to stilbenes alone and may hold greater potential as a natural product drug. Grape seed extract (GSE), which is actively available as a health food supplement, has been shown to have strong antioxidant capabilities [20], cardiac benefits [21,22], neurological effects [23], and cancer preventive and anticancer activities [24–30]. Particularly, it has been shown that GSE has anticancer effects against PCa in vitro and in vivo [24,28,29,31]. Importantly, specific signaling pathways were identified as GSE-regulated, including androgen receptor (AR)-mediated transcription of genes [24] and inhibition of the activation of extracellular signal-regulated kinase 1/2 (ERK 1/2) with associated apoptotic effects [28].

Our interest includes AR-independent pathways that play a role in the progression of PCa. One of these pathways is represented by an overexpression of metastasis-associated protein 1 (MTA1) and the subsequent activation of MTA1-mediated pro-oncogenic signaling associated with the progression of PCa to metastasis [3,11–13,16,32–36]. Clinical studies have demonstrated the correlation of high MTA1 expression in prostate tissues with aggressive clinicopathological characteristics of tumors, signifying MTA1 as a potential therapeutic target in PCa. Therefore, we have intensively investigated and reported on the MTA1-mediated anticancer properties of Res and Pter in PCa in vitro and in vivo [3,4, 7,8,11–14,16].

The present study aimed to investigate the anticancer efficacy and MTA1 targeting ability of grape powder extract (GPE) in PCa cell lines. Grape powder extract consists of seven flavonoids, including resveratrol and three anthocyanidins (Table 1) [37]. We performed cell-based assays with GPE in two PCa cell lines using Res and Pter as reference compounds. Our results indicate that GPE has anticancer and antimetastatic effects in PCa, while stilbenes such as Res and Pter have the strongest MTA1 inhibitory action. Therefore, grape extract enriched for stilbenes through unique extraction procedures may represent an effective dietary agent for chemopreventive and therapeutic activity against PCa.

Table 1. Liquid Chromatography with tandem mass spectrometry (LC-MS/MS) analysis of the GPE (grape powder extract) and chemical structures of its compounds.

Class	Compound	Chemical Structure	Content (ppm)
Phenols	Catechin		4014
	Epicatechin		1268
Flavonols	Quercetin		3429
	Kaempferol		429

Table 1. *Cont.*

Class	Compound	Chemical Structure	Content (ppm)
	Isorhamnetin		346
	Taxifolin		656
Stilbenes	Resveratrol		88.5
	Cyanidin		508
Anthocyanins	Peonidin		5034
	Malvidin		2811

2. Materials and Methods

2.1. Compounds

Grape powder, which is a proportional representation of the different varieties of table grapes grown in California, was obtained from the California Table Grape Commission. The grape powder extract (GPE) was prepared and standardized as described previously [37] and was a generous gift from Dr. Richard van Breemen (Linus Pauling Institute, Oregon State University, Corvallis, OR, USA). Resveratrol and pterostilbene were purchased from Sigma-Aldrich (St. Louis, MO, USA) and were dissolved in dimethyl sulfoxide (DMSO) for the in vitro experiments.

2.2. Cell Culture

Prostate cancer cells, DU145 and PC3M, were maintained in RPMI-1640 media containing 10% FBS in an incubator at 37 °C with 5% CO_2 as described previously [3,6,8–16,33,34,36]. Cells were authenticated using short tandem repeat profiling at Research Technology Support Facility, Michigan State University.

2.3. MTT Assay

Cell viability of DU145 and PC3M cells was measured after treatment with GPE (2–200 µg/mL), Res (5–100 µM), and Pter (5–100 µM) using MTT assay (Sigma-Aldrich, St. Louis, MO, USA) as described previously [6,16]. Briefly, the cells were seeded in 96-well plates and treated with vehicle, GPE, Res, or Pter. Absorbance of the formazan was measured using BioTek Synergy-4 plate reader (BioTek, Winooski, VT, USA) after 72 h of treatment. The % cell viability was calculated assuming 100% viability in vehicle-treated (control) wells.

2.4. Proliferation Assay

DU145 and PC3M cells (2×10^3) were seeded in a 35-mm cell culture dish. The media with appropriate compound (GPE, Res, or Pter) was changed every other day. The proliferation of the cells was determined by counting the cells every other day over a period of 10 days.

2.5. Colony Formation Assay

Colony formation assay was performed as described previously [33]. Briefly, cells (5×10^3) were seeded in a 35 mm cell culture dish for a 21-day observation time. The media with appropriate compound was changed every other day. When colonies were freely visible (>50 cells/colony) in vehicle-treated dish, cells were fixed with formaldehyde and stained with 0.1% crystal violet solution. Colonies were visualized by imaging each dish using Amersham Imager 600 (GE Healthcare Bio-Sciences, Pittsburg, PA, USA). ImageQuant TL software (GE Healthcare Bio-Sciences, Pittsburg, PA, USA) was used for counting the number of colonies in each dish.

2.6. Wound-Healing Assay

Wound-healing assay was performed as described previously [33,36]. Briefly, 95% confluent cells seeded in 6-well plates were starved in low serum media (0.1% serum) overnight, after which three separate wounds were scratched across the well. The media with appropriate compound was changed every other day. The wound was imaged daily until the wounds of vehicle-treated (control) cells were completely closed using the EVOS XL Core microscope (ThermoFisher Scientific, Waltham, MA, USA). Wound area was calculated using the ImageJ software (NIH, Bethesda, MD, USA). % wound area was quantitated assuming 100% for vehicle-treated cells at 0 h.

2.7. Western Blot

Western blot analysis was carried out as previously described [33,36]. Briefly, cells were treated with various concentrations of GPE (25–200 µg/mL), Res (50 µM), or Pter (50 µM) for 24 h, and total protein was extracted. Protein concentration was measured using Bio-Rad protein assay reagent (Bio-Rad Laboratories, Hercules, CA, USA). An equal amount of protein was resolved in 10–15% gels and transferred to a polyvinylidene difluoride (PVDF) membrane. After blocking the membranes for non-specificity, they were probed with MTA1 (1:2000), p21 (1:1000), cleaved caspase 3 (1:1000), PTEN (1:1000), Cyclin D1 (1:1000), and pAkt (1:1000) (Cell Signaling Technology, Danvers, MA, USA) primary antibodies. β-actin antibody (1:2500) (Santa Cruz, Dallas, TX, USA) was used as a loading control. Signals were visualized using enhanced chemoluminescence. Densitometry was performed using Image J software (NIH, Bethesda, MD, USA).

2.8. Statistical Analysis

The differences between the groups were analyzed by one-way analysis of variance (ANOVA). All statistics were performed using GraphPad Prism 7 software (GraphPad Software, La Jolla, CA, USA). The statistical significance was set as $p < 0.05$. All data are cumulative of at least three independent experiments.

3. Results

The cytotoxic effects of GPE were evaluated and compared to those of Res and Pter by MTT cell viability assay in DU145 and PC3M aggressive prostate cancer cell lines. The cells were treated with various concentrations of GPE (5–200 µg/mL), Res (5–100 µM or 1.14–22.8 µg/mL), and Pter (5–100 µM or 1.28–25.6 µg/mL) for 72 h. As shown in Figure 1A, treatment with GPE had a modest cytotoxic effect even at high 200 µg/mL dose, whereas Res and Pter significantly inhibited the DU145 and PC3M cells' viability in relatively low concentrations. The IC_{50} values of Res and Pter in DU145 and PC3M cells were in accordance with our previous reports [10], while GPE showed very low activity in both cell lines, with IC_{50} values of 107 µg/mL in DU145 cells. We were not able to determine IC_{50} values for GPE doses (5–200 µg/mL) used in PC3M cells. To further investigate the inhibition of cell proliferation by GPE, we performed cell-counting assay upon treatment with compounds. We counted cell numbers every other day for 10 days and found that GPE significantly inhibited cell proliferation compared to control untreated cells in all concentrations tested in both DU145 and PC3M cells (Figure 1B). In DU145 cells, higher concentrations of GPE (15 and 100 µg/mL) were significantly more potent at inhibiting cell growth ($p < 0.01$; $p < 0.0001$) than Res but not Pter. In PC3M cells, GPE at high doses (15 and 100 µg/mL) as well as Res and Pter showed significant differences compared to control vehicle-treated cells ($p < 0.001$; $p < 0.0001$).

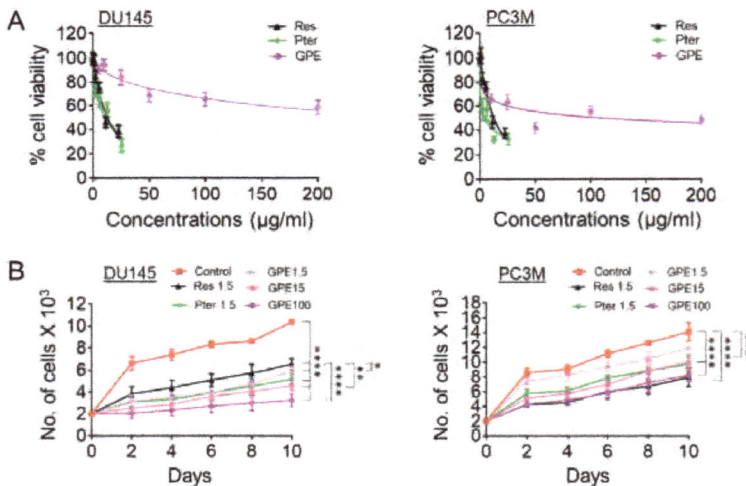

Figure 1. Effects of GPE on cell viability and cell proliferation. (**A**) Cell viability analysis of DU145 (left) and PC3M (right) prostate cancer cells treated with GPE (2–200 µg/mL), Res (1.14–22.8 µg/mL), and Pter (1.28–25.6 µg/mL). Data represent the mean ± scanning electron microscopy (SEM) of three independent sets of experiments. (**B**) Proliferation assay of DU145 (left) and PC3M (right) cells after treatment with GPE (1.5; 15; 100 µg/mL) and Res and Pter (1.5 µg/mL) for 10 days. Data represent the mean ± SEM of three independent sets of experiments. * $p < 0.05$, ** $p < 0.01$, *** $p < 0.001$, and **** $p < 0.0001$ (one-way analysis of variance (ANOVA)) were assessed as significant differences between treated and Ctrl vehicle cells.

Nutrients **2018**, *10*, 1804

To characterize the anti-metastatic capacity of GPE, we examined the effect of GPE on the colony formation and wound healing in DU145 and PC3M cells. As shown in Figure 2A, colony-forming ability was decreased in DU145 cells, with an increased GPE concentration gradient reaching significance at 15 μg/mL ($p < 0.001$) and 100 μg/mL ($p < 0.0001$). In more aggressive PC3M cells, GPE treatment at only a high (100 μg/mL) dose caused a significant reduction of colony-forming ability ($p < 0.0001$) (Figure 2B). However, these results indicated that only the effects of the highest concentration of GPE (100 μg/mL) were comparable with the effects of Res and Pter alone at a relatively low dose (1.5 μg/mL). After this, a wound-healing assay was performed in order to measure the effects of GPE treatment on tumor cell migration. The migration of DU145 and PC3M cells was decreased with an increased GPE concentration gradient (Figure 3A,B). As shown in Figure 3A, reduction in the cell migration of GPE-treated DU145 cells was highly significant ($p < 0.001$) in a dose-dependent manner, compared to control vehicle-treated cells. Interestingly, GPE-treated PC3M cells, which are characterized as more aggressive than DU145 cells, were affected in their migration capabilities by GPE treatment stronger than DU145 cells. These results indicated that GPE could reduce migration of aggressive prostate cancer cells in a dose-dependent manner starting at as low as 1.5 μg/mL dose. Once again, Res and Pter also showed strong ability to reduce migration of prostate cancer cells at 1.5 μg/mL dose.

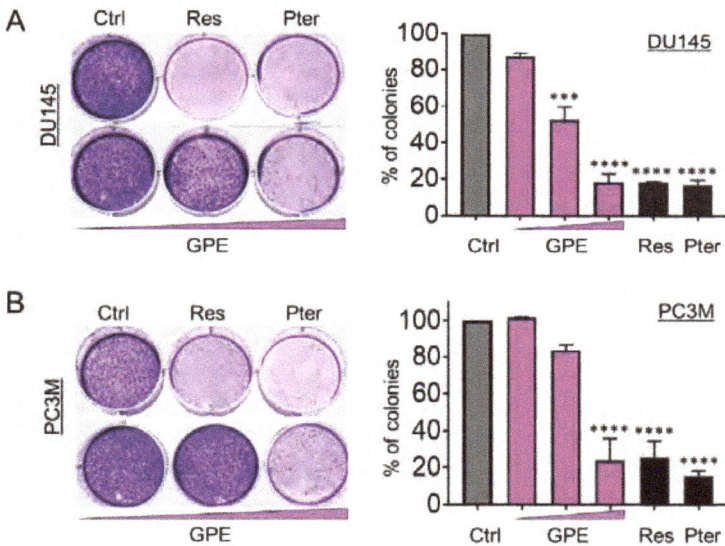

Figure 2. GPE reduces colony formation in DU145 and PC3M prostate cancer cells. Representative images of colony formation ability of (**A**) DU145 and (**B**) PC3M cells after treatment with GPE (1.5; 15; 100 μg/mL) and Res and Pter (1.5 μg/mL). Data represent the mean ± SEM of three independent experiments with duplicate wells. *** $p < 0.001$ and **** $p < 0.0001$ (one-way ANOVA) were assessed as significant differences between treated and Ctrl vehicle cells.

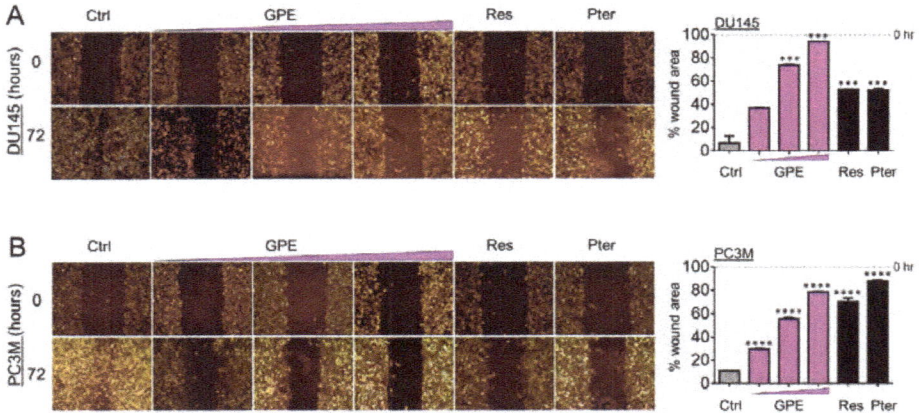

Figure 3. GPE reduces migration of DU145 and PC3M prostate cancer cells. Representative images of migration ability of (**A**) DU145 and (**B**) PC3M cells after treatment with GPE (1.5; 15; 100 µg/mL) and Res and Pter (1.5 µg/mL). Right: quantitation of wound widths, as % wound area is shown for each cell line. Data represent the mean ± SEM of six separate wounds and three independent experiments. *** $p < 0.001$ and **** $p < 0.0001$ (one-way ANOVA) were assessed as significant differences between treated and Ctrl vehicle cells.

We have shown previously that Res and Pter inhibit MTA1-mediated PCa progression in vitro and in vivo [3,7,8,11,13,16]. Therefore, we next measured the effect of GPE treatment on MTA1 protein expression in DU145 and PC3M cells. Cells were treated with GPE at various concentrations (25–200 µg/mL) and with Res and Pter (50 µM~12 µg/mL) for 24 h, after which the total protein was isolated and a western blot was performed. As indicated in Figure 4A,B, GPE downregulated MTA1 in a dose-dependent manner in DU145 cells and PC3M cells, respectively, but with considerably less potency than Res and Pter. We also sought to investigate the effect of GPE on certain MTA1-associated proteins in DU145 and PC3M cells, which we previously identified using ChIP-Seq [11]. We have shown that MTA1 directly regulates CyclinD1 and pAkt and negatively associates with PTEN [11,13]. As seen in Figure 5A,B, there was downregulation of Cyclin D1 and a slight upregulation of PTEN in DU145 cells treated with GPE. pAkt levels were affected by GPE treatment in PC3M cells (Figure 5C,D). Because p21 expression represents an important biomarker of apoptosis, we examined its expression after treatment with GPE. Results show that p21 was induced in a dose-dependent manner upon GPE treatment in PC3M cells (Figure 5C,D).

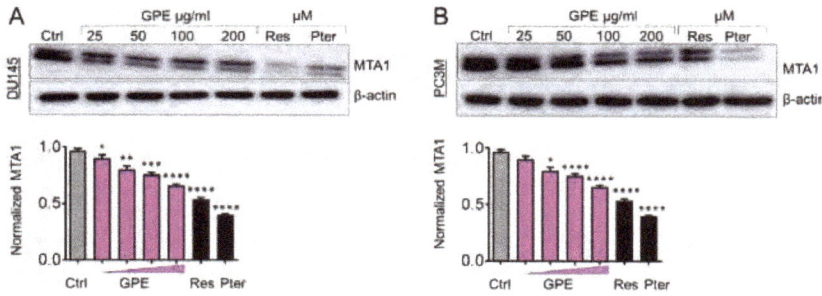

Figure 4. GPE inhibits MTA1 protein expression in a dose-dependent manner in DU145 and PC3M prostate cancer cells. Immunoblots of MTA1 expression in (**A**) DU145 and (**B**) PC3M cells (top panels). β-actin was used as a loading control. Western blots were repeated three times and representative blots are shown. Quantitation of immunoblot signals (lower panels). * $p < 0.05$, ** $p < 0.01$, *** $p < 0.001$, and **** $p < 0.0001$ (one-way ANOVA) were assessed as significant differences between treated and Ctrl vehicle cells.

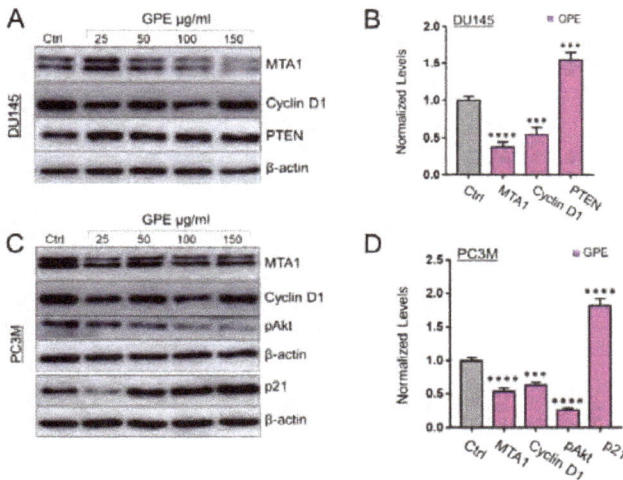

Figure 5. Effects of GPE treatment on MTA1-associated protein levels. (**A**) Immunoblots of MTA1, Cyclin D1, and PTEN expression, in DU145 cells treated with GPE. β-actin was used as a loading control. (**B**) Quantitation of immunoblot signals of MTA1-associated proteins, Cyclin D1, and PTEN, in cells treated with 150 µg/mL GPE. (**C**) Immunoblots of MTA1, Cyclin D1, pAkt, and p21 expression, in PC3M cells treated with GPE. β-actin was used as a loading control. (**D**) Quantitation of immunoblot signals of MTA1-associated proteins, Cyclin D1, pAkt, and p21, in cells treated with 150 µg/mL GPE. Western blots were repeated three times for each protein, and representative blots are shown. *** $p < 0.001$ and **** $p < 0.0001$ (one-way ANOVA) were assessed as significant differences between 150 µg/mL GPE-treated vs. Ctrl vehicle-treated cells.

4. Discussion

Numerous studies have demonstrated that diet is a risk factor for PCa and consumption of plant foods may reduce the incidence of PCa [38–40]. Dietary phytochemicals such as quercetin, curcumin, genistein, selenium, resveratrol, and pterostilbene have been shown to possess anti-inflammatory, antioxidative, cardioprotective, and anticancer activities [4]. These polyphenols individually act through various genetic and epigenetic mechanisms to control numerous biochemical and

Nutrients **2018**, *10*, 1804

molecular pathways, influencing cell growth, differentiation, cell cycle, senescence, apoptosis, epithelial-to-mesenchymal transition, and metastasis. While it is necessary to understand the mechanisms of action for individual bioactive molecules, the composition of dietary sources such as fruits or vegetables consists of various polyphenols, represented by different classes of phytochemicals that provide health benefits in unison. However, at the molecular level, the interaction of these molecules may cause the activation or inhibition of certain molecular pathways.

Published studies have demonstrated the prostate anticancer activity of GSE, which is comprised of high phenolic content. However, the total content might differ with possible active compounds depending on the method of extraction [28]. In the present study, we used grape powder extract (GPE), which is an organic solvent extract of freeze-dried whole table grapes. The varieties of grapes include a proportional representation of table grapes grown in California. Most table grapes grown in California are seedless, but some seeded grapes are produced and were included. After freeze drying, the grape skins and seeds remained and were ground to produce powder.

In this study, we demonstrated that GPE treatment caused growth inhibition and reduced the colony formation and migration ability of DU145 and PC3M prostate cancer cells. Less aggressive DU145 cells showed more sensitivity to the antiproliferative and anti-colony formation effects of GPE than to that of the PC3M cells. Because of our long-standing interest in targeting MTA1 signaling, we asked whether GPE acts through inhibition of MTA1 oncogenic protein in prostate cancer, as we have shown for Res and Pter, which has significant MTA1-mediated anticancer effects [3,7,8,11,13,16]. Our results suggest that although GPE downregulated MTA1 protein levels in a dose-dependent manner (p.6. 11–1128), the inhibition was not significant, possibly due to low nanomolar concentration of Res in GPE. As expected, Res and mainly Pter alone at 50 μM dose showed a marked inhibition of MTA1, suggesting a unique stilbenes–MTA1 relationship.

Taken together, GPE demonstrated anticancer effects in prostate cancer cell lines. Because of strong evidence for the involvement of MTA1 signaling in all stages of PCa progression, we explored a chance of MTA1 inhibition by GPE. Since we detected more potent MTA1 inhibition by stilbenes compared to mixture of polyphenols in GPE, there is a possibility that stilbenes and no other phytochemicals directly bind to MTA1 (unpublished data). Whether or not combination of various stilbenes will be most effective at inhibiting MTA1 and MTA1-guided signaling in PCa is unknown and remains to be elucidated.

In summary, our preclinical in vitro findings support continued interest in GPE as an anticancer agent against PCa. However, in vivo studies and especially clinical trials are needed to explore the chemopreventive and therapeutic effects of GPE. Two recent clinical trials of muscadine grape skin extract containing ellagic acid, quercetin, and resveratrol in men with biochemically recurrent PCa showed the safety of two different doses (500 mg and 4 g) but no significant differences in predictive biomarkers [41,42]. Nevertheless, recent advances in personalized medicine are very promising and may make the translational application of chemoprevention by natural products a distinct possibility in target-stratified patient populations.

Author Contributions: Conceptualization: A.S.L. Methodology: A.K., M.D., and K.D.; Validation: A.K., M.D., K.D., and A.S.L.; Formal analysis: A.K., M.D., and A.S.L.; Writing—Original Draft Preparation: A.K. and A.S.L.; Writing, Review and Editing: A.K and A.S.L.

Funding: Research reported in this publication was supported by the California Table Grape Commission to AS Levenson. It was also partially supported by the National Cancer Institute of the National Institutes of Health under Award Number R15CA216070 to AS Levenson. The content is solely the responsibility of the authors and does not necessarily represent the official views of the National Institutes of Health.

Acknowledgments: We thank Richard van Breemen (Linus Pauling Institute, Oregon State University, Corvallis, OR) for his gracious gift of GPE. We also thank Carmen Fuentealba and Randy Burd (LIU) for their continued support.

Conflicts of Interest: The authors declare no conflict of interest.

References

1. Burns, J.; Yokota, T.; Ashihara, H.; Lean, M.E.; Crozier, A. Plant foods and herbal sources of resveratrol. *J. Agric. Food Chem.* **2002**, *50*, 3337–3340. [CrossRef] [PubMed]
2. Fremont, L. Biological effects of resveratrol. *Life Sci.* **2000**, *66*, 663–673. [CrossRef]
3. Li, K.; Dias, S.J.; Rimando, A.M.; Dhar, S.; Mizuno, C.S.; Penman, A.D.; Lewin, J.R.; Levenson, A.S. Pterostilbene acts through metastasis-associated protein 1 to inhibit tumor growth, progression and metastasis in prostate cancer. *PLoS ONE* **2013**, *8*, e57542. [CrossRef] [PubMed]
4. Kumar, A.; Butt, N.A.; Levenson, A.S. Natural epigenetic-modifying molecules in medical therapy. In *Medical Epigenetics*; Tollefsbol, T., Ed.; Elsevier Inc.: London, UK, 2016; pp. 747–798.
5. Kumar, A.; Rimando, A.M.; Levenson, A.S. Resveratrol and pterostilbene as a microRNA-mediated chemopreventive and therapeutic strategy in prostate cancer. *Ann. N. Y. Acad. Sci.* **2017**, *1403*, 15–26. [CrossRef] [PubMed]
6. Kumar, A.; Lin, S.Y.; Dhar, S.; Rimando, A.M.; Levenson, A.S. Stilbenes Inhibit Androgen Receptor Expression in 22Rv1 Castrate-resistant Prostate Cancer Cells. *J. Med. Active Plants* **2014**, *3*, 1–8.
7. Kumar, A.; Dhar, S.; Rimando, A.M.; Lage, J.M.; Lewin, J.R.; Zhang, X.; Levenson, A.S. Epigenetic potential of resveratrol and analogs in preclinical models of prostate cancer. *Ann. N. Y. Acad. Sci.* **2015**, *1348*, 1–9. [CrossRef] [PubMed]
8. Kai, L.; Samuel, S.K.; Levenson, A.S. Resveratrol enhances p53 acetylation and apoptosis in prostate cancer by inhibiting MTA1/NuRD complex. *Int. J. Cancer* **2010**, *126*, 1538–1548. [CrossRef] [PubMed]
9. Kai, L.; Levenson, A.S. Combination of resveratrol and antiandrogen flutamide has synergistic effect on androgen receptor inhibition in prostate cancer cells. *Anticancer Res.* **2011**, *31*, 3323–3330. [PubMed]
10. Dias, S.J.; Li, K.; Rimando, A.M.; Dhar, S.; Mizuno, C.S.; Penman, A.D.; Levenson, A.S. Trimethoxy-resveratrol and piceatannol administered orally suppress and inhibit tumor formation and growth in prostate cancer xenografts. *Prostate* **2013**, *73*, 1135–1146. [CrossRef] [PubMed]
11. Dhar, S.; Kumar, A.; Zhang, L.; Rimando, A.M.; Lage, J.M.; Lewin, J.R.; Atfi, A.; Zhang, X.; Levenson, A.S. Dietary pterostilbene is a novel MTA1-targeted chemopreventive and therapeutic agent in prostate cancer. *Oncotarget* **2016**, *7*, 18469–18484. [CrossRef] [PubMed]
12. Dhar, S.; Kumar, A.; Rimando, A.M.; Zhang, X.; Levenson, A.S. Resveratrol and pterostilbene epigenetically restore PTEN expression by targeting oncomiRs of the miR-17 family in prostate cancer. *Oncotarget* **2015**, *6*, 27214–27226. [CrossRef] [PubMed]
13. Dhar, S.; Kumar, A.; Li, K.; Tzivion, G.; Levenson, A.S. Resveratrol regulates PTEN/Akt pathway through inhibition of MTA1/HDAC unit of the NuRD complex in prostate cancer. *Biochim. Biophys. Acta* **2015**, *1853*, 265–275. [CrossRef] [PubMed]
14. Dhar, S.; Hicks, C.; Levenson, A.S. Resveratrol and prostate cancer: Promising role for microRNAs. *Mol. Nutr. Food Res.* **2011**, *55*, 1219–1229. [CrossRef] [PubMed]
15. Chakraborty, S.; Kumar, A.; Butt, N.A.; Zhang, L.; Williams, R.; Rimando, A.M.; Biswas, P.K.; Levenson, A.S. Molecular insight into the differential anti-androgenic activity of resveratrol and its natural analogs: In silico approach to understand biological actions. *Mol. Biosyst.* **2016**, *12*, 1702–1709. [CrossRef] [PubMed]
16. Butt, N.A.; Kumar, A.; Dhar, S.; Rimando, A.M.; Akhtar, I.; Hancock, J.C.; Lage, J.M.; Pound, C.R.; Lewin, J.R.; Gomez, C.R.; et al. Targeting MTA1/HIF-1alpha signaling by pterostilbene in combination with histone deacetylase inhibitor attenuates prostate cancer progression. *Cancer Med.* **2017**, *6*, 2673–2685. [CrossRef] [PubMed]
17. Aggarwal, B.B.; Bhardwaj, A.; Aggarwal, R.S.; Seeram, N.P.; Shishodia, S.; Takada, Y. Role of resveratrol in prevention and therapy of cancer: Preclinical and clinical studies. *Anticancer Res.* **2004**, *24*, 2783–2840. [PubMed]
18. Athar, M.; Back, J.H.; Tang, X.; Kim, K.H.; Kopelovich, L.; Bickers, D.R.; Kim, A.L. Resveratrol: A review of preclinical studies for human cancer prevention. *Toxicol. Appl. Pharmacol.* **2007**, *224*, 274–283. [CrossRef] [PubMed]
19. Soleas, G.J.; Yan, J.; Goldberg, D.M. Ultrasensitive assay for three polyphenols (catechin, quercetin and resveratrol) and their conjugates in biological fluids utilizing gas chromatography with mass selective detection. *J. Chromatogr. B Biomed. Sci. Appl.* **2001**, *757*, 161–172. [CrossRef]

20. Shi, J.; Yu, J.; Pohorly, J.E.; Kakuda, Y. Polyphenolics in grape seeds-biochemistry and functionality. *J. Med. Food* **2003**, *6*, 291–299. [CrossRef] [PubMed]

21. Du, Y.; Guo, H.; Lou, H. Grape seed polyphenols protect cardiac cells from apoptosis via induction of endogenous antioxidant enzymes. *J. Agric. Food Chem.* **2007**, *55*, 1695–1701. [CrossRef] [PubMed]

22. National Center for Complementary and Integrative Health. Available online: https://nccih.nih.gov/ (accessed on 22 October 2018).

23. Wang, Y.J.; Thomas, P.; Zhong, J.H.; Bi, F.F.; Kosaraju, S.; Pollard, A.; Fenech, M.; Zhou, X.F. Consumption of grape seed extract prevents amyloid-beta deposition and attenuates inflammation in brain of an Alzheimer's disease mouse. *Neurotox. Res.* **2009**, *15*, 3–14. [CrossRef] [PubMed]

24. Park, S.Y.; Lee, Y.H.; Choi, K.C.; Seong, A.R.; Choi, H.K.; Lee, O.H.; Hwang, H.J.; Yoon, H.G. Grape seed extract regulates androgen receptor-mediated transcription in prostate cancer cells through potent anti-histone acetyltransferase activity. *J. Med. Food* **2011**, *14*, 9–16. [CrossRef] [PubMed]

25. Sharma, S.D.; Meeran, S.M.; Katiyar, S.K. Proanthocyanidins inhibit in vitro and in vivo growth of human non-small cell lung cancer cells by inhibiting the prostaglandin E(2) and prostaglandin E(2) receptors. *Mol. Cancer Ther.* **2010**, *9*, 569–580. [CrossRef] [PubMed]

26. Mao, J.T.; Smoake, J.; Park, H.K.; Lu, Q.Y.; Xue, B. Grape Seed Procyanidin Extract Mediates Antineoplastic Effects against Lung Cancer via Modulations of Prostacyclin and 15-HETE Eicosanoid Pathways. *Cancer Prev. Res. (Phila.)* **2016**, *9*, 925–932. [CrossRef] [PubMed]

27. Iannone, M.; Mare, R.; Paolino, D.; Gagliardi, A.; Froiio, F.; Cosco, D.; Fresta, M. Characterization and in vitro anticancer properties of chitosan-microencapsulated flavan-3-ols-rich grape seed extracts. *Int. J. Biol. Macromol.* **2017**, *104*, 1039–1045. [CrossRef] [PubMed]

28. Agarwal, C.; Sharma, Y.; Agarwal, R. Anticarcinogenic effect of a polyphenolic fraction isolated from grape seeds in human prostate carcinoma DU145 cells: Modulation of mitogenic signaling and cell-cycle regulators and induction of G1 arrest and apoptosis. *Mol. Carcinog.* **2000**, *28*, 129–138. [CrossRef]

29. Kaur, M.; Velmurugan, B.; Rajamanickam, S.; Agarwal, R.; Agarwal, C. Gallic acid, an active constituent of grape seed extract, exhibits anti-proliferative, pro-apoptotic and anti-tumorigenic effects against prostate carcinoma xenograft growth in nude mice. *Pharm. Res.* **2009**, *26*, 2133–2140. [CrossRef] [PubMed]

30. Cheah, K.Y.; Howarth, G.S.; Yazbeck, R.; Wright, T.H.; Whitford, E.J.; Payne, C.; Butler, R.N.; Bastian, S.E. Grape seed extract protects IEC-6 cells from chemotherapy-induced cytotoxicity and improves parameters of small intestinal mucositis in rats with experimentally-induced mucositis. *Cancer Biol. Ther.* **2009**, *8*, 382–390. [CrossRef] [PubMed]

31. Raina, K.; Singh, R.P.; Agarwal, R.; Agarwal, C. Oral grape seed extract inhibits prostate tumor growth and progression in TRAMP mice. *Cancer Res.* **2007**, *67*, 5976–5982. [CrossRef] [PubMed]

32. Levenson, A.S.; Kumar, A.; Zhang, X. MTA family of proteins in prostate cancer: Biology, significance, and therapeutic opportunities. *Cancer Metastasis Rev.* **2014**, *33*, 929–942. [CrossRef] [PubMed]

33. Kumar, A.; Dhar, S.; Campanelli, G.; Butt, N.A.; Schallheim, J.M.; Gomez, C.R.; Levenson, A.S. MTA1 drives malignant progression and bone metastasis in prostate cancer. *Mol. Oncol.* **2018**, *12*, 1596–1607. [CrossRef] [PubMed]

34. Kai, L.; Wang, J.; Ivanovic, M.; Chung, Y.T.; Laskin, W.B.; Schulze-Hoepfner, F.; Mirochnik, Y.; Satcher, R.L., Jr.; Levenson, A.S. Targeting prostate cancer angiogenesis through metastasis-associated protein 1 (MTA1). *Prostate* **2011**, *71*, 268–280. [CrossRef] [PubMed]

35. Dias, S.J.; Zhou, X.; Ivanovic, M.; Gailey, M.P.; Dhar, S.; Zhang, L.; He, Z.; Penman, A.D.; Vijayakumar, S.; Levenson, A.S. Nuclear MTA1 overexpression is associated with aggressive prostate cancer, recurrence and metastasis in African Americans. *Sci. Rep.* **2013**, *3*, 2331. [CrossRef] [PubMed]

36. Dhar, S.; Kumar, A.; Gomez, C.R.; Akhtar, I.; Hancock, J.C.; Lage, J.M.; Pound, C.R.; Levenson, A.S. MTA1-activated Epi-microRNA-22 regulates E-cadherin and prostate cancer invasiveness. *FEBS Lett.* **2017**, *591*, 924–933. [CrossRef] [PubMed]

37. van Breemen, R.B.; Wright, B.; Li, Y.; Nosal, D.; Burton, T. Standardized grape powder for basic and clinical research. In *Grapes and Health*; Pezzuto, J.M., Ed.; Springer International Publishing: Cham, Switzerland, 2016.

38. Lin, P.H.; Aronson, W.; Freedland, S.J. Nutrition, dietary interventions and prostate cancer: The latest evidence. *BMC Med.* **2015**, *13*, 3. [CrossRef] [PubMed]

39. Gathirua-Mwangi, W.G.; Zhang, J. Dietary factors and risk for advanced prostate cancer. *Eur. J. Cancer Prev.* **2014**, *23*, 96–109. [CrossRef] [PubMed]

40. Bommareddy, A.; Eggleston, W.; Prelewicz, S.; Antal, A.; Witczak, Z.; McCune, D.F.; Vanwert, A.L. Chemoprevention of prostate cancer by major dietary phytochemicals. *Anticancer Res.* **2013**, *33*, 4163–4174. [PubMed]

41. Paller, C.J.; Zhou, X.C.; Heath, E.I.; Taplin, M.E.; Mayer, T.; Stein, M.N.; Bubley, G.J.; Pili, R.; Hudson, T.; Kakarla, R.; et al. Muscadine Grape Skin Extract (MPX) in Men with Biochemically Recurrent Prostate Cancer: A Randomized, Multicenter, Placebo-Controlled Clinical Trial. *Clin. Cancer Res.* **2018**, *24*, 306–315. [CrossRef] [PubMed]

42. Paller, C.J.; Rudek, M.A.; Zhou, X.C.; Wagner, W.D.; Hudson, T.S.; Anders, N.; Hammers, H.J.; Dowling, D.; King, S.; Antonarakis, E.S.; et al. A phase I study of muscadine grape skin extract in men with biochemically recurrent prostate cancer: Safety, tolerability, and dose determination. *Prostate* **2015**, *75*, 1518–1525. [CrossRef] [PubMed]

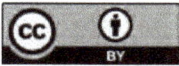

Review

Beneficial Effects of Resveratrol Administration—Focus on Potential Biochemical Mechanisms in Cardiovascular Conditions

Michał Wiciński [1], Maciej Socha [2], Maciej Walczak [1], Eryk Wódkiewicz [1,*], Bartosz Malinowski [1], Sebastian Rewerski [1], Karol Górski [1] and Katarzyna Pawlak-Osińska [3]

[1] Department of Pharmacology and Therapeutics, Faculty of Medicine, Collegium Medicum in Bydgoszcz, Nicolaus Copernicus University, M. Curie 9, 85-090 Bydgoszcz, Poland; wicinski4@wp.pl (M.W.); maciej.walczak5@hotmail.com (M.W.); bartosz.malin@gmail.com (B.M.); srewerski@gmail.com (S.R.); karolgorski-2@gazeta.pl (K.G.)

[2] Department of Obstetrics, Gynecology and Gynecological Oncology, Faculty of Medicine, Collegium Medicum in Bydgoszcz, Nicolaus Copernicus University, Ujejskiego 75, 85-168 Bydgoszcz, Poland; msocha@copernicus.gda.pl

[3] Department of Pathophysiology of Hearing and Balance System, Faculty of Medicine, Collegium Medicum in Bydgoszcz, Nicolaus Copernicus University, M. Curie 9, 85-090 Bydgoszcz, Poland; osinskak1@wp.pl

* Correspondence: eryk.wodkiewicz09@gmail.com; Tel.: +48-696-094-768

Received: 15 October 2018; Accepted: 14 November 2018; Published: 21 November 2018

Abstract: Resveratrol (RV) is a natural non-flavonoid polyphenol and phytoalexin produced by a number of plants such as peanuts, grapes, red wine and berries. Numerous in vitro studies have shown promising results of resveratrol usage as antioxidant, antiplatelet or anti-inflammatory agent. Beneficial effects of resveratrol activity probably result from its ability to purify the body from ROS (reactive oxygen species), inhibition of COX (cyclooxygenase) and activation of many anti-inflammatory pathways. Administration of the polyphenol has a potential to slow down the development of CVD (cardiovascular disease) by influencing on certain risk factors such as development of diabetes or atherosclerosis. Resveratrol induced an increase in Sirtuin-1 level, which by disrupting the TLR4/NF-κB/STAT signal cascade (toll-like receptor 4/nuclear factor κ-light-chain enhancer of activated B cells/signal transducer and activator of transcription) reduces production of cytokines in activated microglia. Resveratrol caused an attenuation of macrophage/mast cell-derived pro-inflammatory factors such as PAF (platelet-activating factor), TNF-α (tumour necrosis factor-α and histamine. Endothelial and anti-oxidative effect of resveratrol may contribute to better outcomes in stroke management. By increasing BDNF (brain-derived neurotrophic factor) serum concentration and inducing NOS-3 (nitric oxide synthase-3) activity resveratrol may have possible therapeutical effects on cognitive impairments and dementias especially in those characterized by defective cerebrovascular blood flow.

Keywords: resveratrol; cardiovascular; inflammation; cytokines; pathways

---

1. Introduction

Resveratrol (3,5,4′-trihydroxy-trans-stilbene) is a natural non-flavonoid polyphenol and phytoalexin produced by a considerable number of plants in response to stress factors such as pathogens or injury [1,2]. The substance can be found in peanuts, grapes, red wine and some berries [3]. It has been proven to be a potent antioxidant [4], antiplatelet [5,6] and anti-inflammatory agent [7] in vitro. Despite numerous studies, mechanisms of resveratrol action have not been clearly identified. According to the results of pharmacokinetic analysis, resveratrol undergoes rapid metabolism in the body, its bioavailability after oral administration is very low despite of absorption reaching

70%, which undermines the physiological significance of the high concentrations used in in vitro studies [6]. Mentioned effects are probably a result of its ability to purify the body from ROS [8,9], inhibition of COX [10,11] and activation of many anti-inflammatory pathways, including among others: SIRT-1 (Sirtuin-1) [12]. SIRT-1 disrupts the TLR4/NF-κB/STAT signal which subsequently leads to the reduction of produced cytokines in activated microglia [13], or macrophage/mast cell-derived pro-inflammatory factors such as platelet-activating factor PAF, TNF-α and histamine [14].

Cardiovascular diseases are the most common cause of death in the world, it is estimated that about 18 million people died because of CVD in 2016. It is 31% of all deaths worldwide. Over 17 million (39%) of premature deaths (under 70 years) due to non-communicable diseases are caused by CVD [15]. Regardless of the significant improvement and great emphasis on CVD treatment, the statistics show that searching for new ways to help cardiovascular patients is essential. Resveratrol has a potential to slow down the development of CVD by influencing on certain risk factors. In this article, the authors present the potential mechanisms of resveratrol's activity (presented in Figure 1).

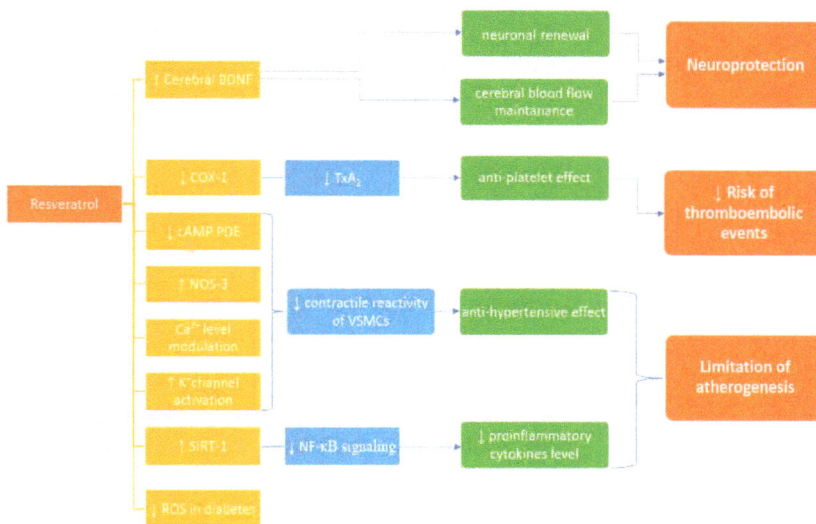

Figure 1. Proposed mechanisms of resveratrol activity. COX-1: cyclooxygenase type 1; cAMP: cyclic adenosine monophosphate; PDE: phosphodiesterase; SIRT-1: sirtuin-1; NOS-3: Nitric oxide synthase, ROS: reactive oxygen species, NF-κB: nuclear factor kappa-light-chain-enhancer of activated B cells; TxA$_2$: thromboxane A$_2$; VSMCs: vascular smooth muscle cells; ↓: a decrease; ↑: an increase.

2. Inflammation

Atherosclerosis is a multifactorial disease of the vascular walls leading to the development of plaques and consequent stenosis of the arteries [16,17]. Current progress in basic science has signified essential role of inflammation in initiation, progression and finally possible thromboembolic complications of the disease. Atherosclerosis-related inflammation is mediated by various cytokines which include among others: TNF-α, interleukin-6 (IL-6), monocyte chemoattractant protein-1 (MCP-1) as well as factors inducing the expression of intercellular adhesion molecule 1 (ICAM-1), vascular cell adhesion molecule 1 (VCAM-1) and E-selectin adhesion molecules. Long-term studies in humans conducted by Tomé Carneiro et al., and Militaru C. et al., imply that resveratrol corrected the lipid profile, inflammatory status and quality of life of patients undergoing primary prevention of CVD [18–20]. It can be connected with its influence in many potential pathways.

Inflammation associated with atherosclerosis is to a large extent regulated by the NF-κB pathway. It is logical to postulate that agents inhibiting or triggering the activation of this factor may play a significant role in atherogenesis [21]. The NF-κB itself is connected to various signalling agents by which can be activated and subsequently provoke inflammatory cascade. Studies in animals implicate that SIRT-1 is a potential target to focus on during the search for new solutions against atherosclerosis. The process of SIRT-1 upregulation may have a substantial impact on the activation of endothelium and its homeostasis [22,23]. SIRT1 is highly expressed in endothelial cells where it exercises control of angiogenesis through a wide variety of transcription regulators.

Resveratrol seems to be promising in its action limiting the inflammatory response at various levels. Experimental studies proved that resveratrol usage elevates the serum concentration of SIRT1 [24]. Pre-treatment of human vascular smooth muscle cells (VSMCs) at a dose 3–100 μM considerably enhanced SIRT1 expression [25]. Kao et al. [26] also noticed an augmentation of SIRT1 mRNA in human umbilical vein endothelial cells after pre-treatment with various doses of resveratrol (10–100 μM). Mechanism of sirtuin's influence at molecular level have been linked to the prevention of atherosclerosis in many proposed models. It is postulated that sirtuin-1 moderates transcription factor RelA/p65 at K310 by deacetylation. What follows is suppression of its binding to naked DNA in human aortic endothelial cells. The changes eventually interfere with NF-κB signalling pathway activation, thereby restraining the expression of genes coding cell adhesion molecules: VCAM-1 and ICAM-1 [26,27]. What is more, SIRT-1-related suppression of NF-κB signalling pathway results in inhibition of synthesis of a number of pro-inflammatory cytokine, including: TNF-α, IL-1β, IL-6 and MCP-1 [28]. Interestingly, SIRT-1 upregulation is also able to lower angiotensin II type I receptor expression in VSMCs. Such changes may cause limitation in vessel contractility contributing to the prevention against hypertension and thereby anti-sclerotic effect [29]. Thus, an increase in SIRT-1 activity has been connected with a decrease in atherosclerotic lesion size and macrophage content in aortic arches [28]. Furthermore, SIRT1 transgenic apolipoprotein E null (apoE−/−) mice had fewer atherosclerotic lesions [30]. Zhang QJ et al., suggested that SIRT-1 overexpression may impede atherogenesis by influencing endothelial function through the alterations involving nitric oxide synthase (NOS-3) [31]. The explicit mechanism of SIRT1 activation by resveratrol remains unspecified, however it is considered that abovementioned polyphenol activates SIRT1 indirectly [31,32]. One of the potential mechanisms is the induction of AMPK (5′ adenosine monophosphate-activated protein kinase). This kinase affects the intracellular AMP-to-ATP concentration ratio, which indirectly increases the level of nicotinamide adenine dinucleotide (NAD+). Increased concentrations of NAD+ are able to enhance SIRT1 activity, considering that NAD+ is substrate for the enzyme [33].

Low levels of adiponectin in serum have been associated with weight gain and visceral fat increase. A noticeable reduction of adiponectin serum concentrations in obese and insulin-resistant states has been observed [34]. Observational human studies imply that a decrease in adiponectin levels may contribute to a development of cardiometabolic disorders [35]. This conclusion may result from certain evidence presenting adiponectin deficit as a risk factor of atherosclerosis [36]. Studies in animals ascribe to adiponectin an ability to restrain formation of atherosclerotic lesions [21,37]. Induction of adiponectin expression by resveratrol was described in animal studies, nevertheless some of the results remain contradicted. On the one hand, month long 10 mg/kg resveratrol pre-treatment of Wistar rats significantly heightened the level of adiponectin in blood serum [24]. Similar results have been obtained by Rivera et al. [38] in obese Zucker rats. They achieved an increase in the adiponectin serum concentrations after 8 weeks of 10 mg/kg resveratrol daily pre-treatment. This escalation was not observed in lean heterozygous littermates [39]. Following studies exploiting experimental rat models proved that 6 weeks of both high-dose resveratrol administration (200 mg/kg daily) and smaller dosage (6 weeks of 15 mg/kg) [40] are able to elevate the adiponectin concentration and its release from adipose tissue (Table 1). On the other hand, Palsamy and Subramanian [41] have not received a significant change of plasma adiponectin levels after 30 days of low-dose resveratrol treatment (5 mg/kg) in a healthy population of Wistar rats, although the raise were noticeable in a diabetic subjects [41]. The exact molecular mechanisms of adiponectin beneficial actions are not fully clarified but it can be assumed that moderating inflammatory response serves a crucial role once again.

Studies show that adiponectin suppresses the nuclear translocation of NF-κB lowering the endothelial synthesis of pro-inflammatory chemokine IL-8 [42], TNF-α-induced expression of adhesion molecules on vascular endothelial cells and prevents monocyte adhesion which constitutes the initial step of atherogenesis [35].

Table 1. Oral administration of resveratrol in vivo trials.

Authors	Subject of Study	Dose	Result
Tomé Carneiro et al. [19]	Human with coronary artery disease	Polyphenolic composition + 8.1 ± 0.5 mg resveratrol per capsule. 1 capsule/day in the morning for the first 6 months and 2 capsules/day for the following 6 months	↑ serum adiponectin ↓ (PAI-1)
Militaru C. et al. [20]	Human with stable angina pectoris	20 mg/day of resveratrol	↓ hs-CRP, ↓ NT-proBNP, ↓ total cholesterol, ↑ quality of life
Bhatt et al. [43]	Human with DM2	250 mg/day of resveratrol	↓ HbA1c, ↓ SBP, ↓ total cholesterol
Brasnyó et al. [44]	Human with DM2	2 × 5mg/day of resveratrol	↓ insulin resistance, ↑ pAkt: Akt
Wiciński et al. [2]	Wistar rats	10 mg/kg of resveratrol per day	↑ serum BDNF
Wiciński et al. [24]	Wistar rats	10 mg/kg of resveratrol per day	↑ serum adiponectin
Rivera et al. [38]	Zucker rats	10 mg/kg of resveratrol per day	↑ serum adiponectin
Beaudoin et al. [39]	Zucker rats	200 mg/kg of resveratrol per day	↑ serum adiponectin and its release
Thirunavukkarasu et al. [45]	streptozotocin induced diabetic rats	2.5 mg/kg of resveratrol per day	↓ glucose level
Dong et al. [46]	Balb/c mice	50 mg/kg of resveratrol per day	↓ infract size after stroke, recover of neurologic function
Huang et al. [47]	Long-Evans rats	10^{-6}–10^{-9} g/kg of resveratrol intravenous	↓ infract size after stroke
Sinha et al. [48]	Wistar rats	20 mg/kg of resveratrol intraperitoneal	prevents motor impairment, ↑ MDA, ↓ glutathione, ↓ infract size after stroke
Fukuda et al. [49]	Rats	10 mg/kg of resveratrol per day	↑ VEGF, ↑ Flk-1,3, ↑ NOS
Della-Morte et al. [50]	Rats	10–100 mg/kg of resveratrol intraperitoneal	↑ SIRT-1, ↓ UCP2
Wang et al. [51]	Mongolian gerbils	30 mg/kg of resveratrol intraperitoneal	↓ DND, ↓ glial activation

Polyphenolic composition is (~25 mg anthocyanins, ~1 mg flavonols, ~40 mg procyanidins and ~0.8 mg hydroxycinnamic acids), ↓—reduction, ↑—increase, PAI-1—Plasminogen activator inhibitor-1, hs-CRP—high-sensitivity C Reactive Protein, NTproBNP—N-terminal prohormone of brain natriuretic peptide, quality of life—measured in the number of angina pectoris episodes and the amount of nitroglycerin used, HbA1c—Glycated haemoglobin A1c, SBP—systolic blood pressure, BDNF—brain-derived neurotrophic factor, MDA—Malondialdehyde, VEGF—vascular endothelial growth factor, Flk-1,3—tyrosine kinase receptor of VEGF , NOS—nitric-oxide synthase, SIRT1—sirtuin 1, DND—delayed neuronal cell death, UCP2—mitochondrial uncoupling protein 2.

Abovementioned aspects contributing to the limitation of inflammatory response by resveratrol may be linked to each other at the transcriptional level. RV is considered to upregulate SIRT1, FoxO1 and adiponectin transcription via interconnecting gene modulation pathways [52]. What is more, adiponectin may be correlated with a SIRT1-independent mechanism acting by induction of the AMPK, or as a FoxO1 activator through phosphoinositide-dependent kinase 1/protein kinase B signalling downregulation. Additionally, resveratrol effects on adiponectin indirectly by altering level of disulphide bond-A oxidoreductase-like protein [53].

3. Anti-Platelets Effect

One of the major causes of cardiovascular diseases such as myocardial infarction, stroke or acute limb ischemia is a thromboembolic event provoked by excessive or abnormal platelet aggregation. Antiplatelet drugs are widely used in the prevention of the above-mentioned diseases [54]. Research conducted on resveratrol suggest its antiplatelet properties both in vitro [5,55] as well as in vivo. It seems that the mechanism of resveratrol activity on platelets is to a large extent focused on the stronger inhibition of COX-1 in relation to COX-2 [56]. Selective inhibition of COX-1 results in reduced synthesis of TxA2 (thromboxane A2), which is a potent triggering factor of platelet aggregation [57]. COX-2, per contra, occurring inter alia in vascular endothelial cells, synthesizes prostacyclin, which is an antiplatelet aggregator [6,58]. In this case, selective COX-1 inhibition appears to be the reason for the antiplatelet action. Interestingly, in Dutra et al.,'s study from 2017 [59] concerning derivatives of resveratrol, researchers created a resveratrol-furoxan hybrid compound able to release NO (nitric oxide) and inhibit platelet aggregation in the ADP agonist, collagen and arachidonic agonist pathway. Administration of this compound was connected with reduced bleeding time compared to acetylsalicylic acid (ASA) and protected up to 80% against thrombotic events in vivo (performed on mice). The above study shows the meaningfulness of further research and efforts to synthesize new resveratrol derivatives with much better properties.

4. Vascular Reactivity

Vascular contractility is a significant factor in atherogenesis, as it is considered clinically relevant that arterial hypertension aggravates atherosclerosis [60]. Peripheral vascular resistance serves an influential role in pathogenesis of primary hypertension (also called essential or idiopathic). Arteries in patients suffering from hypertension often present augmented reactivity to contractive stimulus in comparison to healthy individuals. The exact cause of the phenomenon, however, remains unclear [61,62]. Due to hypertension, oxidative stress in the vascular wall increases which contributes to changes in metabolism and induces endothelium dysfunction, cell migration and proliferation of VSMCs [60]. Furthermore, the level of acute-phase proteins circulating in the bloodstream increases, which have been proven to activate the inflammation process through TLR-4 signalling pathways [61]. In various studies vascular contractile reactivity was evaluated and the mechanisms responsible for the reduction of the aforementioned atherogenic factors were assessed. It has been revealed that resveratrol may inhibit Ca2+/calmodulin cyclic nucleotide PDE (phosphodiesterase) and contribute to diminishment of VSMCs contractile response in partially PDE1 dependent manner.

Research conducted in rat models suggest that hypertension may be correlated with the increase of PDE1 expression and activation [63]. It has been stated that inhibition of PDE1 leads to decrease of arterial contractile response as consequence of intracellular cGMP concentration increase [64]. The subtype 1C of PDE is expressed in proliferating smooth muscle cells and may be potentially involved in atherogenesis [65]. If the inhibition of PDE1C by resveratrol is presented to be relevant in treatment, one additional advantageous effects would be a slowdown of VSMCs proliferation which remains the one of the fundamental elements of atherosclerotic plaque development [66]. Park et al., described resveratrol [67] to be a potent antagonist of cAMP PDEs (including PDE1-4) that inhibits these enzymes directly in a concentration-dependent manner. Kline and Karpinski [68] observed resveratrol's ability to induce NOS-3 in direct and indirect manners through AMPK, SIRT1 and nuclear factor erythroid 2-related factor 2 pathways. Additionally, they noticed that resveratrol acts directly on VSMCs by blocking the L-type calcium channel resulting in limitation of intracellular Ca2+ release.

5. Resveratrol Influence on Diabetes

There exists a close connection between DM (diabetes mellitus) and CVDs, which are the most common causes of morbidity and mortality in diabetic patients. Type 2 diabetes is a condition where persistent hyperglycaemia and hyperinsulinemia are associated with chronic low-grade inflammation. As the consequence, the amount of ROS increases [69] which can have an impact on cell damage. Affected can be also neurons [70]. Bhatt et al. [43] in their studies in a group of 62 patients with type II diabetes compared the use of standard antidiabetic therapy with a combination of this therapy and resveratrol. After three months of treatment, the results in both groups were evaluated. The combination had a statistically significant advantage in positive effect. It caused a decrease in HbA1c (glycated haemoglobin A1c), lowered the systolic blood pressure, as well as total cholesterol level. It did not, however, have a statistically significant effect on body weight and respective lipoprotein fractions. Thirunavukkarasu et al. [45] achieved a reduction in glycaemia in the group of rats with DM2 receiving resveratrol. On the other hand, in a randomized, double-blind study of Bo et al. [71] conducted on a group of 192 people suffering from DM2, the use of resveratrol did not bring any statistically significant changes in biochemical markers such as: CRP (C-reactive-protein), BMI (Body Mass Index), blood pressure, HbA1c and others. In the work of Öztürk et al. [72] which has collected a dozen clinical trials investigating the effect of resveratrol on DM2, researchers have noticed the pleiotropic effects of resveratrol. In attempt to describe potential mechanisms of its profitable actions a broad number of factors have to be considered.

One of the possible mechanisms once more focused on the activation of abovementioned SIRT-1 [73]. Studies have shown a significant reduction in its expression and activity both in vitro and in vivo in the course of DM2 [74,75]. Some of the positive effects of resveratrol may be explained by activation of AMPK. Mentioned kinase regulates intracellular processes such as energy metabolism, mitochondrial functions and cellular homeostasis. AMPK dysregulation correlated with insulin resistance and hyperglycaemia-associated tissue damage suggesting the role of AMPK in DM2 [72,76]. Furthermore, it is hypothesized that the beneficial effect in diabetes can also be explained by the activation by the SIRT-1 of the PGC-1α cascade (peroxisome proliferator-activated receptor gamma coactivator 1-alpha) [76]. PGC-1α, as a transcriptional coactivator, regulates genes involved in energy metabolism. It is one of the main regulators of mitochondrial biogenesis [77]. Mootha et al. [78] in their studies described a reduced level of transcription of the PPARGC1 gene (gene encoding PGC-1α) in calf muscles of diabetic patients. What is more, impaired mitochondrial function (associated with less PGC-1α activity) promoting fatty acid accumulation, as opposed to oxidation, can significantly contribute to intracellular lipid accumulation, which is associated with insulin resistance in DM2 in humans [79]. Based on resveratrol PGC-1α cascade activating abilities, some positive influence od RV may be assumed.

In DM2, pancreatic β-cell damage is related to increased creation of free radicals [80,81]. One possible mechanism of resveratrol usage in DM2 may be its antioxidant effect. In the studies of Brasnyó et al. [44] a decrease in insulin resistance in patients receiving resveratrol has been shown. Researchers linked it to increased activation of the Akt signalling pathway. In addition to direct antioxidative activity, it is suggested that resveratrol may affect the expression of genes regulating pro and antioxidant mechanisms by reducing the expression of enzymes responsible for the production of free radicals and increasing the production of those involved in scavenging of ROS as NADPH oxidase (Nox) and its products: SOD (superoxide dismutase) and GPx1 (glutathione peroxidase 1) [82].

Another potentially advantageous action of resveratrol in DM2 is an attenuation of the NF-κB signalling pathway [83–85]. NF-κB is a protein complex that regulates the immune response and can be considered as prototypical proinflammatory factor in many diseases [86]. Researchers [87] propose a model in which activation of NF-κB results in increased production of IL-6, which induces insulin resistance in hepatocytes [88,89]. In this case, resveratrol reducing the activation of this pathway could affect the decrease of insulin resistance in the tissues. DM2 is often associated with abdominal obesity [90], which can lead to metabolic syndrome, abdominal adiposity and hepatic steatosis (fatty liver). All the states result in persistent low-grade inflammation being a cause of oxidative stress [89]. Cai et al. [89] in their study found that the NF-κB pathway is activated in rodent livers by two obesity models: HFD (High Fat Diet) and genetic hyperphagia.

Chronic hyperglycaemia generates AGEs (advanced glycation end products) and their RAGE receptors [91]. RAGEs activation is another trigger factor of NF-κB transcription cascade [92]. This suggests that activation of NF-κB in diabetic patients correlates with the quality of glycaemic control [93]. The reduction of NF-κB activity by resveratrol in numerous ways provides a potential protection line against lasting hyperglycaemia. Interdependence of described numerous mechanisms is evident, what brings both many opportunities and obstacles.

6. Cerebral Blood Flow

Chronic systemic diseases are thought to impair vasorelaxation with the consequence that cerebral blood flow is diminished [94]. Cognitive impairment and dementia are characterized by defective cerebrovascular blood flow which is considered to be a significant element in their pathogenesis. Moreover, Araya et al., state that cerebrovascular abnormalities, especially in cerebral microvessels, potentially lead to neuronal dysfunction and cognitive impairment [94,95]. Maintenance of cerebral blood flow at both stable and sufficient levels seems to be a potential target in the pharmacological prevention of neurodegeneration. Beneficial effect of resveratrol treatment has been shown in disorders such as Alzheimer's disease, Parkinson's disease, Huntington's disease, amyotrophic lateral sclerosis [96] and vascular dementia [97].

Resveratrol increases BDNF serum concentrations which, according to literature, reflects an increase of BDNF in brain parenchyma. Potentially, the aforementioned neurotrophin constitutes the link in maintaining cerebral blood flow in response to hypoxic stress. Guo et al., suggest that BDNF seems to be serving a major role in the neurovascular unit of brain. Their results confirm that cerebrovascular endothelium can secrete potent neuroprotective agents [98]. BDNF is involved in the differentiation and maturation of nerve cells in the central nervous system. The neurotrophin is also associated with increased ratio of growth, formation of new neuronal connections and nerve branching, as well as induction of synaptic transmission [99–101]. The diminishment of serum BDNF levels may result in aggravation and poor outcome in neurodegenerative diseases [102–105]. Accordingly, agents like resveratrol that induce the expression of BDNF are believed to reproduce the biological effects of the neurotrophin.

Induction of BDNF expression in brain structures following an administration of naturally existing plant-derived polyphenols was previously described by Jeon et al. [106]. Zhang et al., found that resveratrol induces BDNF release from astroglia in rat primary astroglia-enriched cultures suggesting that resveratrol administration may be more efficient than direct treatment with neurotrophic factors [107]. The mechanism of BDNF upregulation by resveratrol has not been explained comprehensively yet. According to Goggi et al., the release of BDNF depends on the concentrations of both extracellular and intracellular calcium. They have also noticed that BDNF release is link to the activation of IP3 (inositol trisphosphate) mediated Ca^{2+} release from intracellular stores. BDNF was also modulated by receptors coupled to adenylate cyclase. Another probable mechanism is activation of the CREB and ERK1/2 signalling pathways which result in an increased production of neurotropic factors [107].

Resveratrol has the ability to induce NOS-3 in both a direct and indirect manner through AMPK, SIRT1 and Nrf2 pathways and, as a result, it positively affects vasorelaxation in cerebral arteries [108]. Results presented in study of Leblais et al., state that resveratrol may directly act on VSMCs promoting pulmonary artery relaxation via different mechanisms including induction of guanylyl cyclase, inhibition of protein kinase C, activation of smooth muscle K+ channels, or acting via Ca2+ [109]. Direct reduction of VSMC contractility by resveratrol may be a meaningful mechanism in neuroprotection since pathogenesis of neurodegenerative diseases is also matched with vasoconstriction [110]

One of the most prevalent CV illness is stroke [111]. During ischemia, the increased production of free radicals by mitochondria becomes responsible for endothelial dysfunction and causes excitation contraction coupling impairment in VSMCs [112]. The direct cell damage resulting from ischemia leads to death, apoptosis or metabolic changes. Insults caused by stroke must be distinguished between primary and secondary. The former cause unavoidable damage in the centre of the ischemic area. Secondary ones result from processes lasting days in the tissues surrounding the primary injury. Induced oedema, release of lethal calcium ions amounts, epigenetic changes and agents created by activated microglia are directly or indirectly toxic to neurons and initiate progressive damage [113,114]. In experimental studies on the mouse model, WenPeng Dong and co-workers assessed the effect of resveratrol on the extent of damage caused by ischemia and reperfusion. [46] (Table 1). The area of ischemia and microcirculatory injuries were significantly smaller compared to the control group not receiving resveratrol. Similar results were obtained by Huang et al., and Sinha K. et al., where resveratrol managed to reduce infarct volume and prevented impairments in motor function in rats. [47–49].

Although mechanisms underlying the beneficial effects are yet still to be elucidated, there exist a supposition that angiogenesis mediated by VEGF and MMP-2 might be responsible for insult limitation [50]. Ischemic cerebral regions showed significantly higher concentrations of abovementioned proteins. [114]. What is more, the alteration of mitochondrial function via SIRT-1 target mitochondrial uncoupling protein 2 (UCP2) caused by RV may be a way to mimic ischemic preconditioning [115]. UCP2–/– mice were described to be less vulnerable to microglia activation and consequent unfavourable effect [116]. Since SIRT 1 inhibitor tended to prevent UCP2 upregulation, the hypothesis of sirtuin involvement in the neuroprotection seems reasonable [115]. Anti-inflammatory effects where presented in work of Wang Q et al., in which RV diminished neuronal cell death and glial activation in the hippocampus of gerbils after artificially induced common carotid artery occlusion [51].

Above all, the most anticipated still remains a perspective of therapeutical application in human. Long-term observation of the influence of the administration of resveratrol on secondary prevention of stroke confirmed its beneficial effects (both in the 100 mg dose and 200 mg/day) on a number of risk factors for recurrence [116]. There was a significant improvement in glucose profile, lipidogram and arterial pressure. During the 12 months of the study, Katalin Fodor et al., they did not detect a single vascular incident [117].

7. Conclusions

The information presented above allows for considering resveratrol as a promising drug in the treatment of cardiovascular conditions. The moderation of free radicals creation and proinflammatory response diminishment may prove to be helpful in slowing down atherosclerosis development as well as in limiting the changes connected to chronic hyperglycaemia. Potential properties stimulating neuronal renewal, if proven, would find application in the treatment of various forms of dementia. If resveratrol is demonstrated to have clinically meaningful anti-sclerotic activity in humans, one potential application may be to reduce the burden of certain neurodegenerative disorders. In perspective of future findings, it is worth to consider the use of not only resveratrol alone but also its derivatives with preferable effects. Studies assessing beneficial effects of RV on cardiovascular system need to be strengthened in order to plausibly evaluate its usability. Wide spread of dosage used with similar effect makes it difficult to determine the proper dose. Additional studies are essential to verify efficacy of resveratrol in conditions specified in the paper.

Author Contributions: M.W. (Michał Wiciński), M.W. (Maciej Walczak) and E.W. contributed to data analysis, interpretation of findings, and drafting the article. M.S., B.M., S.R., K.G. and K.P.-O. participated in data collection, critical revision of the article and final approval.

Funding: The present work was supported by the Department of Pharmacology and Therapeutics, Faculty of Medicine, Collegium Medicum in Bydgoszcz, Nicolaus Copernicus University, Toruń, Poland.

Conflicts of Interest: The authors declare no conflict of interest.

References

1. Higdon, J.; Drake, V.J.; Steward, W.P. *Resveratrol*; Micronutrient Information Center, Linus Pauling Institute, Oregon State University: Corvallis, OR, USA, 2016.
2. Wiciński, M.; Malinowski, B.; Węclewicz, M.M.; Grześk, E.; Grześk, G. Resveratrol increases serum BDNF concentrations and reduces vascular smooth muscle cells contractility via a NOS-3-independent mechanism. *BioMed Res. Int.* **2017**. [CrossRef] [PubMed]
3. Jasiński, M.; Jasińska, L.; Ogrodowczyk, M. Resveratrol in prostate diseases—A short review. *Cent. Eur. J. Urol.* **2013**, *66*, 144.
4. Gülçin, İ. Antioxidant properties of resveratrol: A structure–Activity insight. *Innov. Food Sci. Emerg. Technol.* **2010**, *11*, 210–218. [CrossRef]

5. Bertelli, A.A.; Giovannini, L.; Giannessi, D.; Migliori, M.; Bernini, W.; Fregoni, M.; Bertelli, A. Antiplatelet activity of synthetic and natural resveratrol in red wine. *Int. J. Tissue React.* **1995**, *17*, 1–3. [PubMed]

6. Baur, J.A.; Sinclair, D.A. Therapeutic potential of resveratrol: The in vivo evidence. *Nat. Rev. Drug Discov.* **2006**, *5*, 493. [CrossRef] [PubMed]

7. Frémont, L. Biological effects of resveratrol. *Life Sci.* **2000**, *66*, 663–673. [CrossRef]

8. Mahal, H.S.; Mukherjee, T. Scavenging of reactive oxygen radicals by resveratrol: Antioxidant effect. *Res. Chem. Intermed.* **2006**, *32*, 59–71. [CrossRef]

9. Fibach, E.; Prus, E.; Bianchi, N.; Zuccato, C.; Breveglieri, G.; Salvatori, F.; Finotti, A.; Lipucci di Paola, M.; Brognara, E.; Lampronti, I.; et al. Resveratrol: Antioxidant activity and induction of fetal hemoglobin in erythroid cells from normal donors and β-thalassemia patients. *Int. J. Mol. Med.* **2012**, *29*, 974–982. [PubMed]

10. Subbaramaiah, K.; Chung, W.J.; Michaluart, P.; Telang, N.; Tanabe, T.; Inoue, H.; Jang, M.; Pezzuto, J.M.; Dannenberg, A.J. Resveratrol inhibits cyclooxygenase-2 transcription and activity in phorbol ester-treated human mammary epithelial cells. *J. Biol. Chem.* **1998**, *273*, 21875–21882. [CrossRef] [PubMed]

11. Szewczuk, L.M.; Forti, L.; Stivala, L.A.; Penning, T.M. Resveratrol is a peroxidase mediated inactivator of COX-1 but not COX-2: A mechanistic approach to the design of COX-1 selective agents. *J. Biol. Chem.* **2004**, *279*, 22727–22737. [CrossRef] [PubMed]

12. Saiko, P.; Szakmary, A.; Jaeger, W.; Szekeres, T. Resveratrol and its analogs: Defense against cancer, coronary disease and neurodegenerative maladies or just a fad? *Mutat. Res. Rev. Mutat. Res.* **2008**, *658*, 68–94. [CrossRef] [PubMed]

13. Capiralla, H.; Vingtdeux, V.; Zhao, H.; Sankowski, R.; Al-Abed, Y.; Davies, P.; Marambaud, P. Resveratrol mitigates lipopolysaccharide-and Aβ-mediated microglial inflammation by inhibiting the TLR4/NF-κB/STAT signaling cascade. *J. Neurochem.* **2012**, *120*, 461–472. [CrossRef] [PubMed]

14. Alarcon De La Lastra, C.; Villegas, I. Resveratrol as an anti-inflammatory and anti-aging agent: Mechanisms and clinical implications. *Mol. Nutr. Food Res.* **2005**, *49*, 405–430. [CrossRef] [PubMed]

15. World Health Organization. *World Health Statistics 2016: Monitoring Health for the SDGs Sustainable Development Goals*; World Health Organization: Geneva, Switzerland, 2016.

16. Libby, P. Inflammation in atherosclerosis. *Arterioscler. Thromb. Vasc. Biol.* **2012**, *32*, 2045–2051. [CrossRef] [PubMed]

17. Hansson, G.K.; Hermansson, A. The immune system in atherosclerosis. *Nat. Immunol.* **2011**, *12*, 204–212. [CrossRef] [PubMed]

18. Tomé-Carneiro, J.; Gonzálvez, M.; Larrosa, M.; Yáñez-Gascón, M.J.; García-Almagro, F.J.; Ruiz-Ros, J.A.; Tomás-Barberán, F.A.; García-Conesa, M.T.; Espín, J.C. Resveratrol in primary and secondary prevention of cardiovascular disease: A dietary and clinical perspective. *Ann. N. Y. Acad. Sci.* **2013**, *1290*, 37–51. [CrossRef] [PubMed]

19. Tomé-Carneiro, J.; Gonzálvez, M.; Larrosa, M.; Yáñez-Gascón, M.J.; García-Almagro, F.J.; Ruiz-Ros, J.A.; Tomás-Barberán, F.A.; García-Conesa, M.T.; Espín, J.C. Grape resveratrol increases serum adiponectin and downregulates inflammatory genes in peripheral blood mononuclear cells: A triple-blind, placebo-controlled, one-year clinical trial in patients with stable coronary artery disease. *Cardiovasc. Drugs Ther.* **2013**, *27*, 37–48. [CrossRef] [PubMed]

20. Militaru, C.; Donoiu, I.; Craciun, A.; Scorei, I.D.; Bulearca, A.M.; Scorei, R.I. Oral resveratrol and calcium fructoborate supplementation in subjects with stable angina pectoris: Effects on lipid profles, inflammation markers and quality of life. *Nutrition* **2013**, *29*, 178–183. [CrossRef] [PubMed]

21. Wang, X.; Chen, Q.; Pu, H.; Wei, Q.; Duan, M.; Zhang, C.; Jiang, T.; Shou, X.; Zhang, J.; Yang, Y. Adiponectin improves NF-κB-mediated inflammation and abates atherosclerosis progression in apolipoprotein E-defcient mice. *Lipids Health Dis.* **2016**, *15*, 33. [CrossRef] [PubMed]

22. Ota, H.; Eto, M.; Ogawa, S.; Iijima, K.; Akishita, M.; Ouchi, Y. SIRT1/eNOS axis as a potential target against vascular senescence, dysfunction and atherosclerosis. *J. Atheroscler. Thromb.* **2010**, *17*, 431–435. [CrossRef] [PubMed]

23. Brandes, R.P. Activating SIRT1: A new strategy to prevent atherosclerosis? *Cardiovasc. Res.* **2008**, *80*, 163–164. [CrossRef] [PubMed]

24. Wiciński, M.; Malinowski, B.; Węclewicz, M.M.; Grześk, E.; Grześk, G. Anti-atherogenic properties of resveratrol: 4-week resveratrol administration associated with serum concentrations of SIRT1, adiponectin, S100A8/A9 and VSMCs contractility in a rat model. *Exp. Ther. Med.* **2017**, *13*, 2071–2078. [CrossRef] [PubMed]

25. Thompson, A.M.; Martin, K.A.; Rzucidlo, E.M. Resveratrol induces vascular smooth muscle cell differentiation through stimulation of SirT1 and AMPK. *PLoS ONE* **2014**, *9*, E85495. [CrossRef] [PubMed]

26. Kao, C.L.; Chen, L.K.; Chang, Y.L.; Yung, M.C.; Hsu, C.C.; Chen, Y.C.; Lo, W.L.; Chen, S.J.; Ku, H.H.; Hwang, S.J. Resveratrol protects human endothelium from H(2)O(2)-induced oxidative stress and senescence via SirT1 activation. *J. Atheroscler. Thromb.* **2010**, *17*, 970–979. [CrossRef] [PubMed]

27. Michelsen, K.S.; Wong, M.H.; Shah, P.K.; Zhang, W.; Yano, J.; Doherty, T.M.; Akira, S.; Rajavashisth, T.B.; Arditi, M. Lack of toll-like receptor 4 or myeloid differentiation factor 88 reduces atherosclerosis and alters plaque phenotype in mice defcient in apolipoprotein E. *Proc. Natl. Acad. Sci. USA* **2004**, *101*, 10679–10684. [CrossRef] [PubMed]

28. Stein, S.; Schäfer, N.; Breitenstein, A.; Besler, C.; Winnik, S.; Lohmann, C.; Heinrich, K.; Brokopp, C.E.; Handschin, C.; Landmesser, U.; et al. SIRT1 reduces endothelial activation without affecting vascular function in ApoE−/− mice. *Aging (Albany NY)* **2010**, *2*, 353–360. [CrossRef] [PubMed]

29. Chen, Y.X.; Zhang, M.; Cai, Y.; Zhao, Q.; Dai, W. The Sirt1 activator SRT1720 attenuates angiotensin II-induced atherosclerosis in apoE−/− mice through inhibiting vascular inflammatory response. *Biochem. Biophys. Res. Commun.* **2015**, *465*, 732–738. [CrossRef] [PubMed]

30. Miyazaki, R.; Ichiki, T.; Hashimoto, T.; Inanaga, K.; Imayama, I.; Sadoshima, J.; Sunagawa, K. SIRT1, a longevity gene, downregulates angiotensin II type 1 receptor expression in vascular smooth muscle cells. *Arterioscler. Thromb. Vasc. Biol.* **2008**, *28*, 1263–1269. [CrossRef] [PubMed]

31. Zhang, Q.J.; Wang, Z.; Chen, H.Z.; Zhou, S.; Zheng, W.; Liu, G.; Wei, Y.S.; Cai, H.; Liu, D.P.; Liang, C.C. Endothelium-specifc overexpression of class III deacetylase SIRT1 decreases atherosclerosis in apolipoprotein E-defcient mice. *Cardiovasc. Res.* **2008**, *80*, 191–199. [CrossRef] [PubMed]

32. Higashida, K.; Kim, S.H.; Jung, S.R.; Asaka, M.; Holloszy, J.O.; Han, D.H. Effects of resveratrol and SIRT1 on PGC-1α activity and mitochondrial biogenesis: A reevaluation. *PLoS Biol.* **2013**, *11*, E1001603. [CrossRef] [PubMed]

33. Li, J.; Feng, L.; Xing, Y.; Wang, Y.; Du, L.; Xu, C.; Cao, J.; Wang, Q.; Fan, S.; Liu, Q.; et al. Radioprotective and antioxidant effect of resveratrol in hippocampus by activating Sirt1. *Int. J. Mol. Sci.* **2014**, *15*, 5928–5939. [CrossRef] [PubMed]

34. Cantó, C.; Gerhart-Hines, Z.; Feige, J.N.; Lagouge, M.; Noriega, L.; Milne, J.C.; Elliott, P.J.; Puigserver, P.; Auwerx, J. AMPK regulates energy expenditure by modulating NAD+ metabolism and SIRT1 activity. *Nature* **2009**, *458*, 1056–1060. [CrossRef] [PubMed]

35. Okauchi, Y.; Kishida, K.; Funahashi, T.; Noguchi, M.; Ogawa, T.; Ryo, M.; Okita, K.; Iwahashi, H.; Imagawa, A.; Nakamura, T.; et al. Changes in serum adiponectin concentrations correlate with changes in BMI, waist circumference, and estimated visceral fat area in middle-aged general population. *Diabetes Care* **2009**, *32*, E122. [CrossRef] [PubMed]

36. Lim, S.; Quon, M.J.; Koh, K.K. Modulation of adiponectin as a potential therapeutic strategy. *Atherosclerosis* **2014**, *233*, 721–728. [CrossRef] [PubMed]

37. Shimada, K.; Miyazaki, T.; Daida, H. Adiponectin and atherosclerotic disease. *Clin. Chim. Acta* **2004**, *344*, 1–12. [CrossRef] [PubMed]

38. Rivera, L.; Morón, R.; Zarzuelo, A.; Galisteo, M. Long-term resveratrol administration reduces metabolic disturbances and lowers blood pressure in obese Zucker rats. *Biochem. Pharmacol.* **2009**, *77*, 1053–1063. [CrossRef] [PubMed]

39. Beaudoin, M.S.; Snook, L.A.; Arkell, A.M.; Simpson, J.A.; Holloway, G.P.; Wright, D.C. Resveratrol supplementation improves white adipose tissue function in a depot-specifc manner in Zucker diabetic fatty rats. *Am. J. Physiol. Regul. Integr. Comp. Physiol.* **2013**, *305*, R542–R551. [CrossRef] [PubMed]

40. Gómez-Zorita, S.; Fernández-Quintela, A.; Lasa, A.; Hijona, E.; Bujanda, L.; Portillo, M.P. Effects of resveratrol on obesity-related inflammation markers in adipose tissue of genetically obese rats. *Nutrition* **2013**, *29*, 1374–1380. [CrossRef] [PubMed]

41. Palsamy, P.; Subramanian, S. Resveratrol protects diabetic kidney by attenuating hyperglycemia-mediated oxidative stress and renal inflammatory cytokines via Nrf2-Keap1 signaling. *Biochim. Biophys. Acta* **2011**, *1812*, 719–731. [CrossRef] [PubMed]

42. Kobashi, C.; Urakaze, M.; Kishida, M.; Kibayashi, E.; Kobayashi, H.; Kihara, S.; Funahashi, T.; Takata, M.; Temaru, R.; Sato, A.; et al. Adiponectin inhibits endothelial synthesis of interleukin-8. *Circ. Res.* **2005**, *97*, 1245–1252. [CrossRef] [PubMed]

43. Bhatt, J.K.; Thomas, S.; Nanjan, M.J. Resveratrol supplementation improves glycemic control in type 2 diabetes mellitus. *Nutr. Res.* **2012**, *32*, 537–541. [CrossRef] [PubMed]
44. Brasnyó, P.; Molnár, G.A.; Mohás, M.; Markó, L.; Laczy, B.; Cseh, J.; Mikolás, E.; Szijártó, I.S.; Mérei, Á.; Halmai, R.; et al. Resveratrol improves insulin sensitivity, reduces oxidative stress and activates the Akt pathway in type 2 diabetic patients. *Br. J. Nutr.* **2011**, *106*, 383–389. [CrossRef] [PubMed]
45. Thirunavukkarasu, M.; Penumathsa, S.V.; Koneru, S.; Juhasz, B.; Zhan, L.; Otani, H.; Bagchi, D.; Das, D.K.; Maulik, N. Resveratrol alleviates cardiac dysfunction in streptozotocin-induced diabetes: Role of nitric oxide, thioredoxin, and heme oxygenase. *Free Radic. Biol. Med.* **2007**, *43*, 720–729. [CrossRef] [PubMed]
46. Dong, W.; Li, N.; Gao, D.; Zhen, H.; Zhang, X.; Li, F. Resveratrol attenuates ischemic brain damage in the delayed phase after stroke and induces messenger RNA and protein express for angiogenic factors. *J. Vasc. Surg.* **2008**, *48*, 709–714. [CrossRef] [PubMed]
47. Huang, S.S.; Tsai, M.C.; Chih, C.L.; Hung, L.M.; Tsai, S.K. Resveratrol reduction of infarct size in long-evans rats subjected to focal cerebral ischemia. *Life Sci.* **2001**, *69*, 1057–1065. [CrossRef]
48. Sinha, K.; Chaudhary, G.; Gupta, Y.K. Protective effect of resveratrol against oxidative stress in middle cerebral artery occlusion model of stroke in rats. *Life Sci.* **2002**, *71*, 655–665. [CrossRef]
49. Fukuda, S.; Kaga, S.; Zhan, L.; Bagchi, D.; Das, D.K.; Bertelli, A.; Maulik, N. Resveratrol ameliorates myocardial damage by inducing vascular endothelial growth factor-angiogenesis and tyrosine kinase receptor Flk-1. *Cell Biochem. Biophys.* **2006**, *44*, 43–49. [CrossRef]
50. Della-Morte, D.; Dave, K.R.; DeFazio, R.A.; Bao, Y.C.; Raval, A.P.; Perez-Pinzon, M.A. Resveratrol pretreatment protects rat brain from cerebral ischemic damage via a sirtuin 1–uncoupling protein 2 pathway. *Neurosci.* **2009**, *159*, 993–1002. [CrossRef] [PubMed]
51. Wang, Q.; Xu, J.; Rottinghaus, G.E.; Simonyi, A.; Lubahn, D.; Sun, G.Y.; Sun, A.Y. Resveratrol protects against global cerebral ischemic injury in gerbils. *Brain Res.* **2002**, *958*, 439–447. [CrossRef]
52. Costa Cdos, S.; Rohden, F.; Hammes, T.O.; Margis, R.; Bortolotto, J.W.; Padoin, A.V.; Mottin, C.C.; Guaragna, R.M. Resveratrol upregulated SIRT1, FOXO1, and adiponectin and downregulated PPARγ1-3 mRNA expression in human visceral adipocytes. *Obes. Surg.* **2011**, *21*, 356–361. [CrossRef] [PubMed]
53. Wang, A.; Liu, M.; Liu, X.; Dong, L.Q.; Glickman, R.D.; Slaga, T.J.; Zhou, Z.; Liu, F. Up-regulation of adiponectin by resveratrol: The essential roles of the Akt/FOXO1 and AMP-activated protein kinase signaling pathways and DsbA-L. *J. Biol. Chem.* **2011**, *286*, 60–66. [CrossRef] [PubMed]
54. Behan, M.W.H.; Storey, R.F. Antiplatelet therapy in cardiovascular disease. *Postgrad. Med. J.* **2004**, *80*, 155–164. [CrossRef] [PubMed]
55. Wang, Z.; Huang, Y.; Zou, J.; Cao, K.; Xu, Y.; Wu, J.M. Effects of red wine and wine polyphenol resveratrol on platelet aggregation in vivo and in vitro. *Int. J. Mol. Med.* **2002**, *9*, 77–79. [CrossRef] [PubMed]
56. Jang, M.; Cai, L.; Udeani, G.O.; Slowing, K.V.; Thomas, C.F.; Beecher, C.W.; Fong, H.H.E.; Farnsworth, N.R.; Kinghorn, A.D.; Mehta, R.G.; et al. Cancer chemopreventive activity of resveratrol, a natural product derived from grapes. *Science* **1997**, *275*, 218–220. [CrossRef] [PubMed]
57. FitzGerald, G.A. Mechanisms of platelet activation: Thromboxane A2 as an amplifying signal for other agonists. *Am. J. Cardiol.* **1991**, *68*, B11–B15. [CrossRef]
58. Knebel, S.M.; Sprague, R.S.; Stephenson, A.H. Prostacyclin receptor expression on platelets of humans with type 2 diabetes is inversely correlated with hemoglobin A1c levels. *Prostaglandins Other Lipid Mediat.* **2015**, *116*, 131–135. [CrossRef] [PubMed]
59. Dutra, L.A.; Guanaes, J.F.O.; Johmann, N.; Pires, M.E.L.; Chin, C.M.; Marcondes, S.; Dos Santos, J.L. Synthesis, antiplatelet and antithrombotic activities of resveratrol derivatives with NO-donor properties. *Bioorgan. Med. Chem. Lett.* **2017**, *27*, 2450–2453. [CrossRef] [PubMed]
60. Alexander, R.W. Hypertension and the pathogenesis of atherosclerosis: Oxidative stress and the mediation of arterial inflammatory response: A. new perspective. *Hypertension* **1995**, *25*, 155–161. [CrossRef] [PubMed]
61. Bomfim, G.F.; Dos Santos, R.A.; Oliveira, M.A.; Giachini, F.R.; Akamine, E.H.; Tostes, R.C.; Fortes, Z.B.; Webb, R.C.; Carvalho, M.H. Toll-like receptor 4 contributes to blood pressure regulation and vascular contraction in spontaneously hypertensive rats. *Clin. Sci.* **2012**, *122*, 535–543. [CrossRef] [PubMed]
62. Doyle, A.E.; Fraser, J.R. Vascular reactivity in hypertension. *Circ. Res.* **1961**, *9*, 755–761. [CrossRef] [PubMed]

63. Evgenov, O.V.; Busch, C.J.; Evgenov, N.V.; Liu, R.; Petersen, B.; Falkowski, G.E.; Petho, B.; Vas, A.; Bloch, K.D.; Zapol, W.M.; et al. Inhibition of phosphodiesterase 1 augments the pulmonary vasodilator response to inhaled nitric oxide in awake lambs with acute pulmonary hypertension. *Am. J. Physiol. Lung Cell. Mol. Physiol.* **2006**, *290*, L723–L729. [CrossRef] [PubMed]

64. Giachini, F.R.; Lima, V.V.; Carneiro, F.S.; Tostes, R.C.; Webb, R.C. Decreased cGMP level contributes to increased contraction in arteries from hypertensive rats: Role of phosphodiesterase 1. *Hypertension* **2011**, *57*, 655–663. [CrossRef] [PubMed]

65. Rybalkin, S.D.; Rybalkina, I.; Beavo, J.A.; Bornfeldt, K.E. Cyclic nucleotide phosphodiesterase 1C promotes human arterial smooth muscle cell proliferation. *Circ. Res.* **2002**, *90*, 151–157. [CrossRef] [PubMed]

66. Bischoff, E. Potency, selectivity, and consequences of nonselectivity of PDE inhibition. *Int. J. Impot. Res.* **2004**, *16* (Suppl. 1), S11–S14. [CrossRef] [PubMed]

67. Park, S.J.; Ahmad, F.; Philp, A.; Baar, K.; Williams, T.; Luo, H.; Ke, H.; Rehmann, H.; Taussig, R.; Brown, A.L.; et al. Resveratrol ameliorates aging-related metabolic phenotypes by inhibiting cAMP phosphodiesterases. *Cell* **2012**, *148*, 421–433. [CrossRef] [PubMed]

68. Kline, L.W.; Karpinski, E. The resveratrol-induced relaxation of cholecystokinin octapeptide- or kcl-induced tension in male guinea pig gallbladder strips is mediated through, L-type Ca2+ channels. *J. Neurogastroenterol. Motil.* **2015**, *21*, 62–68. [CrossRef] [PubMed]

69. Lin, Y.; Berg, A.H.; Iyengar, P.; Lam, T.K.; Giacca, A.; Combs, T.P.; Rajala, M.W.; Du, X.; Rollman, B.; Li, W.; et al. The hyperglycemia-induced inflammatory response in adipocytes the role of reactive oxygen species. *J. Biol. Chem.* **2005**, *280*, 4617–4626. [CrossRef] [PubMed]

70. Wiciński, M.; Wódkiewicz, E.; Słupski, M.; Walczak, M.; Socha, M.; Malinowski, B.; Pawlak-Osińska, K. Neuroprotective activity of sitagliptin via reduction of neuroinflammation beyond the incretin effect: Focus on Alzheimer's disease. *BioMed Res. Int.* **2018**. [CrossRef] [PubMed]

71. Bo, S.; Ponzo, V.; Ciccone, G.; Evangelista, A.; Saba, F.; Goitre, I.; Procopio, M.; Pagano, G.F.; Cassader, M.; Gambino, R. Six months of resveratrol supplementation has no measurable effect in type 2 diabetic patients. A randomized, double blind, placebo-controlled trial. *Pharmacol. Res.* **2016**, *111*, 896–905. [CrossRef] [PubMed]

72. Öztürk, E.; Arslan, A.K.K.; Yerer, M.B.; Bishayee, A. Resveratrol and diabetes: A critical review of clinical studies. *Biomed. Pharmacother.* **2017**, *95*, 230–234. [CrossRef] [PubMed]

73. Borra, M.T.; Smith, B.C.; Denu, J.M. Mechanism of human SIRT1 activation by resveratrol. *J. Biol. Chem.* **2005**, *280*, 17187–17195. [CrossRef] [PubMed]

74. Yar, A.S.; Menevse, S.; Alp, E. The effects of resveratrol on cyclooxygenase-1 and-2, nuclear factor kappa beta, matrix metalloproteinase-9, and sirtuin 1 mRNA expression in hearts of streptozotocin-induced diabetic rats. *Genet. Mol. Res.* **2011**, *10*, 2962–2975. [CrossRef] [PubMed]

75. Lagouge, M.; Argmann, C.; Gerhart-Hines, Z.; Meziane, H.; Lerin, C.; Daussin, F.; Messadeq, N.; Milne, J.; Lambert, P.; Elliott, P.; et al. Resveratrol improves mitochondrial function and protects against metabolic disease by activating SIRT1 and PGC-1α. *Cell* **2006**, *27*, 1109–1122. [CrossRef] [PubMed]

76. Oyenihi, O.R.; Oyenihi, A.B.; Adeyanju, A.A.; Oguntibeju, O.O. Antidiabetic effects of resveratrol: The way forward in its clinical utility. *J. Diabetes Res.* **2016**, *2016*, 1–14. [CrossRef] [PubMed]

77. Valero, T. Editorial (thematic issue: Mitochondrial biogenesis: Pharmacological approaches). *Curr. Pharm. Des.* **2014**, *20*, 5507–5509. [CrossRef] [PubMed]

78. Mootha, V.K.; Lindgren, C.M.; Eriksson, K.F.; Subramanian, A.; Sihag, S.; Lehar, J.; Puigserver, P.; Carlsson, E.; Ridderstrale, M.; Laurila, E.; et al. PGC-1α-responsive genes involved in oxidative phosphorylation are coordinately downregulated in human diabetes. *Nature Genet.* **2003**, *34*, 267. [CrossRef] [PubMed]

79. Patti, M.E.; Butte, A.J.; Crunkhorn, S.; Cusi, K.; Berria, R.; Kashyap, S.; Miyazaki, Y.; Kohane, I.; Costello, M.; Saccone, R.; et al. Coordinated reduction of genes of oxidative metabolism in humans with insulin resistance and diabetes: Potential role of PGC1 and NRF1. *Proc. Natl. Acad. Sci. USA* **2003**, *100*, 8466–8471. [CrossRef] [PubMed]

80. Sakuraba, H.; Mizukami, H.; Yagihashi, N.; Wada, R.; Hanyu, C.; Yagihashi, S. Reduced beta-cell mass and expression of oxidative stress-related DNA damage in the islet of Japanese type II diabetic patients. *Diabetologia* **2002**, *45*, 85–96. [CrossRef] [PubMed]

81. Aydın, A.; Orhan, H.; Sayal, A.; Özata, M.; Şahin, G.; Işımer, A. Oxidative stress and nitric oxide related parameters in type II diabetes mellitus: Effects of glycemic control. *Clin. Biochem.* **2001**, *34*, 65–70. [CrossRef]

82. Spanier, G.; Xu, H.; Xia, N.; Tobias, S.; Deng, S.; Wojnowski, L.; Forstermann, U.; Li, H. Resveratrol reduces endothelial oxidative stress by modulating the gene expression of superoxide dismutase 1 (SOD1), glutathione peroxidase 1 (GPx1) and NADPH oxidase subunit (Nox4). *J. Physiol. Pharmacol.* **2009**, *60* (Suppl. 4), 111–116. [PubMed]

83. Manna, S.K.; Mukhopadhyay, A.; Aggarwal, B.B. Resveratrol suppresses TNF-induced activation of nuclear transcription factors NF-κB, activator protein-1, and apoptosis: Potential role of reactive oxygen intermediates and lipid peroxidation. *J. Immunol.* **2000**, *164*, 6509–6519. [CrossRef] [PubMed]

84. Estrov, Z.; Shishodia, S.; Faderl, S.; Harris, D.; Van, Q.; Kantarjian, H.M.; Talpaz, M.; Aggarwal, B.B. Resveratrol blocks interleukin-1β–induced activation of the nuclear transcription factor NF-κB, inhibits proliferation, causes S-phase arrest, and induces apoptosis of acute myeloid leukemia cells. *Blood* **2003**, *102*, 987–995. [CrossRef] [PubMed]

85. Csiszar, A.; Smith, K.; Labinskyy, N.; Orosz, Z.; Rivera, A.; Ungvari, Z. Resveratrol attenuates TNF-α-induced activation of coronary arterial endothelial cells: Role of NF-κB inhibition. *Am. J. Physiol. Heart Circ. Physiol.* **2006**, *291*, H1694–H1699. [CrossRef] [PubMed]

86. Perkins, N.D. Integrating cell-signalling pathways with NF-κB and IKK function. *Nature Rev. Mol. Cell Biol.* **2007**, *8*, 49. [CrossRef] [PubMed]

87. Kanemaki, T.; Kitade, H.; Kaibori, M.; Sakitani, K.; Hiramatsu, Y.; Kamiyama, Y.; Ito, S.; Okumura, T. Interleukin 1β and interleukin 6, but not tumor necrosis factor α, inhibit insulin-stimulated glycogen synthesis in rat hepatocytes. *Hepatology* **1998**, *27*, 1296–1303. [CrossRef] [PubMed]

88. Wilson, D.M.; Binder, L.I. Free fatty acids stimulate the polymerization of tau and amyloid beta peptides. In vitro evidence for a common effector of pathogenesis in Alzheimer's disease. *Am. J. Pathol.* **1997**, *150*, 2181. [PubMed]

89. Cai, D.; Yuan, M.; Frantz, D.F.; Melendez, P.A.; Hansen, L.; Lee, J.; Shoelson, S.E. Local and systemic insulin resistance resulting from hepatic activation of IKK-β and NF-κB. *Nat. Med.* **2005**, *1*, 183. [CrossRef] [PubMed]

90. Klover, P.J.; Zimmers, T.A.; Koniaris, L.G.; Mooney, R.A. Chronic exposure to interleukin-6 causes hepatic insulin resistance in mice. *Diabetes* **2003**, *52*, 2784–2789. [CrossRef] [PubMed]

91. Pugazhenthi, S.; Qin, L.; Reddy, P.H. Common neurodegenerative pathways in obesity, diabetes, and Alzheimer's disease. *Biochim. Biophys. Acta Mol. Basis Dis.* **2017**, *1863*, 1037–1045. [CrossRef] [PubMed]

92. Haslbeck, K.M.; Schleicher, E.; Bierhaus, A.; Nawroth, P.; Haslbeck, M.; Neundörfer, B.; Heuss, D. The AGE/RAGE/NF-κB pathway may contribute to the pathogenesis of polyneuropathy in impaired glucose tolerance (IGT). *Exp. Clin. Endocrinol. Diabetes* **2005**, *113*, 288–291. [CrossRef] [PubMed]

93. Mohamed, A.K.; Bierhaus, A.; Schiekofer, S.; Tritschler, H.; Ziegler, R.; Nawroth, P.P. The role of oxidative stress and NF-κB activation in late diabetic complications. *Biofactors* **1999**, *10*, 157–167. [CrossRef] [PubMed]

94. Araya, R.; Noguchi, T.; Yuhki, M.; Kitamura, N.; Higuchi, M.; Saido, T.C.; Seki, K.; Itohara, S.; Kawano, M.; Tanemura, K.; et al. Loss of M5 muscarinic acetylcholine receptors leads to cerebrovascular and neuronal abnormalities and cognitive defcits in mice. *Neurobiol. Dis.* **2006**, *24*, 334–344. [CrossRef] [PubMed]

95. Gorelick, P.B.; Scuteri, A.; Black, S.E.; Decarli, C.; Greenberg, S.M.; Iadecola, C.; Launer, L.J.; Laurent, S.; Lopez, O.L.; Nyenhuis, D.; et al. Vascular contributions to cognitive impairment and dementia: A statement for healthcare professionals from the American Heart Association/American Stroke Association. *Stroke* **2011**, *42*, 2672–2713. [CrossRef] [PubMed]

96. Tellone, E.; Galtieri, A.; Russo, A.; Giardina, B.; Ficarra, S. Resveratrol: A focus on several neurodegenerative diseases. *Oxid. Med. Cell. Longev.* **2015**, *2015*, 92169. [CrossRef] [PubMed]

97. Ma, X.; Sun, Z.; Liu, Y.; Jia, Y.; Zhang, B.; Zhang, J. Resveratrol improves cognition and reduces oxidative stress in rats with vascular dementia. *Neural Regen. Res.* **2013**, *8*, 2050–2059. [PubMed]

98. Guo, S.; Kim, W.J.; Lok, J.; Lee, S.-R.; Besancon, E.; Luo, B.-H.; Stins, M.F.; Wang, X.Y.; Dedhar, S.; Lo, E.H. Neuroprotection via matrixtrophic coupling between cerebral endothelial cells and neurons. *Proc. Natl. Acad. Sci. USA* **2008**, *105*, 7582–7587. [CrossRef] [PubMed]

99. Cohen-Cory, S.; Kidane, A.H.; Shirkey, N.J.; Marshak, S. Brain-derived neurotrophic factor and the development of structural neuronal connectivity. *Dev. Neurobiol.* **2010**, *70*, 271–288. [CrossRef] [PubMed]

100. Miyake, K.; Yamamoto, W.; Tadokoro, M.; Takagi, N.; Sasakawa, K.; Nitta, A.; Furukawa, S.; Takeo, S. Alterations in hippocampal GAP-43, BDNF, and L1 following sustained cerebral ischemia. *Brain Res.* **2002**, *935*, 24–31. [CrossRef]

101. Binder, D.K.; Scharfman, H.E. Brain-derived neurotrophic factor. *Growth Factors* **2004**, *22*, 123–131. [CrossRef] [PubMed]

102. Weinstein, G.; Beiser, A.S.; Choi, S.H.; Preis, S.R.; Chen, T.C.; Vorgas, D.; Au, R.; Pikula, A.; Wolf, P.A.; DeStefano, A.L.; et al. Serum brainderived neurotrophic factor and the risk for dementia. *JAMA Neurol.* **2014**, *71*, 55–61. [CrossRef] [PubMed]

103. Fumagalli, F.; Racagni, G.; Riva, M.A. Shedding light into the role of BDNF in the pharmacotherapy of Parkinson's disease. *Pharmacogenomics J.* **2006**, *6*, 95–104. [CrossRef] [PubMed]

104. Tongiorgi, E.; Sartori, A.; Baj, G.; Bratina, A.; Di Cola, F.; Zorzon, M.; Pizzolato, G. Altered serum content of brain-derived neurotrophic factor isoforms in multiple sclerosis. *J. Neurol. Sci.* **2012**, *320*, 161–165. [CrossRef] [PubMed]

105. Ventriglia, M.; Zanardini, R.; Bonomini, C.; Zanetti, O.; Volpe, D.; Pasqualetti, P.; Gennarelli, M.; Bocchio-Chiavetto, L. Serum brain-derived neurotrophic factor levels in different neurological diseases. *BioMed Res. Int.* **2013**, *2013*, 901082. [CrossRef] [PubMed]

106. Jeon, S.; Lee, C.-H.; Liu, Q.F.E.; Kim, G.W.O.; Koo, B.-S.; Pak, S.C.H. Alteration in brain-derived neurotrophic factor (BDNF) after treatment of mice with herbal mixture containing Euphoria longana, Houttuynia cordata and Dioscorea japonica. *DARU J. Pharm. Sci.* **2014**, *22*, 77. [CrossRef] [PubMed]

107. Zhang, F.; Lu, Y.-F.; Wu, Q.; Liu, J.; Shi, J.-S. Resveratrol promotes neurotrophic factor release from astroglia. *Exp. Biol. Med.* **2012**, *237*, 943–948. [CrossRef] [PubMed]

108. Xia, N.; Forstermann, U.; Li, H. Resveratrol and endothelial nitric oxide. *Molecules* **2014**, *19*, 16102–16121. [CrossRef] [PubMed]

109. Leblais, V.; Krisa, S.; Valls, J.; Courtois, A.; Abdelouhab, S.; Vila, A.M.; Abdelouhab, S.; Vila, A.M.; Merillon, J.-M.; Muller, B. Relaxation induced by red wine polyphenolic compounds in rat pulmonary arteries: Lack of inhibition by NO-synthase inhibitor. *Fundam. Clin. Pharmacol.* **2008**, *22*, 25–35. [CrossRef] [PubMed]

110. Pires, P.W.; Dams Ramos, C.M.; Matin, N.; Dorrance, A.M. Te effects of hypertension on the cerebral circulation. *Am. J. Physiol. Heart Circ. Physiol.* **2013**, *304*, H1598–H1614. [CrossRef] [PubMed]

111. Jaffer, H.; Morris, V.B.; Stewart, D.; Labhasetwar, V. Advances in stroke therapy. *Drug Deliv. Transl. Res.* **2011**, *1*, 409–419. [CrossRef] [PubMed]

112. Hazell, A.S. Excitotoxic mechanisms in stroke: An update of concepts and treatment strategies. *Neurochem. Int.* **2007**, *50*, 941–953. [CrossRef] [PubMed]

113. Lee, Y.J.; Mou, Y.; Klimanis, D.; Bernstock, J.D.; Hallenbeck, J.M. Global SUMOylation is a molecular mechanism underlying hypothermia-induced ischemic tolerance. *Front. Cell. Neurosci.* **2014**, *8*, 416. [CrossRef] [PubMed]

114. Masel, B.E.; DeWitt, D.S. Traumatic brain injury: A disease process, not an event. *J. Neurotrauma* **2010**, *27*, 1529–1540. [CrossRef] [PubMed]

115. De Bilbao, F.; Arsenijevic, D.; Vallet, P.; Hjelle, O.P.; Ottersen, O.P.; Bouras, C.; Raffin, Y.; Abou, K.; Langhans, W.; Collin, S.; et al. Resistance to cerebral ischemic injury in UCP2 knockout mice: Evidence for a role of UCP2 as a regulator of mitochondrial glutathione levels. *J. Neurochem.* **2004**, *89*, 1283–1292. [CrossRef] [PubMed]

116. O'Donnell, M.J.; Xavier, D.; Liu, L.; Zhang, H.; Chin, S.L.; Rao-Melacini, P.; Rangarajan, S.; Islam, S.; Pais, P.; McQueen, M.J.; et al. Risk factors for ischaemic and intracerebral haemorrhagic stroke in 22 countries (the INTERSTROKE study): A case-control study. *Lancet* **2010**, *376*, 112–123. [CrossRef]

117. Fodor, K.; Tit, D.M.; Pasca, B.; Bustea, C.; Uivarosan, D.; Endres, L.; Iovan, C.; Abdel-Daim, M.M.; Bungau, S. Long-Term Resveratrol supplementation as a secondary prophylaxis for stroke. *Oxid. Med. Cell. Longev.* **2018**, *2018*. [CrossRef] [PubMed]

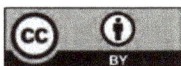

nutrients

MDPI

Article

Study of Potential Anti-Inflammatory Effects of Red Wine Extract and Resveratrol through a Modulation of Interleukin-1-Beta in Macrophages

Pauline Chalons [1,2,†], Souheila Amor [1,†], Flavie Courtaut [1,2], Emma Cantos-Villar [3], Tristan Richard [4], Cyril Auger [5], Philippe Chabert [6], Valérie Schni-Kerth [5], Virginie Aires [1,2] and Dominique Delmas [1,2,*]

1   Université de Bourgogne, F-21000 Dijon, France; paulinechalons@orange.fr (P.C.);
    souheila.amor@u-bourgogne.fr (S.A.); flaviecourtaut@gmail.com (F.C.);
    virginie.aires02@u-bourgogne.fr (V.A.)
2   INSERM Research Center U1231–Cancer and Adaptative Immune Response Team–Bioactive Molecules and
    Health research group, F-21000 Dijon, France
3   Intituto de Investigación y Formación Agraria y Pesquera (IFAPA) Rancho de La Merced, Ctra. Trebujena,
    11.471 Jerez de la Frontera (Cadiz), Spain; flaviecourtaut@gmail.com
4   Université de Bordeaux, Unité de Recherche Œnologie, EA 4577, USC 1366 INRA,
    Equipe Molécules d'Intérêt Biologique-ISVV, F-33882 Villenave d'Ornon, France;
    tristan.richard@u-bordeaux.fr
5   UMR 1260 INSERM Nanomédecine Régénérative, Université de Strasbourg, F-67401 Illkirch, France;
    cyril.auger@unistra.fr (C.A.); valerie.schini-kerth@unistra.fr (V.S.-K.)
6   UMR CNRS 7021-Laboratoire de Bioimagerie et Pathologies-Université de Strasbourg,
    F-67401 Illkirch-Graffenstaden, France; pchabert@unistra.fr
*   Correspondence: dominique.delmas@u-bourgogne.fr; Tel.: +33-380-393226
†   Two coauthors contributed equally of this work.

Received: 30 October 2018; Accepted: 22 November 2018; Published: 1 December 2018

Abstract: Inflammation has been described as an initiator event of major diseases with significant impacts in terms of public health including in cardiovascular disease, autoimmune disorders, eye diseases, age-related diseases, and the occurrence of cancers. A preventive action to reduce the key processes leading to inflammation could be an advantageous approach to reducing these associated pathologies. Many studies have reported the value of polyphenols such as resveratrol in counteracting pro-inflammatory cytokines. We have previously shown the potential of red wine extract (RWE) and the value of its qualitative and quantitative polyphenolic composition to prevent the carcinogenesis process. In this study, we addressed a new effect of RWE in inflammation through a modulation of IL-1β secretion and the NLRP3 inflammasome pathway. NLRP3 inflammasome requires two signals, priming to increase the synthesis of NLRP3 and pro-IL-1β proteins and activation, which activates NLRP3. Inflammasome formation is triggered by a range of substances such as lipopolysaccharide (LPS). Using two different macrophages, one of which does not express the adaptor protein ASC (apoptosis-associated speck-like protein containing a CARD), which is essential to form active inflammasome complexes that produce IL-1β, we show that RWE decreases IL-1 β secretion and gene expression whatever line is used. Moreover, this strong reduction of pro-inflammatory IL-1β is associated with a decrease of NLRP3 and, in J774A, ASC protein expression, which depends on the choice of activator ATP or nigericin.

Keywords: red wine extract; polyphenols; resveratrol; inflammation; interleukins

1. Introduction

For several years, numerous epidemiological studies have maintained that a moderate consumption of wine lowered the risks of mortality, in particular due to coronary diseases, compared to the risk observed with wine abstinence. [1,2]. In France, as compared with other western countries with a fat-containing-diet, the strikingly low incidence of coronary heart diseases is partly attributed to the moderate consumption of red wine [3]. In our previous studies, we have shown an improvement of blood parameters with the decrease in total cholesterol and LDL and the increase in erythrocyte membrane fluidity and antioxidant status on a group of selected post-myocardial infarct patients receiving 250 mL/day of red wine over 2 weeks in comparison to patients receiving water [4]. These cardiovascular benefit effects are commonly attributed to red wine's rich content in polyphenols, particularly resveratrol, as an important source of antioxidants [5]. Interestingly, other epidemiological studies reveal that micronutrients such as resveratrol could protect against cancers [1]. However, resveratrol does not seem to be the only bioactive compound present in wine, which contains numerous other polyphenols [6]. Indeed, some studies have highlighted that other polyphenols of red wine such as quercetin [7], catechin [8], and gallic acid [9] could present potential chemopreventive properties. Various case–control studies have shown that moderate red wine consumption exerts a protective effect on colorectal cancer in both men and women [10,11]. Moreover, other case–control studies have studied the association between wine and the Mediterranean diet, showing a lower risk of colon cancer compared to other diets [12–14]. Nevertheless, one study did not find an inverse association between moderate red wine intake and the risk of colorectal cancer [15] or breast cancer [16]. This controversy may result from the amount and quality of polyphenols present in red wine. Indeed, red wine contains a range of biologically active polyphenols, including phenolic acids, trihydroxystilbenes, and flavonoids. In previous studies, we have shown both that a mixture of polyphenols extracted from vine shoots presents a better antiproliferative activity on colon cancer cells than resveratrol alone due to a synergism between polyphenols [17] and that the quantity and quality of the polyphenols present in the wine also played an important role. We showed that the wine making procedure can increase the quantities of certain polyphenols, especially lengthening the maceration time, which results in an improvement of the biological effects of these red wine extracts, which are then able to slow down the formation of aberrant crypt foci (ACF) [18] and angiogenesis [19]. But very interestingly, some polyphenols do not act in a synergistic manner but rather in an additive manner and in some cases they have opposite effects. These data raise the question of the crucial role of the polyphenol composition of wine where an imbalance between polyphenolic species may increase or conversely reduce their effects. The presence of catechin reduces the synergism effect between resveratrol and quercetin, which could explain the discrepancy between some studies showing a reduction of the risk of colon cancer with moderate red wine consumption in patient [10,11] or in animal models [19,20] while others showed no effect [15,21].

To conduct our previous studies, we investigated the potential effects of a red wine extract (RWE) on a fundamental biological element in the occurrence of various pathologies, in particular cancer, namely inflammation and more particularly the production of IL-1β.

Inflammation can be initially defined as a set of physiological defense reactions put in place by the body and more particularly by the cells of innate immunity. These cells play a role in first-line defense following various traumas caused by infectious agents, chemical substances, physical agents or even post-traumatic tissue lesions. In contrast, inflammation has been described as an initiator event of major diseases with a significant impact in terms of public health such as cardiovascular diseases, autoimmune diseases, eye diseases, age-related diseases, and more particularly neurodegenerative diseases and the occurrence and development of cancers. More particularly, low-level inflammation seems crucial in sustaining these processes. Among polyphenols and flavonoids present in the human diet, resveratrol seems to inhibit NLRP3 inflammasome-derived IL-1β secretion in the J774A.1 murine macrophage cell line and pyroptosis [22]. This point is particularly important because there is a link between activation/controls of NLRP3 and various pathologies, i.e., atherosclerosis [23],

Alzheimer's disease [24], cancers [25], and renal disease [26]. Despite numerous studies showing the impact of polyphenols alone on the inflammation process, there are still very few data on the effect of complex mixtures of polyphenols such as red wine extract (RWE). Some studies have pointed out the potential anti-inflammatory role of RWE in colon cancer cells through a pathway involving both an activation of the nuclear factor-erythroid 2-related factor-2 (Nrf2) pathway and an inhibition of the Janus kinase/signal transducer and activator of transcription (JAK/STAT) pathway [27] or through a disruption of colonic NADPH-oxidase NOX1 activation [28]. These effects lead to a decrease of the pro-inflammatory cytokines Il-6 and IL-8. In view of the importance of the anti-inflammatory potential of RWE, it is therefore essential to better characterize the effects of a polyphenol-enriched extract such as RWE on one of the essential pro-inflammatory cytokines, namely IL-1β, on the mechanisms conducive to its secretion. In this study, we show that RWE was able to strongly decrease IL-1β secretion through a modulation of the expression of key proteins involved in the inflammasome complex, i.e., NLRP3 and apoptosis-associated speck-like protein containing a CARD (ASC). Moreover, we highlight that RWE was able to affect the priming signal and the activating signal leading to inflammasome activation in macrophages.

2. Materials and Methods

2.1. Cells Culture

The murine macrophage cell line J774A.1 and Raw 264.7 were obtained from the European Collection of Authenticated Cell Cultures (ECACC, Salisbury, UK) and from the American Type Culture Collection (ATCC, Manassas, VA, USA), respectively. Raw 264.7 cells were cultured in RPMI 1640 medium supplemented with 10% FBS and 10,000 U/mL penicillin, 10 mg/mL streptomycin, 25 μg/mL amphotericin at 37 °C in a 5% CO_2 incubator; therefore, J774A.1 cells were cultured in DMEM high-glucose medium supplemented with 10% fetal bovine serum (FBS), with 2 mM L-glutamine and 10,000 U/mL penicillin, 10 mg/mL streptomycin, 25 μg/mL amphotericin at 37 °C in a 5% CO_2 incubator. Cells were subcultured twice weekly using standard protocols.

2.2. Preparation of Red Wine Extract

Red wine extract (RWE) was obtained from French red wine, Santenay 1er cru Les Gravières 2012 (EARL Capuano-Ferreri Santenay, Côte-d'Or, France) selected by BIVB (Bureau Interprofessionnel des Vins de Bourgogne, Beaune, France) and provided by CTIVV (Centre Technique Interprofessionnel de la Vigne et du Vin, Beaune, France). Red wine extract dry powder was prepared and analyzed as previously described [19]. Briefly, phenolic compounds were adsorbed on a preparative column, then alcohol desorbed. The alcoholic eluent was gently evaporated, and the concentrated residue was lyophilized and finely sprayed to obtain the phenolic extract dry powder. Briefly, the alcoholic eluent and water were gently evaporated using a rotary evaporator set, and the concentrated residue was deposited on the column (Diainon® HP-20, Supelco, Germany). The reservoir was filled with distilled water and the flow was adjusted to about 20 drops/min. The polyphenol fraction was eluted with an ethanol-0.1% glacial acetic acid solution (flow adjusted to 40 drops/min). The individual eluent fractions were collected and concentrated to dryness using a rotary evaporator set. One liter of red wine produced 104 g of phenolic extract, which contained 5.04 mg/g of total phenolic compounds expressed as gallic acid equivalent.

2.3. HPLC Analysis

The phenolic composition of the wine samples was determined by HPLC analysis following the methods developed by Guererro et al. (2009) [29]. Briefly, HPLC analysis was performed on a HPLC system equipped with a diode array detector, a fluorescence detector and a C18 column (5 μm, 250 mm × 4.6 mm) for compound separation. For anthocyanins and flavonols, the mobile phase consisted of water containing 5% formic acid (v/v) and methanol in various proportions at a flow rate of 1 mL/min. Anthocyanins were quantified at 520 nm as malvidin-3-glucoside and flavonols at 360 nm as quercetin-3-rutinoside. Flavan-3-ols and phenolic acids were analyzed using a gradient containing water with 2% acetic acid (v/v) and methanol–water–acetic acid (90:8:2, v/v/v). Phenolic acids were quantified at 320 nm as caffeic acid, flavan-3-ols as catechin using the fluorescence signal (excitation wavelength, 290 nm; emission wavelength, 320 nm) and stilbenes as resveratrol (excitation wavelength, 330 nm; emission wavelength, 320 nm).

2.4. Reagents

Resveratrol (RSV), LPS (from *Escherichia coli* 0111: B4, L3024), adenosine 5-triphosphate disodium salt solution (A6559) and nigericin sodium salt (N7143) were purchased from Sigma-Aldrich (St. Louis, MO, USA).

2.5. Experimental Protocol

Cells were seeded at the density of 10,000 cells/cm^2 and allowed to recover for 24 h. As usually done, after 24 h, to initiate NLRP3 inflammasome priming, cells were pretreated or not with 100 µg/mL RWE or 60 µM RSV for 30 min and then primed with 1 µg/mL LPS (5.5 h) and finally exposed for an additional 30 min to 10 µM nigericin or 5 mM ATP [22]. For the activation signal analyses, cells were first primed with 1 µg/mL LPS (5.5 h), then treated or not with 100 µg/mL RWE or 60 µM RSV for 30 min and finally with 10 µM of nigericin or 5 mM ATP, as previously described by Chang et al. [22].

Priming and activation are annotated RWE/RSV->LPS->Nig/ATP and LPS->RWE/RSV->Nig/ATP, respectively.

2.6. Cell Proliferation Assay

Cells were seeded in 96-well flat-bottomed microplates and incubated for 24 h. The medium was then removed and replaced with fresh medium containing the RWE or RSV to be tested at increasing concentrations (from 1.9 to 250 µg/mL) at 37 °C for 24 h. Each treatment was performed in sixplicate (in three independent experiments). The activity of compounds was determined using a solution of crystal violet (Sigma-Aldrich, St. Louis, MO, USA). Absorbance at 540 nm was measured by Biochrom Asys UVM 340. IC$_{50}$ (i.e., the half maximum inhibitory concentration representing the concentration of a substance required for 50% in vitro inhibition) values were calculated using GraphPad 6.0 Prism software (GraphPad Software, La Jolla, San Diego, CA, USA).

2.7. Western Blotting

Cells were treated according to the experimental protocol described above, then were harvested for Western blot analysis in RIPA buffer (RadioImmunoPrecipitation Assay buffer; 150 mM sodium chloride, 50 mM Tris-HCl, 0.1% sodium dodecyl sulfate, 1% NP40, 0.5% sodium deoxycholate) supplemented with protease inhibitors such as phosphatase inhibitor cocktail (100 µM, Sigma-Aldrich, St. Louis, MO, USA) and an anti-protease (1x, Roche). The protein concentration of each lysate was determined in a 96-well plate against BSA standards in PBS (range, 0–12 µg), applying the QuantiPro™ BCA Assay Kit (Sigma-Aldrich, St. Louis, MO, USA), and the total amount of proteins per well was calculated. Samples were adjusted into Laemmli gel-loading buffer (50 mM Tris-HCl, pH 6.8, 5% 2-mercaptoethanol, 2% sodium dodecyl sulfate, 0.1% bromphenol blue, 10% glycerol) and then heated for 5 min at 95 °C prior to separation. Denatured proteins were separated by SDS-PAGE and transferred to nitrocellulose membranes (Amershan, GE, Velizy-Villacoublay, France). Membranes were blocked by incubation with skimmed milk (in TBS-Tween 20 0.5%) 1 h at room temperature. The membranes were incubated with the respective primary antibody: NLRP3 (clone cryo2, Adipogen®, Liestal, Switzerland), Asc (clone AL177, Adipogen®, Liestal, Switzerland) overnight at 4 °C according to the manufacturer's recommendations. Afterwards, the membranes were incubated with HRP-conjugated secondary antibody, anti-rabbit and anti-mouse for ASC and NRLP3 (Jackson Immunoresearch Laboratory, Cambridgeshire, UK), respectively, at room temperature for 1 h and developed using the ECL reagents (Supersignal West Femto maximum sensitivity substrate, ThermoFisher Scientific, France). Antibody against housekeeping proteins such as β-actin was used as the loading control (clone AC-15, Sigma-Aldrich, St. Louis, MO, USA). Digital chemiluminescence images were captured and analyzed using the ChemiDocTM XRS + imaging system (BioRad, Marnes-la-Coquette, France). Image processing and analyses were carried out using Image Lab 5.2.1 build 11 Bio-Rad software (Berkeley, CA, USA).

2.8. Imaging

Cells were seeded on chambered coverglass coated with poly-L-lysin and allowed to recover. Cells were treated according to the experimental protocol described above. After the treatment, cells were fixed and permeabilized with 4% PAF for 10 min at 4 °C and then incubated with a blocking buffer (PBS1X-0.2% saponin-3% BSA) for 20 min at room temperature. The blocking buffer was eliminated, and the diluted antibodies were applied. Cells were incubated overnight at 4 °C in a humid light-tight box. Cells were rinsed thrice with PBS1X (5 min each), then incubated with the fluorochrome-conjugated secondary antibodies (Alexa488 and Alexa568 for NRLP3 and ASC, respectively) diluted as indicated on an antibody datasheet for 1 h at room temperature in a humid light-tight box. Cells were then washed thrice with PBS1X (5 min each time) then mounted with mounting medium with DAPI (ProLong® antifade with Dapi, Life Technologies, ThermoFisher Scientific, Strasbourg, France). Confocal imaging was performed using a confocal laser-scanning microscope (Axio Imager M2, Zeiss) coupled with an Apotome.2 with a ×40 objective lens, and Zen software (Carl Zeiss Microscopy GmbH, Germany). The samples were excited using internal microscope lasers and emission intensity was recorded at the appropriate emission wavelength. Image processing and analyses were carried out using ImageJ software. Negative controls were treated with the fluorochrome-conjugated secondary antibodies alone.

2.9. IL-1β Secretion

Cells were treated according to the experimental protocol described above. Then IL-1β in the supernatant was measured using ELISA (Enzyme-Linked Immunosorbent Assay) for Mouse IL-1-beta®/IL-1F2 DuoSet® ELISA (R&D Systems, Minneapolis, MN, USA) according to the manufacturer's protocol.

2.10. Statistical Analysis

Results are shown as means $\pm$ SD for triplicate assay samples (otherwise mentioned), reproduced independently at least three times. Statistical analysis of data was carried out with Prism GraphPad 6.0 Prism Software (GraphPad Software, Inc. La Jolla, San Diego, CA, USA). The significance of the differences between mean values was determined by a one-way ANOVA with Holm-Sidak correction. p-values < 0.05 were considered significant (* $p < 0.05$, ** $p < 0.01$ and *** $p < 0.001$).

3. Results

3.1. RWE Decreases IL-1β Secretion and NLRP3 Expression in Murine Macrophages without Toxicity

The composition of wine is a complex and unique combination due to the various factors such as the vine, the climate, the country and the year, and varies between white and red wines. The amount of polyphenols in wine, although varying greatly, is estimated to be around 190–290 mg/L in white wines and 900–2500 mg/L in red wines. We previously demonstrated that the qualitative and quantitative composition of a wine in bioactive molecules such as polyphenolic compounds is crucial in the biological effects that can be observed and that they are antagonistic or synergistic [18]. Also, we first evaluated the polyphenolic composition of our red wine extract, which contains significant amounts of anthocyanidins, catechins, and a polyphenol emblematic of the vine and wine, resveratrol, which in our experience will serve as a reference compound (Table 1). As compared to our previous studies, it appears that this polyphenolic extract of red wine is richer in caffeic acid and resveratrol [18]. To specify the potential role of RWE in inflammation, we first studied its effects on classical cellular models such as macrophages. To do this, we chose to use two murine macrophage lines, Raw264.7 and J774A.1, derived, respectively, from ascites of a male mouse bearing a tumor induced by murine Abelson leukemia virus and the blood of a tumor-bearing Balb/c female. As we have shown in previous studies that polyphenolic extracts and RWE induce toxicities in various cell lines, in particular against cancer cells [18,19] by disrupting their proliferation, we first evaluated the RWE toxicity (Figure 1a). We observe that after 24 h of treatment with increasing concentrations of RWE, polyphenolic extract has no impact on the cellular viability of Raw264.7 macrophages despite increasing concentrations of up to 250 µg/mL. However, in J774A.1 cells, RWE at 250 µg/mL reduced the number of viable cells by nearly 50%. In the following experiments, RWE was therefore used at 100 µg/mL in both cell lines. This concentration was chosen both because it is noncytotoxic on macrophages and because it significantly inhibited tumor growth and the formation of adenomatous polyps, as we have shown in several in vivo models [18,19]. The experiments were conducted in comparison with the RSV at a concentration of 60 µM, a concentration that is also noncytotoxic on macrophages and for which recent studies have shown an effect on NLRP3 [22].

Table 1. Composition of the red wine extract (RWE) obtained from the 2012 Santenay 1er cru Les Gravières.

	mg/L of Wine	mg/L RWE
Phenolic acids		
Gallic acid	21	5.04
Caftaric acid	53	12.74
Coutaric acid	20	4.80
Caffeic acid	10	2.40
Stilbenes		
Piceid	1	0.24
Resveratrol	7	1.68
Anthocyanidins		
Delphinidin derivatives	15	3.60
Petunidin derivatives	10	2.40
Peonidin derivatives	14	3.36
Malvidin derivatives	78	18.75
Catechins		
Catechin	31	7.45
Epicatechin	8	1.92
Procyanidin dimers	42	10.09
Flavonols		
Quercetin derivatives	4	0.96

Inflammation results from an increased production of pro-inflammatory cytokines. Among them, IL-1β plays a decisive role and its high secretion is responsible for the development of both chronic inflammation and an acute inflammatory response and its maintenance over time. RWE at 100 µg/mL is able to strongly decrease the basal secretion of IL-1β in the two macrophage types in a similar manner of resveratrol (RSV) at 60 µM after 30 min of treatment (Figure 1b). Since IL-1β production results mainly from the activation of NLRP3 inflammasome, we then studied the impact of a treatment with RWE. It appeared that RWE was able to slightly decrease NLRP3 protein expression after 6 h of treatment with 100 µg/mL in Raw264.7 (Figure 1c). Very interestingly, in J774.1, which is the only one of the two lines expressing the apoptosis-associated, speck-like protein containing a CARD domain (ASC), which plays a primordial role in inflammasome formation, RWE treatment strongly decreases ASC protein expression as compared to the control (Figure 1c).

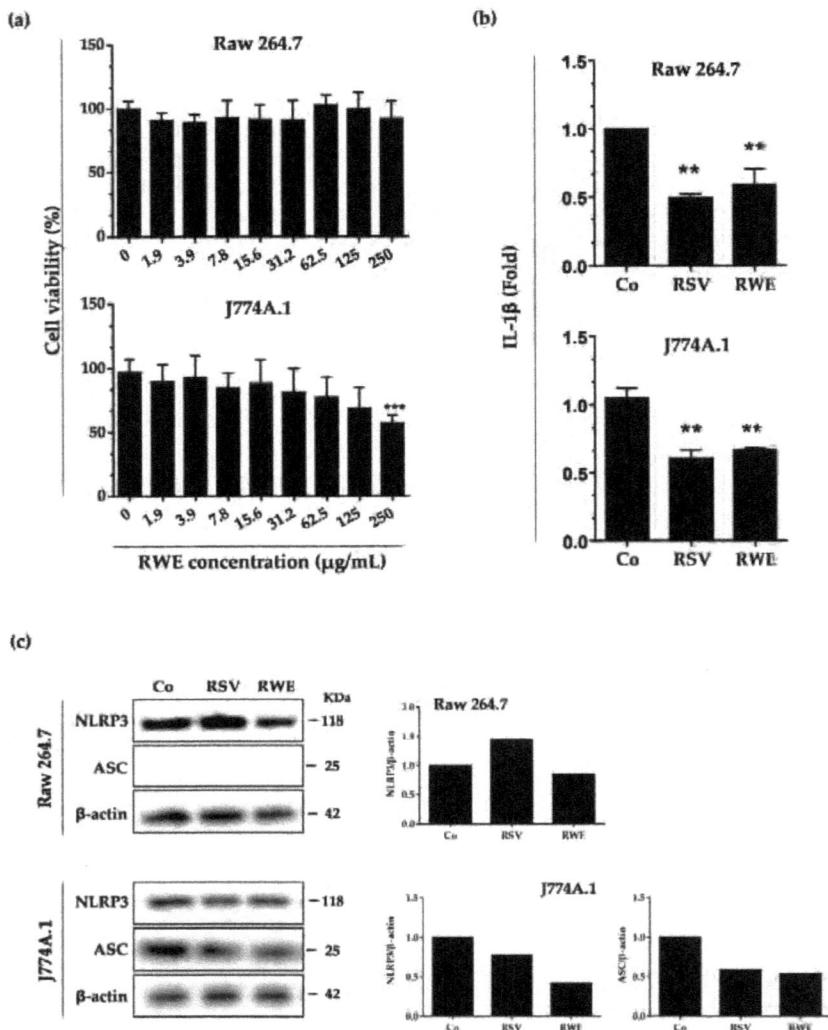

Figure 1. RWE and Resveratrol (RSV) decrease IL-1β secretion in resting conditions through the modulation of the protein expression levels of NLRP3 inflammasome components. (**a**) Cell viability of Raw 264.7 and J774A.1 was determined by crystal violet staining after 24 h of treatment, with concentration ranges of RWE (starting concentration 250 μg/mL, 1:2 serial dilutions). Data are expressed as mean percentages ± s.d. of three independent experiments. *p*-values were determined by a one-way ANOVA with Holm-Sidak correction. *** $p < 0.001$. (**b**) Secreted IL-1β in supernatants was analyzed by ELISA after 6 h of treatment with vehicle (DMSO, Co), RWE (100 μg/mL), or RSV (60 μM). Data are expressed as fold changes in secreted IL-1β levels as compared to vehicle-treated cells (Co) and are mean ± s.d. of three independent experiments. *p*-values were determined by the multiple Student *t* test. ** $p < 0.01$ (**c**) Western blot analysis of NLRP3 and ASC protein expression in Raw 264.7 and J774A.1 macrophages after 6.5 h of treatment with vehicle (DMSO, Co), RWE (100 μg/mL) or RSV (positive control). Left panels: representative blots from three independent experiments are shown. β-actin was used as loading control. Right panels: densitometry quantifications of representative blots. Plotted data are fold changes as compared to vehicle-treated cells (Co).

3.2. RWE Prevents Priming of NLRP3 Inflammasome from LPS in Macrophages

Conventionally, activation of the NLRP3 inflammasome requires two signals: the first a priming signal and the second an activation signal. The priming signal serves to increase the synthesis of NLRP3 and pro-IL-1β proteins. This first signal takes place via the activation of TLR by a multitude of microbial ligands or via the activation of the TNF-α receptor. These activations will trigger the translocation of NF-κB in the nucleus and thus increase the transcription of NLRP3 and pro-IL-1β. This channel can be activated by setting the LPS on toll-like receptor 4 [30]. Consequently, we investigated whether RWE could alter the priming signal from lipopolysaccharides (LPS). To do this, Raw264.7 and J774A.1 cells were pre-incubated for 30 min with 100 µg/mL of RWE then with LPS (1 µg/mL for 5.5 h) to induce a priming end and we then measured IL-1β secretion. Secreted IL-1β in cell supernatants in both experimental conditions was then measured by ELISA. Consistent with the literature, RSV alone significantly decreased IL-1β secretion in macrophage cell lines (Figure 2a). In a manner similar to the RSV-positive control, RWE strongly decreased IL-1β production in J774A.1 and much more slightly in Raw264.7 macrophages (Figure 2a). Since LPS priming controls, at the end of its signaling cascade, pro-inflammatory IL-1β and NLRP3 transcription and finally their protein expression, we evaluated the effect of RWE on inflammasome protein expression in basal and priming conditions. Immunoblotting showed that RSV strongly downregulated NLRP3 protein expression in RAW 264.7, which was not the case in J774.1, but as previously, in the latter cells, RWE strongly reduced ASC protein expression as compared to the control when priming was implemented by the LPS (Figure 2b). We confirm that Raw264.7 macrophages did not express ASC (Figure 2c).

RWE/RSV->LPS

(a) **(b)**

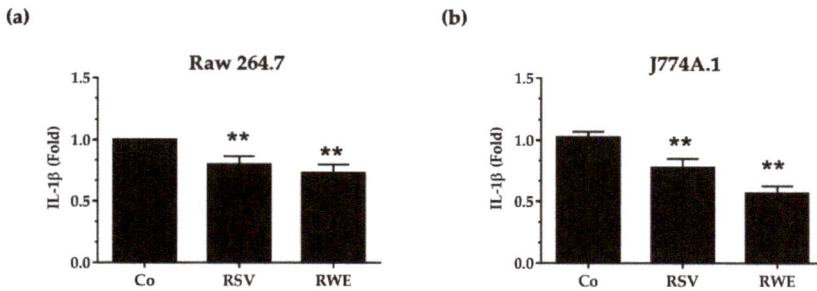

Figure 2. *Cont.*

(c)

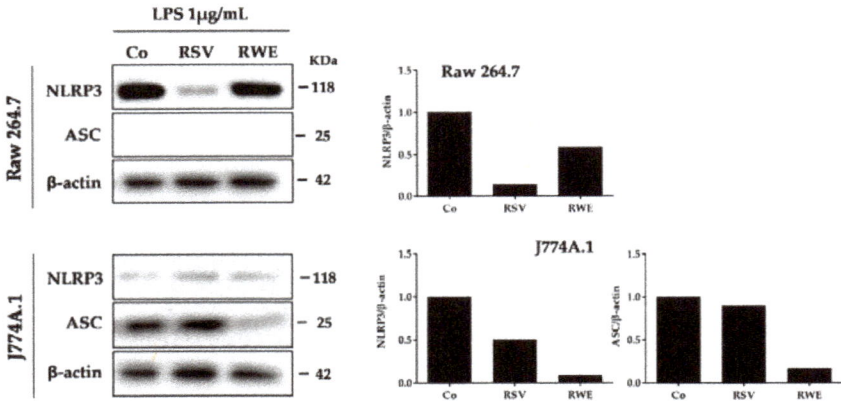

Figure 2. RWE and RSV decrease IL-1β secretion in lipopolysaccharide (LPS)-mediated NLRP3 inflammasome priming conditions. Raw 264.7 (**a**) and J774A.1 (**b**) macrophages were pretreated or not with RWE (100 μg/mL) or RSV (60 μM) for 30 min, prior to NLRP3 inflammasome priming with 1 μg/mL of LPS for 5.5 h. Secreted IL-1β in cell supernatants was analyzed by ELISA at the end of the treatments. Data are expressed as fold changes in secreted IL-1β levels as compared to cells treated with LPS alone (Co) and are mean ± s.d. of three independent experiments. p-values were determined by the multiple Student t test. ** $p < 0.01$ (**c**) Western-blot analysis of NLRP3 and ASC protein expression in Raw 264.7 and J774A.1 macrophages after cell treatments as described above. Left panels: representative blots from three independent experiments are shown. β-actin was used as loading control. Right panels: densitometry quantifications of representative blots. Plotted data are fold changes as compared to LPS-treated cells (Co).

3.3. RWE Decreases IL-1β Secretion after Activation by LPS/Nigericin in Macrophages

After increasing the expression then the synthesis of NLRP3 and pro-IL-1β, the second signal serves to activate NLRP3, which is deubiquitinated while the adapter protein ASC is phosphorylated and ubiquitinated [31]. The permeabilization of membranes by toxins such as nigericin is one of the activation mechanisms of NLRP3 [32]. Therefore, to study the potential effect of RWE on this second signaling process, we treated J77A.1 cells with RWE (100 μg/mL) or RSV (60 μM) for 30 min before treatment with LPS for 5.5 h (LPS priming) following incubation with nigericin (10 μM for 30 min). Very surprisingly, we observed that both RWE and RSV failed to decrease the IL-1β secretion in RAW 264.7 (Figure 3a), which is not the case in J774.1 cells where RWE and RSV completely blocked the production of IL-1β induced by nigericin (Figure 3b). Concerning the expression of protein involved in the inflammasome complex, we observed that RSV and RWE decreased NLRP3 protein expression in RAW 264.7, but only RSV was able to decrease ASC protein expression in J774.1 after nigericin stimulation (Figure 3c). These results differ from previous results wherein priming conditions, RSV and RWE were both able to decrease, in J774.1, the expression of two key proteins NLRP3 and ASC, which was not the case in the second signaling process. It appears from these results that the very large decrease in IL-1β by RWE in J774.1 macrophages is associated with a strong decrease of NLRP3 protein expression.

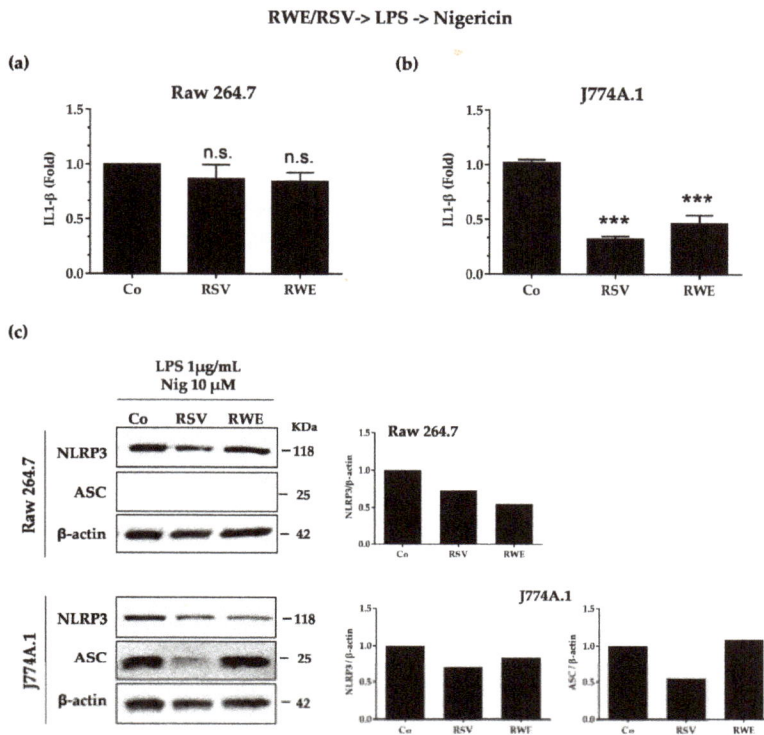

Figure 3. RWE and RSV curtail NLRP3 inflammasome priming and reduce IL-1β secretion, in the nigericin-mediated activation condition. Raw 264.7 (**a**) and J774A.1 (**b**) macrophages were pretreated or not with RWE (100 μg/mL) or RSV (60 μM) for 30 min, prior to NLRP3 inflammasome priming with 1 μg/mL of LPS for 5.5 h and subsequent activation by 10 μM nigericin for 30 min. Secreted IL-1β in cell supernatants was analyzed by ELISA at the end of the treatments. Data are expressed as fold changes in secreted IL-1β levels as compared to cells treated with only LPS + nigericin (Co) and are mean ± s.d. of three independent experiments. *p*-values were determined by the multiple Student *t* test. n.s.: not significant, *** *p* < 0.001. (**c**) Western-blot analysis of NLRP3 and ASC protein expression in Raw 264.7 and J774A.1 macrophages after cell treatments as described above. Left panels: representative blots from three independent experiments are shown. β-actin was used as loading control. Right panels: densitometry quantifications of representative blots. Plotted data are fold changes as compared to LPS-treated cells (Co).

3.4. Crucial Choice of Activators for RWE and RSV Effect on IL-1β Secretion in Macrophages after LPS Priming

Subsequently, we evaluated the ability of RWE to interfere with the second signal "the activation". We first treated macrophages with LPS (1 μg/mL for 5.5 h) and then treated or not with RWE (100 μg/mL) or RSV (60 μM) for 30 min and finally exposed for an additional 30 min to 10 μM nigericin. We surprisingly observed that both RSV and RWE failed to decrease IL-1β production as previously observed (Figure 4a), even though only RWE decreased NLRP3 and ASC protein expression in both types of macrophages as compared to RSV, which presented no effects (Figure 4c).

Given this very surprising lack of an effect of RSV, whereas Chang et al. previously described its ability to block IL-1β secretion when macrophages were pretreated with the LPS before RSV treatment and ATP stimulation [22], we decided to change NLRP3 inflammasome activators. We consequently conducted the same experiment as before by replacing the nigericin with ATP. In this second experiment, macrophages were treated with LPS (1 μg/mL for 5.5 h) and then treated or not with RWE (100 µg/mL) or RSV (60 µM) for 30 min and finally exposed for an additional 30 min to 5 mM ATP. We then observed that RSV was able to decrease NLRP3 protein expression without modulating IL-1β secretion while RWE, in these conditions, both decreased IL-1β production and NRLP3 protein (Figure 5a,b), suggesting that RWE inhibits the ATP-mediated activation signal of the NLRP3 inflammasome. The ability of RWE to inhibit IL-1β production was also found when RAW 264.7 macrophages were pretreated with RSV prior to activation of the NLRP3 inflammasome by LPS/ATP. In accordance with the first results shown in Figure 3, RWE strongly reduced IL-1β production and NLRP3 protein expression (Figure 5c,d). Consequently, RWE was able to prevent priming of NLRP3 inflammasome from LPS in macrophages whether the activator ATP or nigericin was used. These molecular observations were reinforced *in cellulo*, where immunofluorescence imaging revealed that RWE is well able to decrease NLRP3 and ASC expression, as shown by the decrease of fluorescence of these proteins but also of their colocalization when macrophages are pretreated with RWE (Figure 6a). The same observations are highlighted when macrophages were pretreated with LPS before treatment with RWE (Figure 6b).

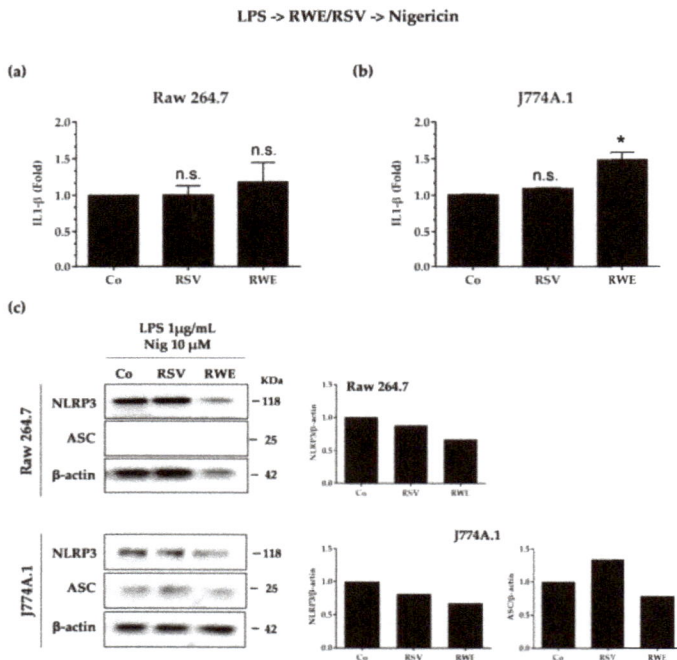

Figure 4. RWE and RSV failed to block IL-1β secretion when added after the NLRP3 priming step. Raw 264.7 (**a**) and J774A.1 (**b**) macrophages were exposed to 1 µg/mL of LPS for 5.5 h, then treated or not with RWE (100 µg/mL) or RSV (60 µM) for 30 min and finally exposed for an additional 30 min to 10 µM nigericin. Secreted IL-1β in cell supernatants was analyzed by ELISA at the end of the treatments. Data are expressed as fold changes in secreted IL-1β levels as compared to cells treated only with LPS + nigericin (Co) and are mean ± s.d. of three independent experiments. *p*-values were determined by the multiple Student *t* test. * *p* < 0.05, n.s.: not significant. (**c**) Western blot analysis of NLRP3 and ASC protein expression in Raw 264.7 and J774A.1 macrophages after cell treatments as described above. Left panels: representative blots from three independent experiments are shown. β-actin was used as loading control. Right panels: quantifications by densitometry of representative blots. Plotted data are fold changes as compared to LPS-treated cells (Co).

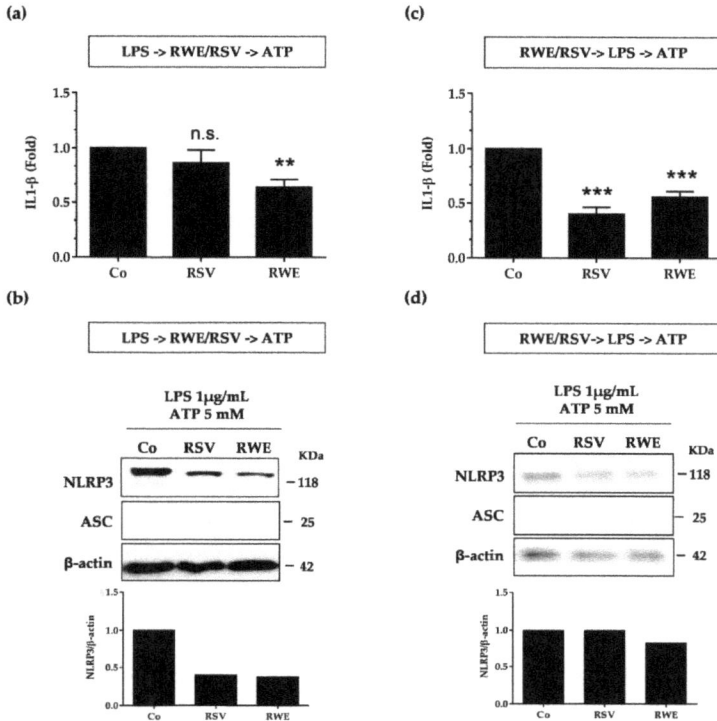

Figure 5. RWE prevents both priming and activation from ATP in macrophages. (**a**) LPS -> RWE/RSV -> ATP sequence: Raw 264.7 cells were exposed to 1 μg/mL of LPS for 5.5 h, then treated or not with RWE (100 μg/mL) or RSV (60 μM) for 30 min and finally exposed for an additional 30 min to 5 mM ATP. Secreted IL-1β in cell supernatants was analyzed by ELISA at the end of the treatments. Data are expressed as fold changes in secreted IL-1β levels as compared to cells treated only with LPS + ATP (Co) and are mean ± s.d. of three independent experiments. *p*-values were determined by the multiple Student *t* test. ** *p* < 0.01, *** *p* < 0.001, n.s.: not significant. (**b**) Western blot analysis of NLRP3 and ASC protein expression in Raw 264.7 macrophages after cell treatments as described in (**a**). Representative blots from three independent experiments are shown. β-actin was used as loading control. Histograms: quantifications by densitometry of representative blots. Plotted data are fold changes as compared to LPS+ATP-treated cells (Co). (**c**) RWE/RSV-> LPS -> ATP sequence: Raw 264.7 cells were pretreated or not with RWE (100 μg/mL) or RSV (60 μM) for 30 min, prior to NLRP3 inflammasome priming with 1 μg/mL of LPS for 5.5 h and subsequent activation by 5 mM nigericin for 30 min. Secreted IL-1β in cell supernatants was analyzed by ELISA at the end of the treatments. Data are expressed as fold changes in secreted IL-1β levels as compared to cells treated only with LPS + ATP (Co) and are mean ± s.d. of three independent experiments. *p*-values were determined by the multiple Student *t* test. ** *p* < 0.01, *** *p* < 0.001. (**d**) Western blot analysis of NLRP3 and ASC protein expression in Raw 264.7 macrophages after cell treatments as described in (**c**). Representative blots from three independent experiments are shown. β-actin was used as loading control. Histograms: densitometry quantifications of representative blots. Plotted data are fold changes as compared to LPS+ATP-treated cells (Co).

(a)

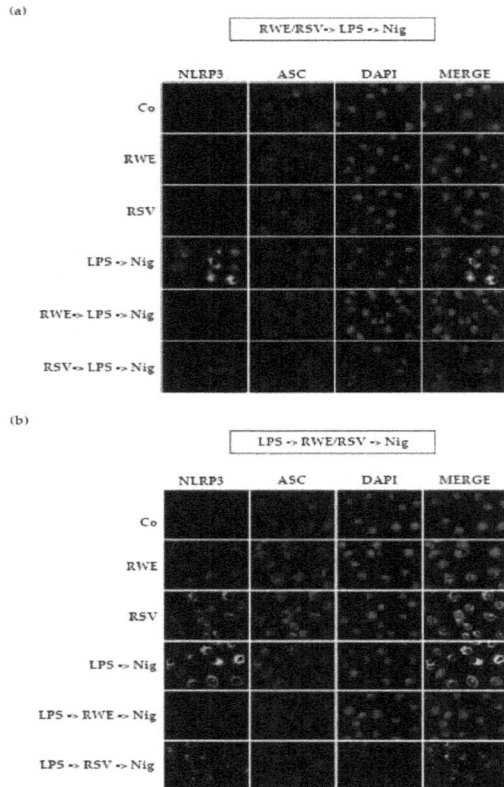

(b)

Figure 6. RWE and RSV decrease NLRP3 and ASC colocalization in both priming and activation conditions. (**a**) RSV and RWE inhibit NLRP3 and ASC formation in priming sequence RWE/RSV-> LPS -> nigericin. J774A.1 macrophages were exposed to 1 μg/mL of LPS for 5.5 h, then treated or not with RWE (100 μg/mL) or RSV (60 μM) for 30 min and finally exposed for an additional 30 min to 10 μM nigericin. (**b**) RSV and RWE inhibit NLRP3 and ASC formation in activating sequence LPS -> RWE/RSV -> nigericin. J774A.1 macrophage cells were exposed to 1 μg/mL of LPS for 5.5 h, then treated or not with RWE (100 μg/mL) or RSV (60 μM) for 30 min and finally exposed for an additional 30 min to 10 μM nigericin. In (**a**) and (**b**) after treatments, cells were fixed and then immunostained for NLRP3 and ASC proteins using Alexa Fluor® 488 (green staining) and Alexa Fluor® 568 (red staining) as secondary antibodies, respectively. Cell nuclei were counterstained with DAPI. Representative confocal images of the staining from three independent experiments are shown (×40 magnification).

4. Discussion and Conclusions

Inflammation can be initially defined as a set of physiological defense reactions put in place by the body and more particularly by the cells of innate immunity. These cells play a role in the first line of defense following various injuries caused by infectious agents, chemical substances, physical agents, or even post-traumatic tissue lesions. In contrast, inflammation has been described as an initiator event of major diseases with significant impact in terms of public health such as cardiovascular diseases, autoimmune diseases, eye diseases, age-related diseases, and more particularly neurodegenerative diseases and the occurrence and development of cancers. A preventive action to reduce the key processes leading to inflammation could, therefore, be very interesting in order to reduce the associated pathologies.

The inflammatory response is often linked to the action of intracellular multiprotein complexes called inflammasomes. These complexes generally consist of a receptor and an adapter allowing the recruitment and activation of pro-inflammatory caspases as well as the maturation and secretion of pro-inflammatory interleukins such as IL-1 [33]. Among these inflammation-inducing complexes, the NLRP3 inflammasome is the most widely studied complex and is responsible for the production of interleukin-1. The activation of this NLRP3 complex results mainly from two signals: signal 1 called priming and signal 2 called activation of NLRP3. The priming step of the NLRP3 inflammasome corresponds to the pretreatment of the macrophages with bacterial compounds such as LPS, capable of greatly increasing its activation [34], which could result from an interaction of NLRP3 with the IRAK1 protein [35]. In this sequence, in a basal condition, without pretreatment by LPS, we first showed that RWE and RSV were able to decrease IL-1β secretion in the two macrophage types associated with strong decreases of NLRP3 and ASC proteins in J774.1 macrophages. When NLRP3 is activated by LPS, we observed that pretreatment with RWE and RSV was able to attenuate IL-1β secretion, more specifically in J774.1, and in all types the key protein expression of NLRP3 and ASC. These first observations show the capacities of RWE to decrease the pro-inflammatory cytokine IL-1β and the NLRP3 complex with a better effect than RSV alone, particularly to downregulate ASC protein expression (Figure 2).

In the second step, we investigated the ability of RWE to modulate the second signal, activation. Activation of NLRP3 will result in aberrant mitochondrial homeostasis, leading to acetylated α-tubulin accumulation. This α-tubulin is responsible for the transport of mitochondria and will allow contact between ASC and NLRP3 [36]. Once formed, the NLRP3 inflammasome causes cleavage of pro-caspase-1 in active caspase-1, which in turn will cleave pro-IL-1β to IL-1β, which will then be excreted [37]. The mechanisms leading to the activation of this are not yet clearly defined, but it seems that some compounds, such as ATP [38] and nigericin [32], could activate the NLRP3 inflammasome. We thus pretreated macrophages with RWE or RSV and then treated them with LPS for the priming signal and with nigericin for the activation signal. It appears that only in J774.1 were RSV and RWE able to decrease IL-1β secretion and NLRP3 inflammasome significantly as compared to RAW macrophages (Figure 3). Very surprisingly, when the activator is changed and substituted by another such as ATP, we observed for the same treatment sequence that RWE and RSV are then able to greatly reduce the production of IL-1β and the expression of NLRP3 proteins (Figure 5c,d). This is much more complicated when studying the effect of RWE and RSV on the second signal and not on the first and second signal sequence. Indeed, we observed that RWE decreased NLRP3 and ASC protein expression, which is not the case for RSV (Figure 4C), but in all cases, both RWE and RSV failed to decrease IL-1β production, when the activator is nigericin. This is not the case when the activator is ATP, where RWE strongly decreases IL-1β production and NLRP3 protein expression (Figure 5a,b). The discrepancies observed between the two results could result from a different mechanism with the two activators. Indeed, it seems that extracellular ATP binds to its P2X7 receptor and then stimulates intracellular proton efflux. The result is the creation of Pannexin-1 membrane protons that may allow extracellular components to enter the cytosol and activate NLRP3 [38]. Some studies have proven that intracellular ATP is required for cellular functions such as the biosynthesis of pro-inflammatory cytokines and the maintenance of mitochondrial membrane potential. Therefore, a decrease in these levels might be a potent signal that activates the NLRP3 inflammasome [39]. According to other studies, the variation in intracellular potassium would be sufficient to induce the activation of NLRP3. In this way, some bacterial toxins such as nigericin leading the formation of ports in the plasma membrane also cause potassium efflux [32]. Further investigations should specify the actors involved in these two distinct mechanisms where one of the activators, namely ATP, does not require the ASC adapter protein for activation and secretion of IL-1β.

In addition to highlighting the effects of RWE on the activation of the inflammasome for the first time, we showed that a complex mixture of polyphenols can exhibit biological effects superior to a single molecule such as RSV. These new findings on inflammation support those obtained in the context of colorectal carcinogenesis where we previously demonstrated that an extract enriched in polyphenols could exhibit synergistic antiproliferative and antineoplastic effects in models of chemo-induced cancers in mice [18]. Qualitative and quantitative polyphenolic compositions are crucial for the determination of biological effects, especially on the occurrence of synergistic effects and additives seen for some antagonists' effects. We previously showed that resveratrol and quercetin combined exhibited a synergistic effect inducing apoptosis, antiproliferative effects, and cell cycle disruption compared to the compounds alone in colon cancer cells. Interestingly, in this same study, the combination of resveratrol+catechin or resveratrol+catechin+quercetin produced only an additive effect on the inhibition of tumor cell proliferation or on cell cycle arrest, and catechin+quercetin did not induce a synergistic effect on apoptosis [18]. In the present study, we observed that RWE presented a greater effect than RSV in various conditions, i.e., decreasing ASC protein expression in basal conditions, decreasing both ASC and NLRP3 protein expression and IL-1β secretion after priming by LPS, and interfering with the second signal to decrease ASC/NLRP3 protein expression and IL-1β secretion when ATP is used as an activator. These better effects can again result from synergies between the various compounds present in the polyphenol red wine extract. Indeed, the analysis of polyphenolic composition reveals the presence of resveratrol, catechin/epicatechin, and quercetin derivatives. These compounds are particularly important since separately they have been shown to exert an action on inflammation. For example, catechin was able to inhibit MSU-IL-1β secretion and NLRP3 inflammasome activation in THP-1 [40]. Similarly, quercetin was able to inhibit NLRP3 activation by interfering with ASC oligomerization and prevented IL-1β secretion in macrophages [41]. A possible mechanism of synergism could result from quercetin. We previously showed that a combination of resveratrol+quercetin increases resveratrol uptake by colon carcinoma cells, and in combination with RWE this combination increases uptake of resveratrol [18]. Similarly, the presence of quercetin in RWE could increase the uptake of RSV as well as others in macrophages to potentiate their effects against inflammasome activation.

In conclusion, many studies have highlighted the value of a polyphenol of the grapevine and wine, resveratrol, to reduce the production of proinflammatory cytokines, especially in the context of cardiovascular pathologies and cancers. However, resveratrol is not the only polyphenol of interest: other polyphenols of nutritional interest could play an important role, including those present in wine. We point out that depending on the activator used, ATP or nigericin, the effects observed can sometimes differ. In view of these results, experiments will have to be conducted to study if the modulation of inflammation by polyphenols of the extract can also be related to a modulation of the immune system, a major player in the production and maintenance of the cytokine balance.

Author Contributions: Formal analysis, E.C.-V.; Investigation, P.C., S.A., F.C., T.R., C.A., V.S.-K. and V.A.; Methodology, P.C.; Project administration, D.D.; Supervision, D.D.; Writing—original draft, V.A. and D.D.

Funding: This research was funded by grants from Bourgogne Franche-Comté Regional Councils (CRBFC), the FEDER and the "Bureau Interprofessionnel des Vins de Bourgogne" (BIVB).

Acknowledgments: The authors thank Linda Northrup for valuable English corrections.

Conflicts of Interest: The authors declare no conflict of interest.

References

1. Renaud, S.C.; Gueguen, R.; Schenker, J.; d'Houtaud, A. Alcohol and mortality in middle-aged men from eastern france. *Epidemiology* **1998**, *9*, 184–188. [CrossRef] [PubMed]
2. Goldberg, D.M.; Soleas, G.J.; Levesque, M. Moderate alcohol consumption: The gentle face of janus. *Clin. Biochem.* **1999**, *32*, 505–518. [CrossRef]
3. St Leger, A.S.; Cochrane, A.L.; Moore, F. Ischaemic heart-disease and wine. *Lancet* **1979**, *1*, 1294. [CrossRef]
4. Rifler, J.P.; Lorcerie, F.; Durand, P.; Delmas, D.; Ragot, K.; Limagne, E.; Mazue, F.; Riedinger, J.M.; d'Athis, P.; Hudelot, B.; et al. A moderate red wine intake improves blood lipid parameters and erythrocytes membrane fluidity in post myocardial infarct patients. *Mol. Nutr. Food Res.* **2012**, *56*, 345–351. [CrossRef] [PubMed]

5. Scalbert, A.; Johnson, I.T.; Saltmarsh, M. Polyphenols: Antioxidants and beyond. *Am. J. Clin. Nutr.* **2005**, *81*, 215S–217S. [CrossRef] [PubMed]

6. Waterhouse, A.L. Wine phenolics. *Ann. N. Y. Acad. Sci.* **2002**, *957*, 21–36. [CrossRef] [PubMed]

7. Wang, P.; Zhang, K.; Zhang, Q.; Mei, J.; Chen, C.J.; Feng, Z.Z.; Yu, D.H. Effects of quercetin on the apoptosis of the human gastric carcinoma cells. *Toxicol. In Vitro* **2012**, *26*, 221–228. [CrossRef] [PubMed]

8. Ebeler, S.E.; Brenneman, C.A.; Kim, G.S.; Jewell, W.T.; Webb, M.R.; Chacon-Rodriguez, L.; MacDonald, E.A.; Cramer, A.C.; Levi, A.; Ebeler, J.D.; et al. Dietary catechin delays tumor onset in a transgenic mouse model. *Am. J. Clin. Nutr.* **2002**, *76*, 865–872. [CrossRef] [PubMed]

9. Angel-Morales, G.; Noratto, G.; Mertens-Talcott, S. Red wine polyphenolics reduce the expression of inflammation markers in human colon-derived ccd-18co myofibroblast cells: Potential role of microrna-126. *Food Funct.* **2012**, *3*, 745–752. [CrossRef] [PubMed]

10. Kontou, N.; Psaltopoulou, T.; Soupos, N.; Polychronopoulos, E.; Xinopoulos, D.; Linos, A.; Panagiotakos, D. Alcohol consumption and colorectal cancer in a mediterranean population: A case-control study. *Dis. Colon Rectum* **2012**, *55*, 703–710. [CrossRef] [PubMed]

11. Crockett, S.D.; Long, M.D.; Dellon, E.S.; Martin, C.F.; Galanko, J.A.; Sandler, R.S. Inverse relationship between moderate alcohol intake and rectal cancer: Analysis of the north carolina colon cancer study. *Dis. Colon Rectum* **2011**, *54*, 887–894. [CrossRef] [PubMed]

12. Magalhaes, B.; Bastos, J.; Lunet, N. Dietary patterns and colorectal cancer: A case-control study from portugal. *Eur. J. Cancer Prev.* **2011**, *20*, 389–395. [CrossRef] [PubMed]

13. Fira-Mladinescu, C.; Fira-Mladinescu, O.; Doroftei, S.; Sas, F.; Ursoniu, S.; Ionut, R.; Putnoky, S.; Suciu, O.; Vlaicu, B. Food intake and colorectal cancers; an ecological study in Romania. *Rev. Med. Chir. Soc. Med. Nat. Iasi* **2008**, *112*, 805–811. [PubMed]

14. Andreatta, M.M.; Navarro, A.; Munoz, S.E.; Aballay, L.; Eynard, A.R. Dietary patterns and food groups are linked to the risk of urinary tract tumors in Argentina. *Eur. J. Cancer Prev.* **2010**, *19*, 478–484. [CrossRef] [PubMed]

15. Chao, C.; Haque, R.; Caan, B.J.; Poon, K.Y.; Tseng, H.F.; Quinn, V.P. Red wine consumption not associated with reduced risk of colorectal cancer. *Nutr. Cancer* **2010**, *62*, 849–855. [CrossRef] [PubMed]

16. Newcomb, P.A.; Nichols, H.B.; Beasley, J.M.; Egan, K.; Titus-Ernstoff, L.; Hampton, J.M.; Trentham-Dietz, A. No difference between red wine or white wine consumption and breast cancer risk. *Cancer Epidemiol. Biomarkers Prev.* **2009**, *18*, 1007–1010. [CrossRef] [PubMed]

17. Colin, D.; Gimazane, A.; Lizard, G.; Izard, J.C.; Solary, E.; Latruffe, N.; Delmas, D. Effects of resveratrol analogs on cell cycle progression, cell cycle associated proteins and 5fluoro-uracil sensitivity in human derived colon cancer cells. *Int. J. Cancer* **2009**, *124*, 2780–2788. [CrossRef] [PubMed]

18. Mazue, F.; Delmas, D.; Murillo, G.; Saleiro, D.; Limagne, E.; Latruffe, N. Differential protective effects of red wine polyphenol extracts (rwes) on colon carcinogenesis. *Food Funct.* **2014**, *5*, 663–670. [CrossRef] [PubMed]

19. Walter, A.; Etienne-Selloum, N.; Brasse, D.; Khallouf, H.; Bronner, C.; Rio, M.C.; Beretz, A.; Schini-Kerth, V.B. Intake of grape-derived polyphenols reduces c26 tumor growth by inhibiting angiogenesis and inducing apoptosis. *FASEB J.* **2010**, *24*, 3360–3369. [CrossRef] [PubMed]

20. Dolara, P.; Luceri, C.; De Filippo, C.; Femia, A.P.; Giovannelli, L.; Caderni, G.; Cecchini, C.; Silvi, S.; Orpianesi, C.; Cresci, A. Red wine polyphenols influence carcinogenesis, intestinal microflora, oxidative damage and gene expression profiles of colonic mucosa in F344 rats. *Mutat. Res.* **2005**, *591*, 237–246. [CrossRef] [PubMed]

21. Caderni, G.; Remy, S.; Cheynier, V.; Morozzi, G.; Dolara, P. Effect of complex polyphenols on colon carcinogenesis. *Eur. J. Nutr.* **1999**, *38*, 126–132. [CrossRef] [PubMed]

22. Chang, Y.P.; Ka, S.M.; Hsu, W.H.; Chen, A.; Chao, L.K.; Lin, C.C.; Hsieh, C.C.; Chen, M.C.; Chiu, H.W.; Ho, C.L.; et al. Resveratrol inhibits nlrp3 inflammasome activation by preserving mitochondrial integrity and augmenting autophagy. *J. Cell Physiol.* **2015**, *230*, 1567–1579. [CrossRef] [PubMed]

23. Duewell, P.; Kono, H.; Rayner, K.J.; Sirois, C.M.; Vladimer, G.; Bauernfeind, F.G.; Abela, G.S.; Franchi, L.; Nunez, G.; Schnurr, M.; et al. Nlrp3 inflammasomes are required for atherogenesis and activated by cholesterol crystals. *Nature* **2010**, *464*, 1357–1361. [CrossRef] [PubMed]

24. Heneka, M.T.; Kummer, M.P.; Stutz, A.; Delekate, A.; Schwartz, S.; Vieira-Saecker, A.; Griep, A.; Axt, D.; Remus, A.; Tzeng, T.C.; et al. Nlrp3 is activated in alzheimer's disease and contributes to pathology in app/ps1 mice. *Nature* **2013**, *493*, 674–678. [CrossRef] [PubMed]

25. Bruchard, M.; Mignot, G.; Derangere, V.; Chalmin, F.; Chevriaux, A.; Vegran, F.; Boireau, W.; Simon, B.; Ryffel, B.; Connat, J.L.; et al. Chemotherapy-triggered cathepsin b release in myeloid-derived suppressor cells activates the nlrp3 inflammasome and promotes tumor growth. *Nat. Med.* **2013**, *19*, 57–64. [CrossRef] [PubMed]

26. Scarpioni, R.; Obici, L. Renal involvement in autoinflammatory diseases and inflammasome-mediated chronic kidney damage. *Clin. Exp. Rheumatol.* **2018**, *36*, 54–60. [PubMed]

27. Nunes, C.; Teixeira, N.; Serra, D.; Freitas, V.; Almeida, L.; Laranjinha, J. Red wine polyphenol extract efficiently protects intestinal epithelial cells from inflammation via opposite modulation of jak/stat and nrf2 pathways. *Toxicol. Res.* **2016**, *5*, 53–65. [CrossRef] [PubMed]

28. Biasi, F.; Guina, T.; Maina, M.; Cabboi, B.; Deiana, M.; Tuberoso, C.I.; Calfapietra, S.; Chiarpotto, E.; Sottero, B.; Gamba, P.; et al. Phenolic compounds present in sardinian wine extracts protect against the production of inflammatory cytokines induced by oxysterols in caco-2 human enterocyte-like cells. *Biochem. Pharmacol.* **2013**, *86*, 138–145. [CrossRef] [PubMed]

29. Guerrero, R.F.; Garcia-Parrilla, M.C.; Puertas, B.; Cantos-Villar, E. Wine, resveratrol and health: A review. *Nat. Prod. Commun.* **2009**, *4*, 635–658. [PubMed]

30. He, Y.; Ou, Z.; Chen, X.; Zu, X.; Liu, L.; Li, Y.; Cao, Z.; Chen, M.; Chen, Z.; Chen, H.; et al. LPS/TLR4 signaling enhances TGF-beta response through downregulating bambi during prostatic hyperplasia. *Sci. Rep.* **2016**, *6*, 27051. [CrossRef] [PubMed]

31. Py, B.F.; Kim, M.S.; Vakifahmetoglu-Norberg, H.; Yuan, J. Deubiquitination of nlrp3 by brcc3 critically regulates inflammasome activity. *Mol. Cell.* **2013**, *49*, 331–338. [CrossRef] [PubMed]

32. Petrilli, V.; Papin, S.; Dostert, C.; Mayor, A.; Martinon, F.; Tschopp, J. Activation of the NALP3 inflammasome is triggered by low intracellular potassium concentration. *Cell Death Differ.* **2007**, *14*, 1583–1589. [CrossRef] [PubMed]

33. Tschopp, J.; Schroder, K. NLRP3 inflammasome activation: The convergence of multiple signalling pathways on ros production? *Nat. Rev. Immunol.* **2010**, *10*, 210–215. [CrossRef] [PubMed]

34. Schroder, K.; Sagulenko, V.; Zamoshnikova, A.; Richards, A.A.; Cridland, J.A.; Irvine, K.M.; Stacey, K.J.; Sweet, M.J. Acute lipopolysaccharide priming boosts inflammasome activation independently of inflammasome sensor induction. *Immunobiology* **2012**, *217*, 1325–1329. [CrossRef] [PubMed]

35. Fernandes-Alnemri, T.; Kang, S.; Anderson, C.; Sagara, J.; Fitzgerald, K.A.; Alnemri, E.S. Cutting edge: Tlr signaling licenses IRAK1 for rapid activation of the NLRP3 inflammasome. *J. Immunol.* **2013**, *191*, 3995–3999. [CrossRef] [PubMed]

36. Misawa, T.; Takahama, M.; Kozaki, T.; Lee, H.; Zou, J.; Saitoh, T.; Akira, S. Microtubule-driven spatial arrangement of mitochondria promotes activation of the NLRP3 inflammasome. *Nat. Immunol.* **2013**, *14*, 454–460. [CrossRef] [PubMed]

37. Baroja-Mazo, A.; Martin-Sanchez, F.; Gomez, A.I.; Martinez, C.M.; Amores-Iniesta, J.; Compan, V.; Barbera-Cremades, M.; Yague, J.; Ruiz-Ortiz, E.; Anton, J.; et al. The NLRP3 inflammasome is released as a particulate danger signal that amplifies the inflammatory response. *Nat. Immunol.* **2014**, *15*, 738–748. [CrossRef] [PubMed]

38. Kanneganti, T.D.; Lamkanfi, M.; Kim, Y.G.; Chen, G.; Park, J.H.; Franchi, L.; Vandenabeele, P.; Nunez, G. Pannexin-1-mediated recognition of bacterial molecules activates the cryopyrin inflammasome independent of toll-like receptor signaling. *Immunity* **2007**, *26*, 433–443. [CrossRef] [PubMed]

39. Nomura, J.; So, A.; Tamura, M.; Busso, N. Intracellular ATP decrease mediates NLRP3 inflammasome activation upon nigericin and crystal stimulation. *J. Immunol.* **2015**, *195*, 5718–5724. [CrossRef] [PubMed]

40. Jhang, J.J.; Lu, C.C.; Ho, C.Y.; Cheng, Y.T.; Yen, G.C. Protective effects of catechin against monosodium urate-induced inflammation through the modulation of NLRP3 inflammasome activation. *J. Agric. Food Chem.* **2015**, *63*, 7343–7352. [CrossRef] [PubMed]

41. Domiciano, T.P.; Wakita, D.; Jones, H.D.; Crother, T.R.; Verri, W.A., Jr.; Arditi, M.; Shimada, K. Quercetin inhibits inflammasome activation by interfering with asc oligomerization and prevents interleukin-1 mediated mouse vasculitis. *Sci. Rep.* **2017**, *7*, 41539. [CrossRef] [PubMed]

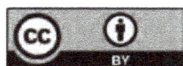

nutrients

MDPI

Review

Health Effects of Resveratrol: Results from Human Intervention Trials

Sonia L. Ramírez-Garza [1,2], Emily P. Laveriano-Santos [1], María Marhuenda-Muñoz [1,2], Carolina E. Storniolo [1,2], Anna Tresserra-Rimbau [3], Anna Vallverdú-Queralt [1,2] and Rosa M. Lamuela-Raventós [1,2,*]

[1] Department of Nutrition, Food Science and Gastronomy, School of Pharmacy and Food Sciences XaRTA, Institute of Nutrition and Food Safety (INSA-UB), University of Barcelona, 08921 Santa Coloma de Gramenet, Spain; sonialrmz@gmail.com (S.L.R.-G.); elaversa21@alumnes.ub.edu (E.P.L.-S.); mmarhuendam@ub.edu (M.M.-M.); carolina.e.storniolo@gmail.com (C.E.S.); avallverdu@ub.edu (A.V.-Q.)
[2] CIBER Physiopathology of Obesity and Nutrition (CIBEROBN), Institute of Health Carlos III, 28029 Madrid, Spain
[3] Human Nutrition Unit, University Hospital of Sant Joan de Reus, Department of Biochemistry and Biotechnology, Faculty of Medicine and Health Sciences, Pere Virgili Health Research Center, University Rovira i Virgili, 43201 Reus, Tarragona, Spain; anna.tresserra@iispv.cat
* Correspondence: lamuela@ub.edu; Tel.: +34-934-034-843; Fax: +34-934-035-931

Received: 30 October 2018; Accepted: 27 November 2018; Published: 3 December 2018

Abstract: The effect of resveratrol (RV) intake has been reviewed in several studies performed in humans with different health status. The purpose of this review is to summarize the results of clinical trials of the last decade, in which RV was determined in biological samples such as human plasma, urine, and feces. The topics covered include RV bioavailability, pharmacokinetics, effects on cardiovascular diseases, cognitive diseases, cancer, type 2 diabetes (T2D), oxidative stress, and inflammation states. The overview of the recent research reveals a clear tendency to identify RV in plasma, showing that its supplementation is safe. Furthermore, RV bioavailability depends on several factors such as dose, associated food matrix, or time of ingestion. Notably, enterohepatic recirculation of RV has been observed, and RV is largely excreted in the urine within the first four hours after consumption. Much of the research on RV in the last 10 years has focused on its effects on pathologies related to oxidative stress, inflammatory biomarkers, T2D, cardiovascular diseases, and neurological diseases.

Keywords: bioavailability; antioxidant; obesity; metabolic diseases

---

1. Introduction

In the last decades, lifestyle changes, especially in dietary patterns, have been increasingly seen as a means of preventing and treating chronic diseases. In this context, polyphenols have emerged as natural compounds with wide-ranging beneficial effects against cardiovascular diseases (CVD) and cancer [1,2]. Polyphenols are metabolized by the intestine, hepatic cells, or intestinal microbiota. The intestinal absorption, bioavailability, and pharmacokinetics of polyphenols are conditioned by the food matrix in which they are ingested [3,4].

Resveratrol (RV), a naturally occurring polyphenol (*trans*-3,4′,5-trihydroxystilbene), possesses anti-inflammatory, anti-tumorigenic, and antioxidant properties, which may be harnessed in strategies against chronic diseases. The main sources of RV include, above all, grapes (*Vitis vinifera* L.), a variety of berries, peanuts, medicinal plants such as Japanese knotweed [5], and red wine.

Studies on the health benefits of RV have reported a reduction in age-associated symptoms and the prevention of early mortality in obese animals [6–8]. The life expectancy of some small organisms has been extended by RV via the stimulation of caloric restriction [9] and the delay of specific age-related phenotypes, e.g., abnormal glucose metabolism [10]. RV is also associated with a slowing down or prevention of cognitive deterioration [11].

The potential mechanisms of action responsible for the health effects of RV are numerous [5]. As RV triggers the expression of a wide range of antioxidant enzymes, determining the contribution of each mechanism to an overall decrease in oxidative stress is a complex task [12]. Additionally, a large number of receptors, kinases, and other enzymes interact with RV, which may influence its biological effects.

The activities of sirtuin 1 (SIRT1) and adenosine monophosphate-activated protein kinase (AMPK), enzymatic regulators of metabolism in multiple tissues, are stimulated by RV in vivo [5,13,14]. Some of the beneficial effects of RV are due to the overexpression of SIRT1 [15]. Moreover, RV has been reported to be a potent inhibitor of quinone reductase 2 activity, which is associated with neurological disorders, although more research is required to confirm this hypothesis [16]. The determination of all effects of RV in humans remains a major challenge.

After oral ingestion, RV is metabolized in the liver to glucuronide and sulphate forms and in the intestine by hydrogenation of the aliphatic double bond [17,18]. RV has been found in urine samples of subjects who have drunk a glass of wine per week or three glasses per week three or five days after the last consumption, respectively [19].

The aim of this review is to summarize the health effects of RV in humans as reported by studies carried out in the last decade, including the determination of plasma, urine, and feces RV and its metabolites. The information is presented in two sections: bioavailability and pharmacokinetics of RV and the effects of RV in different health status.

2. Bioavailability and Pharmacokinetics of Resveratrol

After oral administration, RV is absorbed by passive diffusion or by forming complexes with membrane transporters followed by release into the bloodstream, where it can be found mainly as a glucuronide, sulfate, or free [20]. Phase II metabolism of RV or metabolites occurs in the liver, after an enterohepatic transport in the bile that may lead to some RV return to the small intestine [1].

Human clinical trials with RV showed its rapid metabolism [20,21]; it occurs in the liver and promotes the production of conjugated glucuronides and sulfate metabolites, which have biological activity [20]. The metabolites identified were measured by high-performance liquid chromatography analysis, followed by mass spectrometry.

Different clinical trials have found that the majority of plasma RV metabolites are RV-3-*O*-sulfate, RV-4′-*O*-glucuronide, and RV-3-*O*-glucuronide. RV-3-*O*-sulfate circulating levels showed the highest peak concentration compared to the other conjugated RV metabolites [22–25], except in one study where RV-3-*O*-glucuronide presented the highest peak concentration when the dose of RV was 2.5 g [25]. Pharmacokinetic studies revealed that RV concentration in plasma depends on the doses ingested [22,25–27].

In this section, we address research on the bioavailability and pharmacokinetics of RV in human clinical trials during the last 10 years. The subsections are organized according to the effects of different factors.

2.1. Effect of Pharmaceutical Formulation and Particle Size

Different strategies have been developed to improve RV efficacy [28], including pharmaceutical manipulation. A novel soluble formulation of *trans*-RV (caplets) was administered to 15 healthy subjects; the same amount of *trans*-RV (single dose of 40 mg) was also administered in dry powder (capsules). There were significant differences in bioavailability between the formulations, being the Cmax (maximum concentration) in plasma 8.8-fold higher for the soluble formulation [29].

RV can be absorbed, metabolized, and excreted in urine, in which up to 21 metabolites of RV have been identified [30]. The intake of 4.7 mg of RV in grape extract tablets (as a nutraceutical) resulted in a delay of the urinary excretion of RV metabolites up to 4-fold higher compared with the intake of 6.3 mg of RV in red wine [31]. This indicates a delayed absorption of RV when it is ingested in grape extract tablets. As a consequence, RV stays longer in the gut and could be metabolized by the gut microbiota. Therefore, RV supplementation can be a good source of this polyphenol.

Furthermore, reducing the size of the chemical particles can increase their absorption and kinetics [32]. The daily intake of 5 g microparticulate RV with a particle size of less than 5 mm (SRT501) for 14 days produced a higher peak plasma concentration than the equivalent dose of non-micronized RV [33], therefore a small particle size improves RV bioavailability.

2.2. Matrix Effect

The food matrix is important for RV bioavailability and pharmakocinetics. The bioavailability of RV was assessed when it was consumed together with food, quercetin, or ethanol in a study where 2000 mg of *trans*-RV were administered twice daily for seven days to eight healthy subjects. In this clinical trial, the combined intake with other phenols such as quercetin and alcohol did not influence *trans*-RV pharmacokinetics. However, when RV was ingested within a high-fat breakfast compared with a standard breakfast, the area under the plasma concentration–time curve and the maximum plasma concentration were lower (45% and 46% decrease, respectively) [34]. In a two-way crossover study, 24 healthy subjects were administered 400 mg of *trans*-RV with a high-fat content meal or in fasting conditions [35], and it was concluded that the presence of high-fat food delayed the rate of absorption of *trans*-RV but not the extent of absorption.

The solubility of *trans*-RV in water containing dextrose, fructose, ribose, sucrose, or xylitol was analyzed and compared. The best result was obtained with the ribose solution. A mixture of ribose and 146 ± 5.5 mg *trans*-RV was administered to two healthy human participants, leading to a higher and quicker RV release than that obtained with traditional free RV capsules [36]. A similar result was demonstrated when 250 mg *trans*-RV doses were administered with 20 mg of piperine to 23 healthy adults [23]. In this context, it is possible that the affinity for or the solubility of *trans*-RV in the presence of different substances such as soluble formulations, ribose, and piperine improves RV bioavailability when compared to the classic formulations (capsules).

Furthermore, a study with 36 healthy males ingesting capsules containing 800 mg polyphenols with protein-rich dairy, soy, fruit-flavored drinks, or water, showed that the intake of polyphenols incorporated in protein-rich drinks did not change significantly the bioavailability of polyphenols or their metabolites [37].

A similar result was obtained when 59 high-risk adult subjects at high cardiovascular risk drank 272 mL of red wine (RW, 30 g ethanol/day) or dealcoholized red wine (DRW) every day for four weeks. The RV effect was independent of the alcohol in the red wine [38].

2.3. Effects of Other Factors

Repeated oral supplementation of *trans*-RV may influence pharmacokinetic variables. In this context, 13 doses of 25, 50, 100, or 150 mg *trans*-RV were administered six times/day to four groups of eight healthy adults. Differences were observed between the peak *trans*-RV plasma concentrations after ingestion of the 1st and 13th dose, demonstrating the highest peak concentration for the latter. Moreover, *trans*-RV pharmacokinetic values were higher at 8 am and 12 pm [39], meaning that circadian variation and repeated doses affected the bioavailability.

It is important to remember that a wide range of factors such as gut microbiota composition, hormones, gender, and other interindividual differences can modify the structure of RV [40,41]. The gut microbiota plays an important role in the structure of RV, which can affect human health. In feces of healthy humans, *Slackia Equolifaciens* sp. and *Adlercreutzia Equolifaciens* sp. have been identified as dihydroresveratrol producers [40].

2.4. Is It Safe to Consume Resveratrol?

Clinical trials have shown that RV and *trans*-RV supplementation is safe and well tolerated at different doses [25,29,33,39,42–45]. However, some participants reported one or more adverse events, such as gastrointestinal symptoms including nausea, flatulence, bowel motions, abdominal discomfort, loose stools, and diarrhea, after ingesting a dose of 2.5 to 5 g of RV [22,25,34,42,43].

On the other hand, *trans*-RV half-life was one to three hours following single doses and two to five hours following repeated dosing [39]. It is noteworthy that the most important phase of RV excretion occurs in the first four hours after ingestion. Moreover, there exists a relationship between RV levels in plasma and in stools, indicating an enterohepatic recirculation [43].

For the above-mentioned reasons, the bioavailability and pharmacokinetics of RV depend on the doses ingested, the ingestion of food matrix, the particle size, and the role of the gut microbiota in the metabolism of RV. Last, RV intake is safe at a dose of up to 5 g; however, adverse reactions have been observed at higher doses, which should be considered in future studies.

Figure 1 recapitulates the bioavailability and pharmacokinetics of RV. The image schematizes the results of different studies in which RV was identified in urine and blood. Additionally, Table 1 presents the details of the bioavailability and pharmacokinetics of RV in each study considered; it is organized according to health status and year of publication.

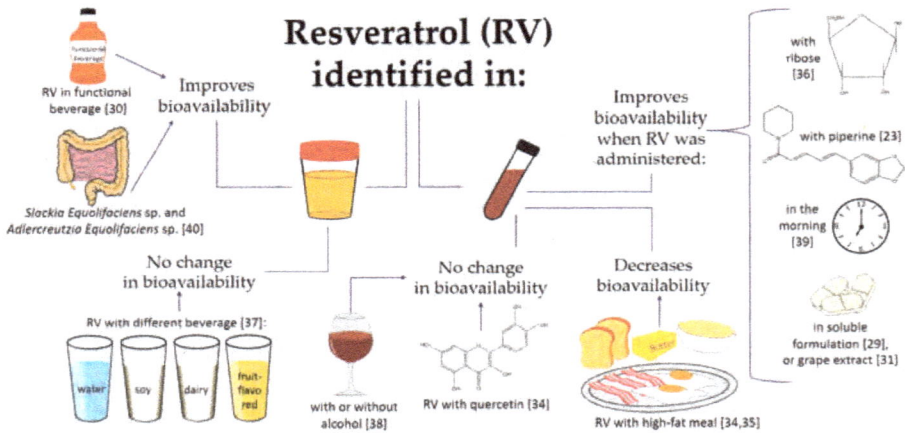

Figure 1. Bioavailability and pharmacokinetics. The image summarizes the results of different studies that identified resveratrol (RV) in urine and blood.

Table 1. Studies of resveratrol bioavailability and pharmacokinetics in the last 10 years *.

Metabolite (form of RV)	Sample	Type of Study	(n)	Dose	Participants' Health Status	Effect	Ref.
RV and six metabolites: two monosulfates, one disulfate, two monoglucuronides, and one glucuronide-sulfate	Urine and feces	Clinical trial	40	After a five-day washout, 10 subjects received a 0.5 g dose, which was escalated sequentially to 1, 2.5, and 5 g	Healthy	An intake of up to one dose of 5 g of RV was safe, with minor adverse events in some cases; 77% of urinary excretion of RV and its metabolites occurred within four hours after the lowest dose. RV underwent enterohepatic recirculation.	[43]
tRV	Plasma	Randomized, crossover, open-label, and single-dose Phase I,	24	Two treatments with a single dose of 400 mg tRV after a high-fat meal or eight hours without breakfast, separated by a washout of seven days or more.	Healthy	The rate of absorption of tRV was reduced by the presence of a meal	[35]
tRV	Plasma	randomized, double-blind, placebo-controlled, and single-center	40	25, 50, 100, or 150 mg, administered at four hours intervals (six times/day) for 48 h (13 doses in total)	Healthy	High daily doses of tRV were well tolerated but produced low plasma tRV levels; tRV bioavailability was higher when it was administered in the morning.	[39]
tRV	Plasma	Open-label and single-arm	8	tRV 2000 mg twice daily for seven days and tRV 2000 mg with quercetin 500 mg twice daily for seven days, with a two-week washout period	Healthy	tRV 2000 g twice daily had adequate exposure and was well tolerated by subjects. Moreover, combined intake with quercetin did not influence its exposure	[34]
RV glucuronide and sulfate conjugates, RV glucoside, piceid glucuronides, sulfates, DHR, glucuronide, and sulfate conjugates	Plasma and urine	Randomized and crossover	10	After a three-day washout period, three people were chosen for the pilot study in which they consumed 15 grape extract tablets (total RV 4.72 ± 0.07 mg) with 400 mL of water within 10 min. In parallel, seven people were selected randomly to drink 375 mL of red wine (total RV 6.30 ± 0.09 mg) with 400 mL of water consumed within 10 min.	Healthy	Statistically significant differences between grape extract tablets and red wine treatments were obtained for some metabolites, mainly due to the different composition of RV and piceid from both sources. The grape extract tablets delayed RV absorption compared to the red wine treatment.	[31]
Free RV and conjugated RV (monosulfate, disulfate, and glucoronide)	Plasma	Clinical trial	15	Single dose (40 mg) of tRV in soluble formulation or dry powder	Healthy	Bioavailability was higher with soluble formulation compared to dry powder.	[29]

Table 1. Cont.

Metabolite (form of RV)	Sample	Type of Study	(n)	Dose	Participants' Health Status	Effect	Ref.
*t*RV, DHR, 3,4′-dihydroxy-*trans*-stilbene, and 3,4′-dihydroxybibenzyl (lunularin).	24 h urine and feces	Controlled intervention	12	Following a washout period, all the subjects received a single oral dose of 0.5 mg *t*RV/kg body weight in the form of a grapevine-shoot supplement (7.7% *t*RV as well as other stilbene mono- and oligomers [14.6% *ε*-viniferin, 3.4% ampelopsin A, 1.8% hopeaphenol, 0.6% *trans*-piceatannol, 1.6% r-2-viniferin (vitisin A), 2.5% miyabenol C, 2.5% r-viniferin (vitisin B), and 2.4% iso-*trans*-ε-viniferin].	Healthy	The human gut microbiota produced pronounced interindividual differences in *t*RV. *Slackia Equolifaciens* sp. and *Adlercreutzia Equolifaciens* sp. were identified as DHR producers, but the bacteria that produce dehydroxylated metabolites were not determined.	[40]
*t*RV	Plasma	Pilot study	2	146 +/− 5.5 mg *t*RV per 2000 mg of lozenge mass, containing about 46% ribose, 46% (fructose/sucrose mixture), and 8% *t*RV	Healthy	A mixture of ribose and RV oral transmucosal administration achieved a much higher and quicker RV release compared to the reported traditional free RV capsules.	[36]
Free and conjugated RV	Plasma	Randomized and three-way crossover	15	Oral doses equivalent to 50 mg or 150 mg of *t*RV or plant-derived RV (150 mg) on three occasions separated by seven-day washout periods.	Healthy	150 mg dose of *t*RV showed higher total and free levels than 50 mg dose	[46]
*t*RV, RV, 3-*O*-sulphate, RV 4′-*O*-glucuronide, and RV 3-*O*-glucuronide	Plasma	Randomized, double-blind, and placebo-controlled	23	250 mg of *t*RV or 250 mg of *t*RV with 20 mg of piperine on separate days at least a week apart.	Healthy	Piperine co-supplementation with 250 mg of RV or 250 mg of *t*RV; piperine enhanced the absorption of the polyphenol leading to an increase in cerebral blood flow.	[23]
*t*R4G, *c*R4G, *t*R3G, *c*R3G, *t*R4S, *c*R4S, *t*R3S, *c*R3S, *t*R34dS, RV-SG, *t*piceid, *c*piceid, Pic-G, Pic-S1, Pic-S2, DHR, DHR-G1, DHR-G2, DHR-S1, DHR-S2, and DHR-SG	24 h urine	Randomized, double-blind, placebo-controlled, crossover, and intervention study	26	Consumed twice a day (with breakfast and dinner) for 15 days (per each phase) 187 mL of: a control placebo and a functional beverage (4280 g/L of hydroxycinnamic acids, 16 mg/L of anthocyanins, 96 mg/L of flavanols, 83 mg/L of hydroxybenzoic acids, and 5.7 mg/L of stilbenes)	Healthy	The whole profile of the 21 RV metabolites increased after acute and chronic consumption of the functional beverage with respect to the control-placebo beverage and to the baseline.	[30]

Table 1. *Cont.*

Metabolite (form of RV)	Sample	Type of Study	(n)	Dose	Participants' Health Status	Effect	Ref.
Phenolic acids including, 3-hydroxyphenylacetic acid, 3-hydroxyhippuric acid, 4-hydroxyhippuric acid, and Hippuric Acid,	24 h urine	Randomized, placebo-controlled, and crossover	35	Six placebo gelatin capsules consumed with 200 mL of water (control) Six capsules containing 800 mg polyphenols (141 mg anthocyanins, 24 mg flavan-3-ols, 16 mg procyanidins, 10 mg phenolic acids, 9 mg flavonols, and 1 mg stilbenes) derived from red wine and grape extracts, or the same dose of polyphenols incorporated into one of the following: 200 mL of water (positive control). 200 g of dairy drink, 200 g of soy drink, 200 g fruit-flavored drink, or protein-free drink.	Healthy	Bioavailability of polyphenols and the excretion of their phenolic metabolites were not significantly affected when polyphenols were consumed in protein-rich soy or dairy drinks.	[37]
Total RV	Plasma	Randomized and double-blind	9	5 g/day of SRT501 for approximately 14 days	IV colorectal cancer and hepatic metastasis subjects scheduled to undergo hepatectomy.	RV treatment was well tolerated by the patients. The peak plasma after ingestion of SRT501 was 1.942 ng/m, higher than that of an equivalent dose of non-micronized RV supplementation.	[33]
tR4G, cR4G, tR3G, cR3G, tR4S, cR4S, tR3S, cR3S, tR34dS, RV-SG, tpiceid, cpiceid, Pic-G, Pic-S1, Pic-S2, DHR, DHR-G1, DHR-G2, DHR-S1, DHR-S2, and DHR-SG	24 h urine	Randomized, crossover, and controlled clinical trial	59	15-day run-in period in which they consumed neither grape-derived products nor alcoholic beverages. Afterwards, they consumed every day for four weeks: 272 mL of RW (red wine) with 30 g ethanol/day or 272 mL of DRW (dealcoholized red wine), following the same background diet.	High cardiovascular risk	The whole profile of the 21 RV metabolites increased after RW and DRW consumption, and no differences between them were presented	[38]

cpiceid: *cis*-3,4′,5-trihydroxystilbene-3-β-D-glucopyranoside, cR3G: *cis*-RV-3-*O*-glucuronide, cR3S: *cis*-RV-3-*O*-sulfate, cR4G: *cis*-RV-4′-*O*-glucuronide, cR4S: *cis*-RV-4′-*O*-sulfate, DHR: Dihydroresveratrol, DHR-G1: DHR glucuronide 1, DHR-G2: DHR glucuronide 2, DHR-S1: DHR sulfate 1, DHR-S2: DHR sulfate 2, DHR-SG: DHR sulfoglucuronide, Pic-G: piceid-glucuronide, Pic-S1: Piceid sulfate 1, Pic-S2: Piceid sulfate 2, RV: resveratrol, RV-SG: RV sulfoglucuronide, SRT501: microparticular RV of particle size less than 5um, tpiceid: *trans*-3,4′,5-trihydroxystilbene-3-β-D-glucopyranoside, tRV: *trans*-RV, tR3G: *trans*-RV-3-*O*-glucuronide, tR3S: *trans*-RV-3-*O*-sulfate, tR4G: *trans*-RV-4′-*O*-glucuronide, tR4S: *trans*-RV-4′-*O*-sulfate, and tR34dS: *trans*-RV-3,4′-*O*-disulfate. * Studies which identified resveratrol or some metabolite of resveratrol in plasma, urine, and/or feces.

193

3. Different Health Effects of Resveratrol

This section addresses research on the effect of RV in human clinical trials in the last 10 years. The subsections are organized according to the different health status or diseases under research.

3.1. Effects of Resveratrol on Neurological Diseases and Cognitive Performance

RV is associated with a slowing down or prevention of cognitive deterioration [11]. Although few clinical trials have focused on the effect of RV on Alzheimer's disease (AD), two studies suggest that RV may change some AD biomarkers. Both studies are rated class II because more than two primary outcomes were designated. A dose of 500 mg RV/day was administered to patients with mild to moderate AD, with 500 mg increments every 13 weeks up to 52 weeks, ending with 1000 mg twice daily. In one of the studies, the brain volume decreased in the RV group; however, the mechanisms of this event were unclear, and cognitive deterioration was not indicated. Both the RV and placebo group showed a decline of Aβ40 (beta amyloid) levels in the cerebrospinal fluid (CSF) or plasma at 52 weeks [24]. A subsequent study reported similar results for CSF Aβ40 compared to baseline, whereas a greater reduction of CSF Aβ42 occurred in the placebo group when compared to the group receiving the RV treatment, indicating that RV could attenuate the progressive decline of this biomarker of AD. In plasma, RV increased MMP10 (matrix metalloproteinase) and reduced IL-12P40 (interleukin) and IL-12P70. Compared to the placebo, the RV treatment reduced MMP9 in CSF [47]. From the evidence described above, RV may regulate neuro-inflammation in AD patients; however, more studies are needed to draw conclusions about RV efficacy in AD.

In 36 adult patients with type 2 diabetes (T2D), a single dose of 75 mg of RV ingested at weekly intervals showed significant changes, enhancing neurovascular coupling capacity and improving cognitive performance [27].

On the other hand, single doses of 250 and 500 mg *trans*-RV in two different days, in healthy subjects, improved cerebral blood flow variables, with increases of total hemoglobin (Hb) and oxygenated Hb (oxy-Hb) and a reduction of deoxy-Hb concentration; nevertheless, it did not produce any change in cognitive performance variables [48]. In a consecutive study, a similar result was reported with 23 healthy adults who ingested two capsules with a dose of 250 mg *trans*-RV and 20 mg of piperine (a pepper-derived alkaloid) in three different days. A significant increase in total-Hb and oxy-Hb was observed, but without any improvement in cognitive functioning [23].

A possible explanation for the contrasting results could be that a different methodology to evaluate cognitive performance was used in these studies. When a more objective measure is used, such as near-IR spectroscopy, the results are not as clear as when the results are based on cognitive test batteries. Likewise, it could be interesting to know the capsule composition, because it could contribute to the observed different effect.

The effects of RV have been observed in other neurological diseases such as Friedreich ataxia. The effect of 5 g of RV ingested daily for 12 weeks was studied in patients diagnosed with the aforementioned disease, showing an improvement in neurologic function, audiologic and speech measures, and oxidative stress marker plasma F2-isoprostane [25].

3.2. Effects of Resveratrol on Diabetes Mellitus

RV enhances the endothelial function, increases liver fatty acid oxidation, and decreases oxidative stress [49], leading to an improvement in insulin sensitivity [50]. A study in which 10 overweight individuals with impaired glucose tolerance were administered 1, 1.5, or 2 g of RV per day for four weeks, showed that insulin sensitivity and postprandial glucose levels were improved by RV intake [45]. In another clinical study, 17 volunteers with T2D were treated with 150 mg/day of RV for 30 days, after which, intrahepatic lipid content and systolic blood pressure decreased. Similarly, when overweight and obese men were administered RV for two weeks, 1 g in the first week and 2 g in the second, a reduction in intestinal and hepatic lipoprotein particle production was observed.

RV diminished the production rate of ApoB-48 and both the production and fractional catabolic rates of ApoB-100, compared to a placebo [51].

Nevertheless, RV did not enhance hepatic and peripheral insulin sensitivity, which could be explained by a negative interaction with metformin in the patients receiving this kind of treatment [52]. Similar results were reported in 20 overweight or obese men with non-alcoholic fatty liver disease when given a daily dose of 3 g RV for eight weeks. No reduction in insulin resistance, steatosis, abdominal fat distribution, plasma lipids, or antioxidant activity was observed. However, an increase of alanine and aspartate aminotransferases with RV supplementation was observed, due to RV increased hepatic stress [42].

Some studies have analyzed the effect of RV on obesity. A daily dose of 150 mg/day of RV for four weeks was given to 10 slightly obese adults. RV supplementation suppressed postprandial glucagon, which may be important for the treatment of T2D because an excess of this hormone contributes to patient hyperglycemia [53]. Contrasting results can be explained by the effect of the pharmacokinetics of different medications on RV or by liver's health, because both RV and other medications could be metabolized in the liver; nevertheless, the main reason could be the dose taken.

3.3. Effect of Resveratrol on Cancer

The insulin-like growth factor (IGF) signaling pathway, including IGFs, IGF-binding proteins (IGFBP), and IGF receptors, is related to the anticarcinogenic effects linked to dietary restriction. In parallel, RV can act as a chemopreventive agent and a calorie-restriction mimetic in humans [9,54]. Related to these effects, RV decreased IGF-I and IGFBP-3 in 40 healthy volunteers who consumed RV at 0.5, 1.0, 2.5, or 5.0 g daily for 29 days, leading to a reduction of cancer risk. The highest reduction was observed with a 2.5 g dose. Therefore, it was concluded that the IGF system could act as a biomarker of RV chemopreventive action in humans [22].

3.4. Effect of Resveratrol on Cardiovascular Diseases

Flow-mediated dilatation (FMD) of the brachial artery is a biomarker of endothelial function and cardiovascular health, with notable importance as an indicator of structural and functional endothelium changes [55,56]. A 270 mg dose of RV administered weekly for four weeks to 14 overweight or obese men or five post-menopausal women with untreated borderline hypertension significantly increased FMD [26]. In another study, RV in red wine was associated with improved levels of glucose and triglycerides, as well as a lower heart rate, whereas no effect was observed for total cholesterol, HDL, LDL, and high blood pressure [57]. However, in overweight individuals, the intake of 150 mg per day of RV for four weeks did not influence metabolic risk markers such as endothelial function or inflammation, which are related to cardiovascular health risk [58,59]. A possible reason for the contrasting results could be related to the ingested dose of RV, because a positive effect of RV in higher doses on other diseases has been observed. However, it is important to note that the first mentioned work [26] had a significantly lower number of participants than the last one [58,59].

3.5. Effect of Resveratrol on Obesity

In a crossover study with 11 subjects, RV mimicked the effect of calorie restriction, reducing the metabolic rate, activating AMPK in muscle, and increasing the levels of SIRT1 and peroxisome proliferator-activated receptor gamma coactivator 1 alpha protein. RV also increased the activity of citrate synthase and decreased the lipid content inside the liver, the levels of circulating glucose, triglycerides, alanine aminotransferase, and other inflammation markers. The homeostatic model assessment index was also improved after the intervention [60].

To analyze the longer-term effect of some polyphenols on the metabolic profile, RV and epigallocatechin-3-gallate supplements (80 and 282 mg/day, respectively) were administered during a period of 12 weeks to 38 overweight or obese subjects. An increase in mitochondrial capacity and fat oxidation stimulation was observed, together with a better skeletal muscle oxidative capacity and a preservation of fasting and postprandial fat oxidation. Consequently, triacylglycerol concentration remained unchanged after the RV treatment, unlike in the placebo group, but no improvement of insulin resistance was found in peripheral, hepatic, or adipose tissue [61].

3.6. Effect of Resveratrol on Other Health Conditions Associated with Oxidative Stress and Inflammation

The antioxidant effects of RV have been widely studied. In a study with 10 healthy individuals, a single dose of 5 g of RV was given, and a significant increase of tumor necrosis factor-alpha (TNF-α) in plasma was found after 24 h. This enhanced production, as well as the inhibition of IL-10, was confirmed by analysis of peripheral blood mononuclear cells (PBMC), which were activated with different toll-like receptor agonists [62].

In a different trial with nine healthy men and women, who ingested 1 g/day RV capsules for 28 days, RV effect on immune cells was assessed. The results showed that RV induced an increase in circulating T cells and was consequently able to reduce the plasma levels of proinflammatory cytokines TNF-α and monocyte chemoattractant protein 1; moreover, RV significantly increased the plasma antioxidant capacity with a resulting decrease of oxidative stress markers involved in DNA damage [63].

A study consisting in the administration of 75 mg/day of RV per 12 weeks to non-obese, postmenopausal women with normal glucose tolerance, did not observe any change in inflammatory markers, body composition, resting metabolic rate, plasma lipids, liver, skeletal muscle, and adipose tissue volumes, or insulin sensitivity [44].

Lastly, in a study with patients undergoing peritoneal dialysis, the daily consumption of 450 mg of RV over 12 weeks improved urinary ultrafiltration and decreased vascular endothelial growth factor, fetal liver kinase-1, and angiopoietin-2 (angiogenesis markers) when the highest dose was ingested [64].

A possible reason for the contrasting results could be that low doses [44] or a single but higher dose [62] do not have positive health effects and, furthermore, they may cause an acute metabolic stress. On the other hand, a moderate (>450 mg) but continuing intake [63,64] has demonstrated an improved effect of RV. These results suggest that a repeated and moderate administration of RV is better than a single, higher dose administration. Figure 2 schematizes the results of different studies from the last 10 years in which RV had a healthy effect. Additionally, Table 2 presents the details of the effect of RV in each study analyzed. The table is organized according to the participants' health status.

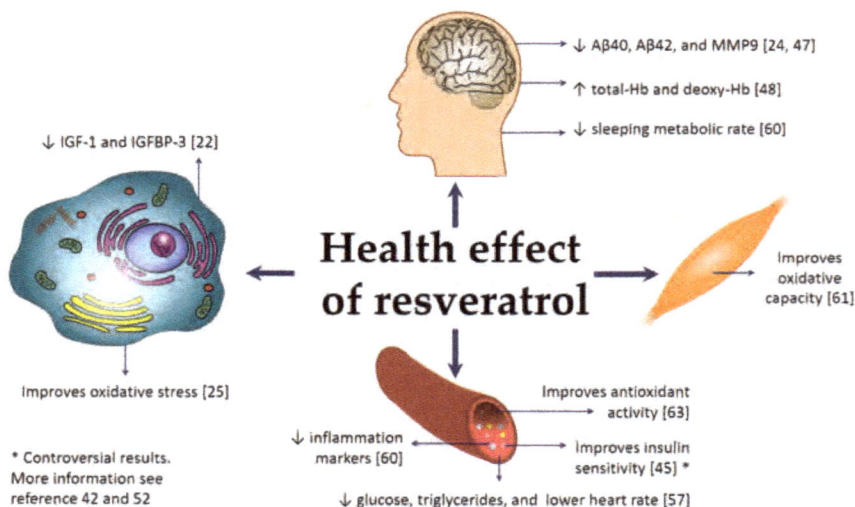

↓ IGF-1 and IGFBP-3 [22]

↓ Aβ40, Aβ42, and MMP9 [24, 47]

↑ total-Hb and deoxy-Hb [48]

↓ sleeping metabolic rate [60]

Health effect of resveratrol

Improves oxidative capacity [61]

Improves oxidative stress [25]

Improves antioxidant activity [63]

↓ inflammation markers [60]

Improves insulin sensitivity [45] *

* Controversial results. More information see reference 42 and 52

↓ glucose, triglycerides, and lower heart rate [57]

Figure 2. Health effects of resveratrol. A summary of the results of different studies reporting a positive effect of RV on health.

Table 2. Effects of resveratrol on individuals with different health status reported in the last 10 years *.

Metabolite (form of RV)	Sample	Type of Study	(n)	Dose	Participants' Health Status	Effect	Ref.
RV 3-O-glucuronidated-RV, 4-O-glucuronidated-RV, and 3-sulfated-RV	Plasma	Phase II, randomized, double-blind, placebo-controlled, and multi-center	119	500 mg/day RV with 500 mg increments every 13 weeks up to 52 weeks, ending with 1000 mg twice daily	Alzheimer	RV was safe and well tolerated, decreased Aβ40 and MMP9 in CSF, modulated neuroinflammation, and induced adaptive immunity.	[24,47]
RV, RV-3-glucuronide, RV-4′-glucuronide, and RV-3-sulfate RV-4′-sulfate	Plasma	Non-randomized, and open-label	24	Low-dose RV (1 g daily) or high-dose RV (5 g daily) over a 12-week period	Friedreich ataxia	PBMC frataxin protein levels were not affected. High-dose RV treatment showed a beneficial effect on both oxidative stress and some clinical outcome measures.	[25]
Total tRV	Plasma	Randomized, double-blind, and placebo-controlled	36	0, 75, 150, and 300 mg at weekly intervals	T2D	A 75 mg dose of RV correlated with an increase in plasma RV concentration, enhanced the cerebrovascular responsiveness to selected stimuli in T2DM adults.	[27]
RV and dehydro RV (aglycones and glucuronide conjugates)	Plasma	Randomized, double-blind, and crossover	17	150 mg/day of resVida (RV) for 30 days	T2D	Intrahepatic lipid content correlated negatively with the plasma RV content. RV plasma levels might be affected by metformin treatment; RV did not improve insulin sensitivity. Total urinary RV metabolites were directly associated with lower concentrations of fasting	[52]
TRM: tR3G, cR4G, cR3G, tR4S, tR3S, cR4S, and cR3S	Urine	Randomized, parallel-group, multi-center, and controlled clinical trial	1000	Exploratory study of the baseline data of PREDIMED study	T2D or at less three major cardiovascular risk factors	blood glucose and triglycerides, and also with lower heart rate. No significant associations were observed between TRM and total cholesterol, HDL, and LDL concentrations, or blood pressure. Therefore, RV may help to decrease cardiovascular risk.	[57]
Total RV	Plasma	Randomized	10	1, 1.5, and 2 g/day RV, taken in divided doses for four weeks	Overweight or obese and insulin resistant.	Fasting glucose was unchanged, but postprandial glucose and three-hour glucose area under the curve decreased significantly. Insulin sensitivity (using the Matsuda index) improved. Fasting lipid profile, CRP, and adiponectin were unchanged.	[45]
Total RV	Plasma	Randomized, double-blind, and placebo-controlled	20	3000 mg/day RV for eight weeks	Overweight or obese with non-alcoholic fatty liver disease	RV did not improve insulin sensitivity, plasma lipids, antioxidant activity, and IGF-1, but it increased ALT and AST, liver enzymes that indicate hepatic stress.	[42]
Total RV	Plasma	Randomized, double-blind, placebo-controlled, and crossover	19	A single dose of RV (30, 90, and 270 mg) administered at one-week intervals over four weeks	Overweight and obese individuals or postmenopausal women with untreated borderline hypertension	Significant linear relationship between RV dose intake and plasma RV concentration. Higher plasma RV concentration was associated with acute flow-mediated dilatation response.	[26]

197

Table 2. *Cont.*

Metabolite (form of RV)	Sample	Type of Study	(n)	Dose	Participants' Health Status	Effect	Ref.
Total conjugated, unconjugated RV, and DHR	Plasma	Randomized, double-blind, and crossover	11	150 mg/day RV for 30 days	Obese	RV supplementation modestly mimicked the beneficial effects of calorie restriction. It reduced sleeping metabolic rate, affected the AMPK–SIRT1–PGC1α axis, decreased hepatic lipid accumulation. and reduced inflammation markers.	[50]
Epigallocatechin-3-gallate, RV, and DHR	Plasma	Randomized, double-blind, placebo-controlled, and parallel intervention	38	Epigallocatechin-3-gallate + RV 282 and 80 mg/day, respectively for 12 weeks	Overweight and obese	The supplementation improved skeletal muscle oxidative capacity, preserved fasting and postprandial fat oxidation, and prevented an increase in triacylglycerol concentrations.	[61]
Total RV and DHR (both free and conjugated)	Plasma	Randomized, placebo-controlled, and crossover	45	150 mg/day RV capsule for four weeks, with a four-week wash-out period	Overweight and slightly obese	RV did not have an effect on cardiovascular risk metabolic markers, endothelial function, or inflammation.	[58,59]
Total RV and DHR (free and conjugated forms)	Plasma	Randomized, double-blind, and placebo-controlled	45	75 mg/day (99% pure *t*RV), for 12 weeks.	Lean and overweight, postmenopausal	RV supplementation did not change plasma substrates and hormones (glucose, plasma lipids, and insulin), adiponectin, leptin, CRP, and IL-6.	[44]
Total RV, RV glucuronide, and RV sulfate	Plasma	Randomized, double-blind, placebo-controlled, and crossover	22	250 and 500 mg *t*RV on separate days. On three visits, the participants received two single-dose capsules. The capsules were combined to give the following treatments: 1) inert placebo, 2) 250 mg *t*RV, and 3) 500 mg *t*RV.	Healthy	RV intake increased total-Hb and deoxy-Hb concentration, variables related to cerebral blood flow.	[48]
*t*R4G, *t*RDS, *t*R3G, *t*R4S, and *t*R3S	Plasma	Pilot study, randomized, open-label, single-dose, and parallel-group	10	Single 5 g dose	Healthy	RV increased TNF-α level 24 h after supplementation, by an average of 3.5 pg/mL, compared with placebo. High levels of sulfo- and glucuronide-conjugated RV compounds.	[62]

Table 2. *Cont.*

Metabolite (form of RV)	Sample	Type of Study	(n)	Dose	Participants' Health Status	Effect	Ref.
RV	Plasma	Phase I and randomized	9	1000 mg/day RV for 28 days	Healthy	RV was associated with an increase in the number of circulating γδ T cells and regulatory T cells and higher plasma antioxidant activity.	[63]
RV-3-O-sulfate, RV-4'-O-glucuronide, RV-3-O-glucuronide,	Plasma	Clinical trial	40	0.5, 1.0, 2.5, or 5.0 g/day RV for 29 days	Healthy	Treatment with 2.5 g RV decreased IGF-1 and IGFBP-3 levels in all volunteers; RV might contribute to cancer chemoprevention.	[22]

Aβ40: beta amyloid 40, ALT: alanine aminotransferase, AMPK: adenosine monophosphate-activated protein kinase, AST: aspartate aminotransferase, CRP: C reactive protein, cR3G: *cis*-RV-3-O-glucuronide, cR3S: *cis*-RV-3-O-sulfate, cR4G: *cis*-RV-4'-O-glucuronide, cR4S: *cis*-RV-4'-O-sulfate, CSF: cerebrospinal fluid, deoxy-Hb: deoxygenated Hb, DHR: Dihydroresveratrol, Hb: hemoglobin, IGF-1: insulin-like growth factor 1, IGFBP-3: insulin-like growth factor binding protein 3, IL-6: interleukin-6, MMP9: matrix metalloproteinase 9, PBMC: peripheral blood mononuclear cells, PGC1α: peroxisome proliferator-activated receptor gamma coactivator 1 alpha, RV: resveratrol, SIRT1: sirtuin 1, T2D: type 2 diabetes, TNF-α: tumour necrosis factor alpha, TRM: total RV metabolites, tR3G: *trans*-RV-3-O-glucuronide, tR3S: *trans*-RV-3-O-sulfate, tR4G: *trans*-RV-4'-O-glucuronide, tR4S: *trans*-RV-4'-O-sulfate, tRV: *trans*-RV, and tRDS: *trans*-RV-disulfate. * Studies which identified resveratrol or some metabolite of resveratrol in plasma, urine, and/or feces.

4. Conclusions

In this review, we have described the human clinical trials held in the last decade in which RV was determined in human plasma, urine, or feces. On the one hand, we conclude that the bioavailability and pharmacokinetics of RV depend on the doses ingested, the concomitant ingestion of food matrix, the particle size, the gut microbiota, and the circadian variation.

The results suggest that a repeated and moderate administration of RV is better than the administration of a single, higher dose. A safe and efficient dose is 1 g or more per day; however, RV intake is safe at a dose of up to 5 g, although everyone may experience different adverse effects. Furthermore, the studies showed that RV excretion occurs mainly within the first four hours after ingestion.

On the other hand, RV could have positive effects such as improved antioxidant capacity and modulated neuroinflammation. However, there is disagreement about its positive effects in type 2 diabetes patients and on endothelial function, inflammation, and cardiovascular markers. Contrasting results may be due to the effects of the dose ingested, the gut microbiota status, the health status, and the bioavailability and pharmacokinetics of RV.

It is important to note that the contrasting effects of RV in the different works can be explained by factors such as the number of participants, health status of the gut microbiota, age, gender, lifestyle, dose, administration medium (with or without food), and type of administration (caplet, tablet, powder, gel caps, etc.). For this reason, future studies on RV effects should take into consideration these variables. In addition, further research should be conducted to study in more depth the mechanisms of action of RV in neurological diseases. This review supports the necessity to conduct of larger studies to further investigate the effects of RV on metabolism and neurological functions.

Author Contributions: Conceptualization, R.M.L.-R. and A.V.-Q.; writing, S.L.R.-G., E.P.L.-S., M.M.-M., C.E.S., A.T.-R., and A.V.-Q.; visualization, S.L.R.-G. and E.P.L.-S.; review, R.M.L.-R., A.V.-Q., and S.L.R.-G.

Funding: This work was supported in part by CICYT (AGL2016-75329-R), the Instituto de Salud Carlos III—ISCIII (CIBEROBN CB12/03/30020) from the Ministerio de Ciencia, Innovación y Universidades (AEI/FEDER, UE), and Generalitat de Catalunya (GC) 2017 SGR 196.

Acknowledgments: A.V.-Q. thanks the Ministry of Science, Innovation and Universities for the Ramon y Cajal contract. M.M.-M. thanks the Ministerio de Ciencia, Innovación y Universidades FPU17/00513. A.T.-R. was supported by a Juan de la Cierva Formación postdoctoral fellowship (FJCI-2016-28694) from the Ministerio de Economía, Industria y Competitividad.

Conflicts of Interest: R.M.L.-R. is receiving lecture fees from Cerveceros de España and lecture fees and travel support from Adventia. The other authors declare no conflict of interest.

References

1. Crozier, A.; Jaganath, I.B.; Clifford, M.N. Dietary phenolics: Chemistry, bioavailability and effects on health. *Nat. Prod. Rep.* **2009**, *26*, 1001–1043. [CrossRef] [PubMed]
2. Del Rio, D.; Rodriguez-Mateos, A.; Spencer, J.P.E.; Tognolini, M.; Borges, G.; Crozier, A. Dietary (Poly)phenolics in Human Health: Structures, Bioavailability, and Evidence of Protective Effects Against Chronic Diseases. *Antioxid. Redox Signal.* **2013**, *18*, 1818–1892. [CrossRef] [PubMed]
3. Stockley, C.; Teissedre, P.-L.; Boban, M.; Di Lorenzo, C.; Restani, P. Bioavailability of wine-derived phenolic compounds in humans: A review. *Food Funct.* **2012**, *3*, 995–1007. [CrossRef] [PubMed]
4. Martínez-Huélamo, M.; Vallverdú-Queralt, A.; Di Lecce, G.; Valderas-Martínez, P.; Tulipani, S.; Jáuregui, O.; Escribano-Ferrer, E.; Estruch, R.; Illan, M.; Lamuela-Raventós, R.M. Bioavailability of tomato polyphenols is enhanced by processing and fat addition: Evidence from a randomized feeding trial. *Mol. Nutr. Food Res.* **2016**, *60*, 1578–1589. [CrossRef] [PubMed]
5. Baur, J.A.; Pearson, K.J.; Price, N.L.; Jamieson, H.A.; Lerin, C.; Kalra, A.; Prabhu, V.V.; Allard, J.S.; Lopez-Lluch, G.; Lewis, K.; et al. Resveratrol improves health and survival of mice on a high-calorie diet. *Nature* **2006**, *444*, 337–342. [CrossRef] [PubMed]

6. Miller, R.A.; Harrison, D.E.; Astle, C.M.; Baur, J.A.; Boyd, A.R.; de Cabo, R.; Fernandez, E.; Flurkey, K.; Javors, M.A.; Nelson, J.F.; et al. Rapamycin, but not resveratrol or simvastatin, extends life span of genetically heterogeneous mice. *J. Gerontol. Ser. A Biol. Sci. Med. Sci.* **2011**, *66*, 191–201. [CrossRef] [PubMed]

7. Pearson, K.J.; Baur, J.A.; Lewis, K.N.; Peshkin, L.; Price, N.L.; Labinskyy, N.; Swindell, W.R.; Kamara, D.; Minor, R.K.; Perez, E.; et al. Resveratrol delays age-related deterioration and mimics transcriptional aspects of dietary restriction without extending lifespan. *Cell Metab.* **2008**, *8*, 157–168. [CrossRef]

8. Barger, J.L.; Kayo, T.; Vann, J.M.; Arias, E.B.; Wang, J.; Hacker, T.A.; Wang, Y.; Raederstorff, D.; Morrow, J.D.; Leeuwenburgh, C.; et al. A low dose of dietary resveratrol partially mimics caloric restriction and retards aging parameters in mice. *PLoS ONE* **2008**, *3*, e2264. [CrossRef]

9. Baur, J.A.; Sinclair, D.A. Therapeutic potential of resveratrol: The in vivo evidence. *Nat. Rev. Drug Discov.* **2006**, *5*, 493–506. [CrossRef]

10. Poulsen, M.M.; Vestergaard, P.F.; Clasen, B.F.; Radko, Y.; Christensen, L.P.; Stødkilde-Jørgensen, H.; Møller, N.; Jessen, N.; Pedersen, S.B.; Jørgensen, J.O.L. High-dose resveratrol supplementation in obese men: An investigator-initiated, randomized, placebo-controlled clinical trial of substrate metabolism, insulin sensitivity, and body composition. *Diabetes* **2013**, *62*, 1186–1195. [CrossRef]

11. Ranney, A.; Petro, M.S. Resveratrol protects spatial learning in middle-aged C57BL/6 mice from effects of ethanol. *Behav. Pharmacol.* **2009**, *20*. [CrossRef] [PubMed]

12. Halliwell, B. Dietary polyphenols: Good, bad, or indifferent for your health? *Cardiovasc. Res.* **2007**, *73*, 341–347. [CrossRef] [PubMed]

13. Lagouge, M.; Argmann, C.; Gerhart-hines, Z.; Meziane, H.; Lerin, C.; Daussin, F.; Messadeq, N.; Milne, J.; Lambert, P.; Elliott, P.; et al. Resveratrol Improves mitochondrial function and protects against metabolic disease by activating SIRT1 and PGC-1 a. *Cell* **2006**, *127*, 1109–1122. [CrossRef] [PubMed]

14. Zang, M.; Xu, S.; Maitland-Toolan, K.A.; Zuccollo, A.; Hou, X.; Jiang, B.; Wierzbicki, M.; Verbeuren, T.J.; Cohen, R.A. Polyphenols stimulate AMP-activated protein kinase, lower lipids, and inhibit accelerated atherosclerosis in diabetic LDL receptor–deficient mice. *Diabetes* **2006**, *55*, 2180. [CrossRef] [PubMed]

15. Bordone, L.; Cohen, D.; Robinson, A.; Motta, M.C.; Van Veen, E.; Czopik, A.; Steele, A.D.; Crowe, H.; Marmor, S.; Luo, J.; et al. SIRT1 transgenic mice show phenotypes resembling calorie restriction. *Aging Cell* **2007**, *6*, 759–767. [CrossRef] [PubMed]

16. Buryanovskyy, L.; Fu, Y.; Boyd, M.; Ma, Y.; Hsieh, T.; Wu, J.M.; Zhang, Z. Crystal structure of quinone reductase 2 in complex with resveratrol. *Biochemistry* **2004**, *43*, 11417–11426. [CrossRef]

17. Soleas, G.J.; Yan, J.; Goldberg, D.M. Ultrasensitive assay for three polyphenols (catechin, quercetin and resveratrol) and their conjugates in biological fluids utilizing gas chromatography with mass selective detection. *J. Chromatogr. B Biomed. Sci. Appl.* **2001**, *757*, 161–172. [CrossRef]

18. Meng, X.; Maliakal, P.; Lu, H.; Lee, M.-J.; Yang, C.S. Urinary and plasma levels of resveratrol and quercetin in humans, mice, and rats after ingestion of pure compounds and grape juice. *J. Agric. Food Chem.* **2004**, *52*, 935–942. [CrossRef]

19. Zamora-Ros, R.; Urpí-Sardà, M.; Lamuela-Raventós, R.M.; Estruch, R.; Vázquez-Agell, M.; Serrano-Martínez, M.; Jaeger, W.; Andres-Lacueva, C. Diagnostic performance of urinary resveratrol metabolites as a biomarker of moderate wine consumption. *Clin. Chem.* **2006**, *52*, 1373–1380. [CrossRef]

20. Gambini, J.; Inglés, M.; Olaso, G.; Lopez-Grueso, R.; Bonet-Costa, V.; Gimeno-Mallench, L.; Mas-Bargues, C.; Abdelaziz, K.M.; Gomez-Cabrera, M.C.; Vina, J.; Borras, C. Properties of resveratrol: In vitro and in vivo studies about metabolism, bioavailability, and biological effects in animal models and humans. *Oxid. Med. Cell. Longev.* **2015**, *2015*, 1–13. [CrossRef]

21. Walle, T.; Hsieh, F.; DeLegge, M.H.; Oatis, J.E.J.; Walle, U.K. High absorption but very low bioavailability of oral resveratrol in humans. *Drug Metab. Dispos.* **2004**, *32*, 1377–1382. [CrossRef] [PubMed]

22. Brown, V.A.; Patel, K.R.; Viskaduraki, M.; Crowell, J.A.; Perloff, M.; Booth, T.D.; Vasilinin, G.; Sen, A.; Schinas, A.M.; Piccirilli, G.; et al. Repeat dose study of the cancer chemopreventive agent resveratrol in healthy volunteers: Safety, pharmacokinetics, and effect on the insulin-like growth factor axis. *Cancer Res.* **2010**, *70*, 9003–9011. [CrossRef] [PubMed]

23. Wightman, E.L.; Reay, J.L.; Haskell, C.F.; Williamson, G.; Dew, T.P.; Kennedy, D.O. Effects of resveratrol alone or in combination with piperine on cerebral blood flow parameters and cognitive performance in human subjects: A randomised, double-blind, placebo-controlled, cross-over investigation. *Br. J. Nutr.* **2014**, *112*, 203–213. [CrossRef] [PubMed]

24. Turner, R.S.; Thomas, R.G.; Craft, S.; van Dyck, C.H.; Mintzer, J.; Reynolds, B.A.; Brewer, J.B.; Rissman, R.A.; Raman, R.; Aisen, P.S. A randomized, double-blind, placebo-controlled trial of resveratrol for Alzheimer disease. *Neurology* **2015**, *85*, 1383–1391. [CrossRef] [PubMed]

25. Yiu, E.M.; Tai, G.; Peverill, R.E.; Lee, K.J.; Croft, K.D.; Mori, T.A.; Scheiber-Mojdehkar, B.; Sturm, B.; Praschberger, M.; Vogel, A.P.; et al. An open-label trial in Friedreich ataxia suggests clinical benefit with high-dose resveratrol, without effect on frataxin levels. *J. Neurol.* **2015**, *262*, 1344–1353. [CrossRef] [PubMed]

26. Wong, R.H.X.; Howe, P.R.C.; Buckley, J.D.; Coates, A.M.; Kunz, I.; Berry, N.M. Acute resveratrol supplementation improves flow-mediated dilatation in overweight/obese individuals with mildly elevated blood pressure. *Nutr. Metab. Cardiovasc. Dis.* **2011**, *21*, 851–856. [CrossRef] [PubMed]

27. Wong, R.H.X.; Raederstorff, D.; Howe, P.R.C. Acute resveratrol consumption improves neurovascular coupling capacity in adults with type 2 diabetes mellitus. *Nutrients* **2016**, *8*, 425. [CrossRef]

28. Amri, A.; Chaumeil, J.C.; Sfar, S.; Charrueau, C. Administration of resveratrol: What formulation solutions to bioavailability limitations? *J. Control. Release* **2012**, *158*, 182–193. [CrossRef]

29. Amiot, M.J.; Romier, B.; Dao, T.A.; Fanciullino, R.; Ciccolini, J.; Burcelin, R.; Pechere, L.; Emond, C.; Savouret, J.; Seree, E. Optimization of trans -Resveratrol bioavailability for human therapy. *Biochimie* **2013**, *95*, 1233–1238. [CrossRef]

30. Rotches-Ribalta, M.; Urpi-Sarda, M.; Martí, M.M.; Reglero, G.; Andres-Lacueva, C. Resveratrol metabolic fingerprinting after acute and chronic intakes of a functional beverage in humans. *Electrophoresis* **2014**, *35*, 1637–1643. [CrossRef]

31. Rotches-Ribalta, M.; Andres-Lacueva, C.; Estruch, R.; Escribano, E.; Urpi-Sarda, M. Pharmacokinetics of resveratrol metabolic profile in healthy humans after moderate consumption of red wine and grape extract tablets. *Pharmacol. Res.* **2012**, *66*, 375–382. [CrossRef] [PubMed]

32. Hintz, R.; Johnson, K. The effect of particle size distribution on dissolution rate and oral absorption. *Int. J. Pharm.* **1989**, *51*, 9–17. [CrossRef]

33. Howells, L.M.; Berry, D.P.; Elliott, P.J.; Jacobson, E.W.; Hoffmann, E.; Hegarty, B.; Brown, K.; Steward, W.P.; Gescher, A.J. Phase I randomized, double-blind pilot study of micronized resveratrol (SRT501) in patients with hepatic metastases—Safety, pharmacokinetics, and pharmacodynamics. *Cancer Prev. Res.* **2011**, *4*, 1419–1425. [CrossRef] [PubMed]

34. La Porte, C.; Voduc, N.; Zhang, G.; Seguin, I.; Tardiff, D.; Singhal, N.; Cameron, D.W. Steady-State Pharmacokinetics and Tolerability of Trans-Resveratrol 2000 mg Twice Daily with Food, Quercetin and Alcohol (Ethanol) in Healthy Human Subjects. *Clin. Pharmacokinet.* **2010**, *49*, 449–454. [CrossRef] [PubMed]

35. Vaz-da-Silva, M.; Loureiro, A.I.; Falcao, A.; Nunes, T.; Rocha, J.-F.; Fernandes-Lopes, C.; Soares, E.; Wright, L.; Almeida, L.; Soares-da-Silva, P. Effect of food on the pharmacokinetic profile of trans-resveratrol. *Int. J. Clin. Pharmacol. Ther.* **2008**, *46*, 564–570. [CrossRef] [PubMed]

36. Blanchard, O.L.; Friesenhahn, G.; Javors, M.A.; Smoliga, J.M. Development of a lozenge for oral transmucosal delivery of trans-resveratrol in humans: Proof of concept. *PLoS ONE* **2014**, *9*, e90131. [CrossRef] [PubMed]

37. Draijer, R.; Van Dorsten, F.A.; Zebregs, Y.E.; Hollebrands, B.; Peters, S.; Duchateau, G.S.; Grün, C.H. Impact of proteins on the uptake, distribution, and excretion of phenolics in the human body. *Nutrients* **2016**, *8*, 814. [CrossRef]

38. Rotches-Ribalta, M.; Urpi-Sarda, M.; Llorach, R.; Boto-Ordoñez, M.; Jauregui, O.; Chiva-Blanch, G.; Perez-Garcia, L.; Jaeger, W.; Guillen, M.; Corella, D.; et al. Gut and microbial resveratrol metabolite profiling after moderate long-term consumption of red wine versus dealcoholized red wine in humans by an optimized ultra-high-pressure liquid chromatography tandem mass spectrometry method. *J. Chromatogr. A* **2012**, *1265*, 105–113. [CrossRef]

39. Almeida, L.; Vaz-da-Silva, M.; Falcão, A.; Soares, E.; Costa, R.; Loureiro, A.I.; Fernandes-Lopes, C.; Rocha, J.; Nunes, T.; Wright, L.; Soares-da-Silva, P. Pharmacokinetic and safety profile of trans-resveratrol in a rising multiple-dose study in healthy volunteers. *Mol. Nutr. Food Res.* **2009**, *53*, 7–15. [CrossRef]

40. Bode, L.M.; Bunzel, D.; Huch, M.; Cho, G.; Ruhland, D.; Bunzel, M.; Bub, A.; Franz, C.M.A.P.; Kulling, S.E. In vivo and in vitro metabolism of trans -resveratrol by human gut. *Am. J. Clin. Nutr.* **2013**, *97*, 295–309. [CrossRef]

41. Most, J.; Penders, J.; Lucchesi, M.; Goossens, G.H.; Blaak, E.E. Gut microbiota composition in relation to the metabolic response to 12-week combined polyphenol supplementation in overweight men and women. *Eur. J. Clin. Nutr.* **2017**, *71*, 1040–1045. [CrossRef] [PubMed]

Nutrients 2018, 10, 1892

42. Chachay, V.S.; Macdonald, G.A.; Martin, J.H.; Whitehead, J.P.; O'Moore–Sullivan, T.M.; Lee, P.; Franklin, M.; Klein, K.; Taylor, P.J.; Ferguson, M.; et al. Resveratrol Does Not Benefit Patients With Nonalcoholic Fatty Liver Disease. *Clin. Gastroenterol. Hepatol.* **2014**, *12*, 2092–2103.e6. [CrossRef] [PubMed]
43. Boocock, D.J.; Faust, G.E.S.; Patel, K.R.; Schinas, A.M.; Brown, V.A.; Ducharme, M.P.; Booth, T.D.; Crowell, J.A.; Perloff, M.; Gescher, A.J.; et al. Phase i dose escalation pharmacokinetic study in healthy volunteers of resveratrol, a potential cancer chemopreventive agent. *Cancer Epidemiol. Biomark. Prev.* **2007**, *16*, 1246–1253. [CrossRef]
44. Yoshino, J.; Conte, C.; Fontana, L.; Mittendorfer, B.; Imai, S.I.; Schechtman, K.B.; Gu, C.; Kunz, I.; Fanelli, F.R.; Patterson, B.W.; et al. Resveratrol supplementation does not improve metabolic function in nonobese women with normal glucose tolerance. *Cell Metab.* **2012**, *16*, 658–664. [CrossRef] [PubMed]
45. Crandall, J.P.; Oram, V.; Trandafirescu, G.; Reid, M.; Kishore, P.; Hawkins, M.; Cohen, H.W.; Barzilai, N. Pilot study of resveratrol in older adults with impaired glucose tolerance. *J. Gerontol. Ser. A* **2012**, *67*, 1307–1312. [CrossRef] [PubMed]
46. Azachi, M.; Yatuv, R.; Katz, A.; Hagay, Y.; Danon, A. A novel red grape cells complex: Health effects and bioavailability of natural resveratrol. *Int. J. Food Sci. Nutr.* **2014**, *65*, 848–855. [CrossRef]
47. Moussa, C.; Hebron, M.; Huang, X.; Ahn, J.; Rissman, R.A.; Aisen, P.S.; Turner, R.S. Resveratrol regulates neuro-inflammation and induces adaptive immunity in Alzheimer's disease. *J. Neuroinflamm.* **2017**, *14*, 1. [CrossRef] [PubMed]
48. Kennedy, D.O.; Wightman, E.L.; Reay, J.L.; Lietz, G.; Okello, E.J.; Wilde, A.; Haskell, C.F. Effects of resveratrol on cerebral blood flow variables and cognitive performance in humans: A double-blind, placebo-controlled, crossover. *Am. J. Clin. Nutr.* **2010**, *91*, 1590–1597. [CrossRef]
49. Bakker, G.C.M.; Van Erk, M.J.; Pellis, L.; Wopereis, S.; Rubingh, C.M.; Cnubben, N.H.P.; Kooistra, T.; Van Ommen, B.; Hendriks, H.F.J. An antiinflammatory dietary mix modulates inflammation and oxidative and metabolic stress in overweight men: A nutrigenomics approach 1–4. *Am. J. Clin. Nutr.* **2010**, *91*, 1044–1059. [CrossRef] [PubMed]
50. Brasnyó, P.; Molnár, G.A.; Mohás, M.; Markó, L.; Laczy, B.; Cseh, J.; Mikolás, E.; Szijártó, I.A.; Mérei, Á.; Halmai, R.; Mészáros, L.G.; et al. Resveratrol improves insulin sensitivity, reduces oxidative stress and activates the Akt pathway in type 2 diabetic patients. *Br. J. Nutr.* **2011**, *106*, 383–389. [CrossRef] [PubMed]
51. Dash, S.; Xiao, C.; Morgantini, C.; Szeto, L.; Lewis, G.F. High-dose resveratrol treatment for 2 weeks inhibits intestinal and hepatic lipoprotein production in overweight/obese men. *Arterioscler. Thromb. Vasc. Biol.* **2013**, *33*, 2895–2901. [CrossRef] [PubMed]
52. Timmers, S.; de Ligt, M.; Phielix, E.; van de Weijer, T.; Hansen, J.; Moonen-Kornips, E.; Schaart, G.; Kunz, I.; Hesselink, M.K.C.; Schrauwen-Hinderling, V.B.; et al. Resveratrol as add-on therapy in subjects with well-controlled type 2 diabetes: A randomized controlled trial. *Diabetes Care* **2016**, *39*, 2211–2217. [CrossRef] [PubMed]
53. Knop, F.K.; Konings, E.; Timmers, S.; Schrauwen, P.; Holst, J.J.; Blaak, E.E. Thirty days of resveratrol supplementation does not affect postprandial incretin hormone responses, but suppresses postprandial glucagon in obese subjects. *Diabet. Med.* **2013**, *30*, 1214–1218. [CrossRef] [PubMed]
54. Grifantini, K. Understanding pathways of calorie restriction: A way to prevent cancer? *J. Natl. Cancer Inst.* **2008**, *100*, 619–621. [CrossRef] [PubMed]
55. Caramori, P.R.; Zago, A.J. Endothelial dysfunction and coronary artery disease. *Arq. Bras. Cardiol.* **2000**, *75*, 163–182. [CrossRef] [PubMed]
56. Grassi, G.; Seravalle, G.; Scopelliti, F.; Dell'Oro, R.; Fattori, L.; Quarti-Trevano, F.; Brambilla, G.; Schiffrin, E.L.; Mancia, G. Structural and functional alterations of subcutaneous small resistance arteries in severe human obesity. *Obesity* **2010**, *18*, 92–98. [CrossRef] [PubMed]
57. Zamora-Ros, R.; Urpi-Sarda, M.; Lamuela-Raventós, R.M.; Martínez-González, M.Á.; Salas-Salvadó, J.; Arós, F.; Fitó, M.; Lapetra, J.; Estruch, R.; Andres-Lacueva, C. High urinary levels of resveratrol metabolites are associated with a reduction in the prevalence of cardiovascular risk factors in high-risk patients. *Pharmacol. Res.* **2012**, *65*, 615–620. [CrossRef]
58. Van Der Made, S.M.; Plat, J.; Mensink, R.P. Resveratrol does not influence metabolic risk markers related to cardiovascular health in overweight and slightly obese subjects: A randomized, placebo-controlled crossover trial. *PLoS ONE* **2015**, *10*, 1–13. [CrossRef]

59. Van der Made, S.M.; Plat, J.; Mensink, R.P. Trans-resveratrol supplementation and endothelial function during the fasting and postprandial phase: A randomized placebo-controlled trial in overweight and slightly obese participants. *Nutrients* **2017**, *9*, 596. [CrossRef]
60. Timmers, S.; Konings, E.; Bilet, L.; Houtkooper, R.H.; van de Weijer, T.; Goossens, G.H.; Hoeks, J.; van der Krieken, S.; Ryu, D.; Kersten, S.; et al. Calorie restriction-like effects of 30 days of resveratrol supplementation on energy metabolism and metabolic profile in obese humans. *Cell Metab.* **2011**, *14*, 612–622. [CrossRef]
61. Most, J.; Timmers, S.; Warnke, I.; Jocken, J.W.; van Boekschoten, M.; de Groot, P.; Bendik, I.; Schrauwen, P.; Goossens, G.H.; Blaak, E.E. Combined epigallocatechin-3-gallate and resveratrol supplementation for 12 wk increases mitochondrial capacity and fat oxidation, but not insulin sensitivity, in obese humans: A randomized controlled trial. *Am. J. Clin. Nutr.* **2016**, *104*, 215–227. [CrossRef] [PubMed]
62. Gualdoni, G.A.; Kovarik, J.J.; Hofer, J.; Dose, F.; Doberer, D.; Steinberger, P.; Wolzt, M.; Zlabinger, G.J. Resveratrol enhances TNF-α production in human monocytes upon bacterial stimulation. *Biochim. Biophys. Acta Gen. Subj.* **2014**, *1840*, 95–105. [CrossRef] [PubMed]
63. Espinoza, J.L.; Trung, L.Q.; Inaoka, P.T.; Yamada, K.; An, D.T.; Mizuno, S.; Nakao, S.; Takami, A. The Repeated Administration of Resveratrol Has Measurable Effects on Circulating T-Cell Subsets in Humans. *Oxid. Med. Cell. Longev.* **2017**, *2017*, 6781872. [CrossRef] [PubMed]
64. Lin, C.; Sun, X.; Lin, A. Supplementation with high-dose trans-resveratrol improves ultrafiltration in peritoneal dialysis patients: A prospective, randomized, double-blind study. *Ren. Fail.* **2016**, *38*, 214–221. [CrossRef] [PubMed]

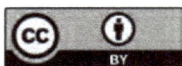

Article

Solid Dispersion of Resveratrol Supported on Magnesium DiHydroxide (Resv@MDH) Microparticles Improves Oral Bioavailability

Roberto Spogli [1], Maria Bastianini [1], Francesco Ragonese [2,3], Rossana Giulietta Iannitti [4], Lorenzo Monarca [2], Federica Bastioli [2], Irina Nakashidze [5], Gabriele Brecchia [6], Laura Menchetti [6], Michela Codini [7], Cataldo Arcuri [3], Loretta Mancinelli [2] and Bernard Fioretti [2,*]

[1] Prolabin & Tefarm, Spin-Off Un. of University of Perugia, Via Dell'Acciaio 9, Ponte Felcino, 06134 Perugia, Italy; roberto.spogli@prolabintefarm.com (R.S.); maria.bastianini@prolabintefarm.com (M.B.)
[2] Department of Chemistry, Biology and Biotechnologies, University of Perugia, Via Elce di Sotto 8, 06123 Perugia, Italy; francesco.ragonese@studenti.unipg.it (F.R.); lorenzo.monarca@unipg.it (L.M.); federica.bastioli@unipg.it (F.B.); loretta.mancinelli@unipg.it (L.M.)
[3] Department of Experimental Medicine, Perugia Medical School, University of Perugia, Piazza Lucio Severi 1, 06132 Perugia, Italy; cataldo.arcuri@unipg.it
[4] S&R Farmaceutici S.p.A Bastia Umbra, 08063 Perugia Italy; r.iannitti@srfarmaceutici.com
[5] Department of Biology, Faculty of Natural Science and Health Care, Batumi Shota Rustaveli State University, 6010 Batumi, Georgia; irina.nakashidze@bsu.edu.ge
[6] Department of Veterinary Science, University of Perugia, Via San Costanzo 4, 06126 Perugia, Italy; gabriele.brecchia@unipg.it (G.B.); laura.menchetti7@gmail.com (L.M.)
[7] Department of Pharmaceutical Sciences, University of Perugia, Via A. Fabretti 48, 06123 Perugia, Italy; michela.codini@unipg.it
* Correspondence: bernard.fioretti@unipg.it

Received: 24 October 2018; Accepted: 26 November 2018; Published: 5 December 2018

Abstract: Resveratrol, because of its low solubility in water and its high membrane permeability, is collocated in the second class of the biopharmaceutical classification system, with limited bioavailability due to its dissolution rate. Solid dispersion of resveratrol supported on Magnesium DiHydroxide (Resv@MDH) was evaluated to improve solubility and increase bioavailability of resveratrol. Fluorimetric microscopy analysis displays three types of microparticles with similar size: Type 1 that emitted preferably fluorescence at 445 nm with bandwidth of 50 nm, type 2 that emitted preferably fluorescence at 605 nm with bandwidth of 70 nm and type 3 that is non-fluorescent. Micronized pure resveratrol displays only microparticles type 1 whereas type 3 are associated to pure magnesium dihydroxide. Dissolution test in simulated gastric environment resveratrol derived from Resv@MDH in comparison to resveratrol alone displayed better solubility. A 3-fold increase of resveratrol bioavailability was observed after oral administration of 50 mg/kg of resveratrol from Resv@MDH in rabbits. We hypothesize that type 2 microparticles represent magnesium dihydroxide microparticles with a resveratrol shell and that they are responsible for the improved resveratrol solubility and bioavailability of Resv@MDH.

Keywords: resveratrol; magnesium dihydroxide; solubility; bioavailability; dissolution rate; microparticles

---

1. Introduction

Resveratrol (trans-3,5,4′-tri-hydroxic-stilbene) is a stilbenic structure polyphenol, initially isolated from the root of the white hellebore (*Veratrum Grandiflorum O. Loes*) and later from the root of the *Polygonum cuspidatum*, a plant used in traditional Chinese and Japanese medicine. Resveratrol became popular in 1992 when it was suggested that it could be the reason behind red wine's cardio-protective effects (French paradox; [1]), and its popularity increased in 1997 when it was proven that resveratrol was able to prevent colorectal cancer in mice [1]. Resveratrol based compounds present anti-oxidant, anti-inflammatory, anti-viral, cardio-protective, neuro-protective, anti-cancer and anti-angiogenetic activities [1–3]. It has been recently observed in obese human subjects that treatment with trans-resveratrol reduces glucose, triglycerides and inflammatory marker levels with a similar effect to the one induced by caloric restriction [4]. The mechanism of action of resveratrol has not been completely defined yet, and for this reason recently studies have been carried out in order to understand the aspects that are still not clear [4].

Resveratrol is poorly bioavailable because of reduced absorption mainly due to its low solubility and fast metabolism that converts it into glucuronide and sulfates compounds [1,5]. In humans resveratrol can be detected in plasma about 30 min after oral administration, meaning that its absorption already starts at the gastric level and reaches a plasmatic submicromolar concentration peak. Such peak is variable and hardly related to the used dose. For example, by administrating a 25 mg dose of resveratrol a 10 ng/mL plasmatic concentration is obtained, while increasing such dose by 20 times (500 mg/day) its plasma level increases only seven times (72.6 ng/mL) [6]. Differences in resveratrol absorption have been demonstrated by clinical trials based on the oral administration of 150 mg/day of resveratrol for a prolonged period of time. It has been observed that the same dose produces different plasmatic concentrations: 231 ng/mL [4] and 24.8 ng/mL [7]. Several strategies have been performed to increase its bioavailability and improve its potential health properties. A recent revision of the literature highlights how the increased bioavailability of resveratrol is a necessary element in order to evaluate the real pharmaceutical and health potential of this well-known polyphenol [5]. According to the biopharmaceutical classification system (BCS) [8,9], resveratrol belongs to the second class which means that it is characterized by low solubility in water (about 30 mg/L), while it shares a high membrane permeability (log P~3.1) [10]. Among the different strategies, new formulations have been developed that are able to increase its apparent solubility for example by using a lipophilic vehicle or through various processes such as the complexation with cyclodextrins, nanopreparation, or micellar solubilization with biliary acid [10–12]. It has been demonstrated, in in vitro studies, that the increase of apparent resveratrol solubility allows a partial saturation of the mechanisms that are involved in its metabolism (conjugation) with a subsequent increase of resveratrol's bioavailability [13]. This is in accordance with BCS for molecules class II that increasing resveratrol apparent solubility produces a bioavailability improvement [8,9,14], but in a dedicated study the increased solubility with cyclodextrins doesn't modify its bioavailability [12].

In the present study we investigated that the solid dispersion of resveratrol on magnesium dihydroxide increases its solubility and bioavailability indicating that in some instance this approach could be exploited to enhance biological properties of resveratrol. Although resveratrol does not display chelating properties, some studies have shown its ability to interact with heavy metals such as copper, zinc and aluminum [15,16]. In this work we report that resveratrol interacts with magnesium dihydroxide at the microparticle level and that this is able to modify its bioavailability.

2. Material and Methods

2.1. Solid Dispersion of Resveratrol on Magnesium Dihydroxide Preparation

Magnesium dihydroxide and resveratrol (from *Polygomun cuspidatum,* 98% pure) solid dispersion was performed by modified co-precipitation method of Biswicka et al. [17]. Magnesium dihydroxide on resveratrol solid dispersion and pure micronized resveratrol described in this study was obtained by Good Manufacturing Practice (GMP) chain by Prolabin & Tefarm, Ponte Felcino (PG) and distributed by S&R Farmaceutici SpA, Via dei Pioppi 2, 06083 Bastia Umbra (PG), with the trade name, Revifast®(produced by the manufacturer La Sorgente del Benessere, Via Prenestina, 141 -02014 Fiuggi (FR) Italy on behalf of S&R Farmaceutici S.p.A) The resveratrol content in the solid dispersion was evaluated using the HPLC method (see below). The mean value obtained in the three samples was about 30% and 70% of total weight of resveratrol and magnesium dihydroxide, respectively.

2.2. Particle Size Analysis

The size of the particles was determined using a Malvern Mastersizer 2000, a laser diffraction particle size analyzer, for the dried powders.

2.3. Dissolution Assays

A weighed amount of RSV@MDH or resveratrol were placed in series of closed flat-bottomed glass vessels containing 250 mL of Simulated Gastric Fluid (SGF). The composition of SGF was 35 mM of NaCl, pH 1.2 with HCl. The vessels were inserted in shaking water bath (Nuve ST 30) at 37 °C and 110 rpm for 2 h. At appropriate times (1, 3, 5, 10, 15, 20, 30, 45, 60, 90 and 120 min) 2 mL samples were withdrawn and replaced by fresh dissolution medium, then filtered (Spartan 13/02 RC, Whatman GmbH, Dassel, Germany) and analyzed. The drug concentration was determined by HPLC (see below).

2.4. Field Emission Scanning Electron Microscopy

The morphology of the samples was investigated with a FEG LEO 1525 scanning electron microscope (FE-SEM). FE-SEM micrographs were collected by depositing the samples on a stub holder and after sputter coating with chromium for 20 s.

2.5. Fluorescence Microscopy

Microscopic fluorescence analysis of powders was performed using an Axio Esaminer (Zeiss, Jena, Germany) fluorescence microscope with a CCD digital camera Axio Cam 502 Mono. Samples have been observed with DAPI filter (G 365, FT 395, BP 445/50), and with Rhodamine (BP 545/25, FT 570, BP 605/70) using for excitation mercury lamp (HXP 120V). Image acquisition and analysis was performed with Zen 2 software (Zeiss, Jena, Germany).

2.6. In Vivo Absorption Test

The trial was carried out at the experimental farm of the University of Batumi, Georgia. Rabbits were exposed to a continuous photoperiod of 16 h light per day at 40 lx. Room temperature ranged from 18 to 27 °C. Fresh water was always available. Animals were fed with 130 g/day of a standard diet. The experimental protocol was approved by the Local Ethical Committee for Animal Experimentation at the University Batumi, Georgia. All efforts were made to minimize animal distress and to use only the number of animals necessary to produce reliable results. The tests were conducted on New Zealand White hybrid rabbits (4.5–5 kg weight range). Two groups of four animals each were prepared for the comparative treatment of resveratrol (pure resveratrol versus Resv@MDH). The rabbits were fasted for 24 h before administration of a suspension containing 50 mg/kg of pure resveratrol or 50 mg/kg of resveratrol from Resv@MDH according to Jaisamut et al., 2017 [18]. The powders were suspended in 10 mL of a glucose solution and orally administered to a conscious animal by a syringe (0 min). At 0, 5, 15, 30, 45, 90, 120 and 180 min, blood samples were taken (about 2 mL) through the auricular artery and put in heparinized tubes. The samples were centrifuged at 2500 g for 5 min and the plasma was recovered. Acetonitrile was added to the plasma samples (v:v 1:1 ratio) and left for 5 min in order to precipitate plasma proteins. After centrifugation the supernatant was recovered for the dosage of resveratrol by HPLC.

2.7. HPLC Analysis

The measurements were performed by an Agilent HPLC 1200 series equipped with an Agilent Zorbax SB C18 4.6 × 250 mm 5-µm Agilent P/N 880975-902 column. Elution was carried out under isocratic conditions using as mobile phase (Water + 0.1% *v*/*v* Trifluoroacetic acid)/(Acetonitrile + 0.1% *v*/*v* Trifluoroacetic acid) = 65/35, with a flow of 1mL/min and a column temperature of 30 °C. A total of 20 μL of samples were injected, after 0.2 μm Nylon membrane filtration, and the analytes were detected by VWD Detector, λ = 306 nm. For the quantification of resveratrol a calibration was performed to detect the polyphenol at a retention time of 5.6 min with a detection limit of 4 ng/mL. All the plasma concentrations were multiplied by 2 to take into account the dilution in acetonitrile during sample preparation and by 3.6 to take into account the yield of extraction of resveratrol from plasma (28%) [19].

2.8. Statistical Analysis

All results are expressed as the mean ± SE. Differences between two related parameters were assessed by Student's *t*-test. Differences were considered significant at $p < 0.05$. The number of animals used in the current experimental trial is based on the work by Jaisamut et al., 2017 [18].

3. Results

3.1. Microscopic Analysis of Solid Dispersion of Resveratrol on Magnesium Dihydroxide

RSV@MDH powder was dispersed in glycerol and was observed by bright-field microscopy. The presence of particles with different scattering profiles in a narrow size range of a few micrometers was observed (Figure 1A). Fluorescence analysis of the samples with DAPI filter showed that about 10–20% of the microparticles emitted fluorescence. These microparticles were defined as type 1 (Figure 1B). The mean size of type 1 microparticles was 1.8 ± 0.1 μm, *n* = 40 in diameter (given the non-spherical morphology of the particles, the longest diameter has been taken into account). When the sample was analyzed with the rhodamine filter, a comparable population of particles was visualized with a mean size of 2.0 ± 0.2 μm, *n* = 34 and was named type 2 (Figure 1C). Type 1 microparticles displayed very scant signals when observed with the rhodamine filter similar to the type 2 particles with the DAPI filter. Finally, the majority of the microparticles didn't display any fluorescence in either filter and were defined as type 3 and had medium size similar to others (Figure 1D).

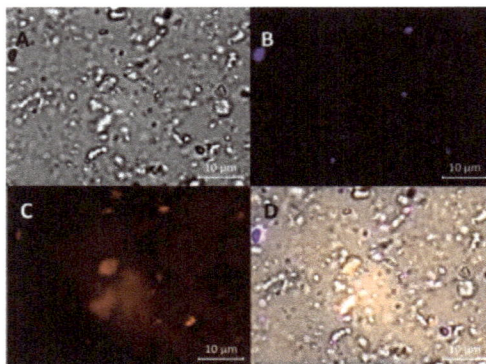

Figure 1. Image of Resv@MDH powder dispersed in glycerol under different excitation sources. (**A**) Bright-field; (**B**) DAPI (4',6-diamidino-2-phenylindole) fluorescence filter; (**C**) Rhodamine fluorescence filter; (**D**) merging of the Bright-field, DAPI and Rhodamine images.

Thus, the solid dispersion of resveratrol on magnesium dihydroxide was composed by three distinct populations of microparticles based on the fluorescence profile. When we similarly analyzed the dry powder without dispersion in glycerol we observed aggregates of size around 5 μm were present as a possible consequence of the interaction of the three types of microparticles (Figure 2A).

In accordance, that the aggregates are based on different types of microparticles, they displayed fluorescence signals from every channel. Granulometric and SEM analysis showed two distinct population sizes, one with size around 1 μm and the second population with size around 6 μm of diameter (Figure 2B,C).

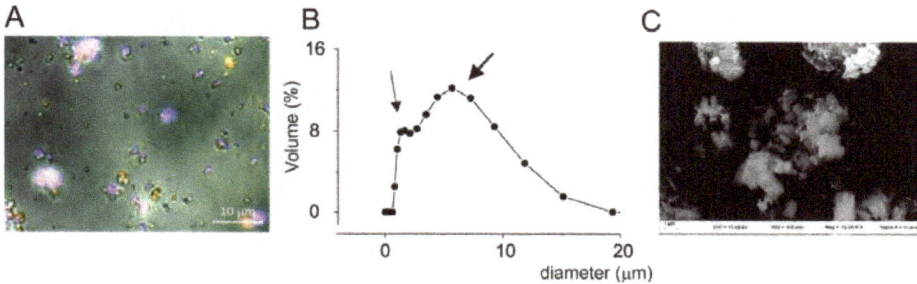

Figure 2. Properties of Resv@MDH dry powder. (**A**) Image created by digital merging of bright-field and DAPI/Rhodamine fluorescence illumination. (**B**) Granulometric analysis of Resv@MDH dry powder. (**C**) SEM image of Resv@MDH dry powder.

3.2. Molecular Nature of Microparticles of Solid Dispersion of Resveratrol on Magnesium Dihydroxide

To define the molecular nature of the different types of microparticles, we studied a powder of pure micronized resveratrol with similar distribution size of solid dispersion. Granulometric analysis confirmed that micronized resveratrol have the size of 1–6 μm in diameter (Figure 3A) similar to the particles size of RSV@MDH (see Figure 1 for comparison). Fluorescence microscopy analysis of the micronized resveratrol displayed all the microparticles emitted fluorescence intensity as type 1 particles (Figure 3B,C), whereas the presence of microparticles that showed fluorescent properties as type 2 and 3 were not observed (Figure 3D,E). No fluorescence was observed (DAPI and Rhodamine filters) during microscopic analysis of pure magnesium dihydroxide, indicating that type 3 microparticles could be constituted by only magnesium dihydroxide. These data suggested that the type 1 microparticles were microparticles of pure resveratrol, whereas the type 3 microparticles represented magnesium dihydroxide. Since the fluorescence properties were due to resveratrol, type 2 macroparticles could be distinguished from type 3 microparticles by presence of resveratrol. The type 2 microparticles were further investigated to define the morphological features. In fact, it was possible to see a shell of fluorescence around a non-fluorescent core and this was due to resveratrol surrounding the core of magnesium hydroxide microparticles (Figure S1). All the features of the microparticles are stated in Table 1.

Table 1. Principle features of microparticles of RSV@MDH.

Characteristic	Type 1 Microparticles	Type 2 Microparticles	Type 3 Microparticles
DAPI filter (G 365, FT 395, BP 445/50)	High intensity	Low intensity	none
Rhodamine (BP 545/25, FT 570, BP 605/70)	Low intensity	High intensity	none
Particles size	~1.8 ± 0.1 μm	~2.0 ± 0.2 μm	~1.7 ± 0.1 μm
Resveratrol contents	High	Low (shell distribution)	none
Dissolution rate	Low	High	n.d.

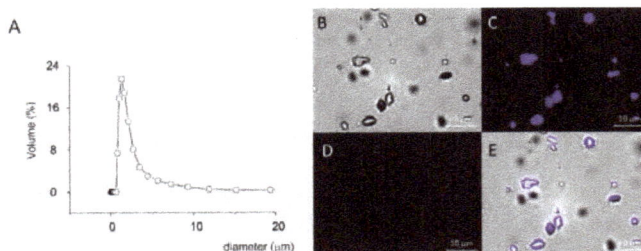

Figure 3. Properties of pure micronized resveratrol. (**A**) Granulometric analysis of microcrystalline resveratrol. (**B–E**) Image of crystalline resveratrol powder dispersed in glycerol under different excitation sources. (**B**) Bright-field; (**C**) DAPI fluorescence filter; (**D**) Rhodamine fluorescence filter. (**E**) Merging of the Bright-field, DAPI and Rhodamine images.

3.3. Dissolution of Solid Dispersion of Resveratrol on Magnesium Dihydroxide.

In Figure 4 dissolution profiles of Resv@MDH (red squares) and pure resveratrol (black squares) are presented (mg/L in function of time). The experimental data was fit with exponential equation $C(t) = Cmax (1 - \exp(-t/\tau))$, where Cmax = maximum solubility value; t = time; τ = time in which dissolution reaches about 63% of maximum process. The equation represents a form studying the dissolution profiles according to Weibull's models [20]. The best data fit is for Cmax: 40.8 and 13 mg/L for Resv@MDH and resveratrol respectively while τ was 0.4 and 2.2 min for Resv@MDH and resveratrol respectively. These data indicated that Resv@MDH showed a dissolution rate five times higher than resveratrol (compared to τ) and a maximum solubility three times as big (compared to Cmax). To assess the importance of particles size in dissolution rate, we compared the solubility profile of pure micronized resveratrol with similar size particles of Resv@MDH (Figures 3 and 4). It was possible to see (compare black and green squares in Figure 4A) the reduction of particles size modified only dissolution kinetic according to the Noise-Witting law, but did not modify the maximal solubility [21].

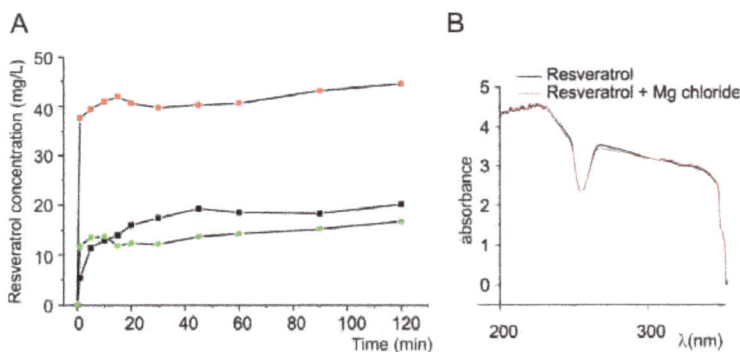

Figure 4. Solubility of resveratrol from Resv@MDH and its interaction with magnesium ion. (**A**) dissolution test of pure resveratrol powder (black MDH square) versus solid dispersion on magnesium dihydroxide (Resv@MDH, red square) and pure micronized resveratrol (green square). (**B**) UV/Vis Absorbance spectroscopy for the study of Resveratrol. Black: 0.008 mM Resveratrol in ethanol:water (75:25, v/v) in 100 mM HCl; Red: 0.008 mM Resveratrol in ethanol:water (75:25, v/v) in 100 mM HCl + 0.008 mM of MgCl.

To verify if magnesium ion participates in major solubility (Cmax) of resveratrol by forming a complex, we verified the interaction between them by performing spectrophotometric profile of resveratrol alone or in presence of magnesium ion in acid environment. It is possible to see in Figure 4B, that the addition of magnesium does not significantly modify the UV absorption spectra, suggesting that the magnesium does not interact with resveratrol and that the major solubility was dependent on other factors.

3.4. Pharmacokinetic Profile of Solid Dispersion of Resveratrol on Magnesium Dihydroxide

The rabbit animal model is excellent to perform pharmacokinetic studies [20] and recently was used to evaluate the bioavailability of a new resveratrol formulation [18]. The mean plasma concentration of resveratrol following oral administration of 50 mg/kg of Resv@MDH and pure resveratrol was investigated in the rabbit animal model. Resveratrol plasma concentration versus time curves from administration is displayed in Figure 5. Pharmacokinetic variables derived from this pharmacokinetic profile are summarized in Table 2. Resveratrol is virtually absent in animal plasma prior to oral administration (0 min) but it seemed to be rapidly absorbed with a peak of maximal concentrations (C_{max}) between 15 and 30 min post-dose. The C_{max} of resveratrol was 76.3 ng/mL and 101.3 ng/mL for resveratrol and Resv@MDH respectively. At 30 up to 90 min from the administration, the resveratrol plasma concentration of Resv@MDH treated animals results statistically greater as compared to resveratrol treated animal, while at 180 min the resveratrol is no longer detectable in the plasma of both groups of animals. The values of Area Under Curve (AUC) of the plasma concentration profile until the 3-h time point was 2698 ng min/mL and 8944 ng min/mL or resveratrol and Resv@MDH respectively. This data demonstrates an enhancement of resveratrols bioaviability by 3.3-fold (ratio of $AUC_{Resv@MDH}/AUC_{resveratrol}$, Table 2).

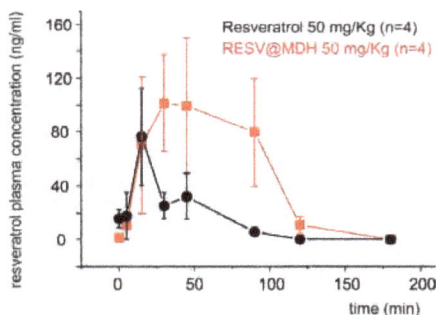

Figure 5. Pharmacokinetic profiles of resveratrol after oral administration in rabbits. Groups of 4 animals each were treated with resveratrol (50 mg/Kg of pure resveratrol versus Resv@MDH). Blood samples taken at 0, 5, 15, 30, 45, 90, 120 and 180 min.

Table 2. Pharmacokinetic parameters of oral administration of 50 mg/Kg of resveratrol from pure resveratrol and from Resv@MDH.

Parameters	Resveratrolo 50 mg/Kg	Resv@MDH (Resveratrol 50 mg/Kg)	Increase %
AUC (Area Under Curve)	2698 ng min/mL	8944 ng min/mL	330
Time to plasmatic peak	15 min	30 min	200
Peak duration	25 min	105 min	420
Cmax	76.3 ng/mL	101.3 ng/mL	130

4. Discussion

Solid dispersion of resveratrol on magnesium dihydroxide (Resv@MDH) represents a new formulation that possesses an increased solubility of resveratrol (spring form). Resv@MDH is able to solubilize itself faster and in greater amounts with respect to resveratrol, with remarkable advantages in biopharmaceutical terms and therefore of bioavailability. From the physical point of view it is a polydisperse granular material, where the active is supported by inorganic material with a high safety level (magnesium hydroxide). Furthermore, this improves its performance without chemically modifying the natural product's structure. Resv@MDH allows to obtain an apparent solubility much higher with respect to resveratrol as a consequence of an increased dissolution rate and of the establishment of over-saturation phenomena due to different energetic states of resveratrol (Figure 6). This dispersion is formed by three types of microparticles that we define as type 1, 2 and 3. Based on our results we hypothesized that microparticles type 1 and 3 represent resveratrol and magnesium dihydroxide crystals, respectively. The unexpected result is the presence of microparticles type 2 that probably represent the form responsible for enhanced properties of the solid dispersion. Based on the evidence of change of its fluorescence, we suggest that a fraction of resveratrol forms a shell around magnesium dihydroxide microparticles. The better solubility of resveratrol displayed by solid dispersion could be explained by the coexistence of two energetic states of resveratrol related to the two types of microparticles observed (type 1 and 2, Figure 6). It is possible to exclude the involvement of free magnesium ions (Mg^{2+}) in improving the solubility of resveratrol since their absorbance spectrum was not modified by the presence of metals in acidic environment (Figure 4B). The state of over-saturation could lead to the major absorption (increase of the gradient concentration) and therefore increased bioavailability [22].

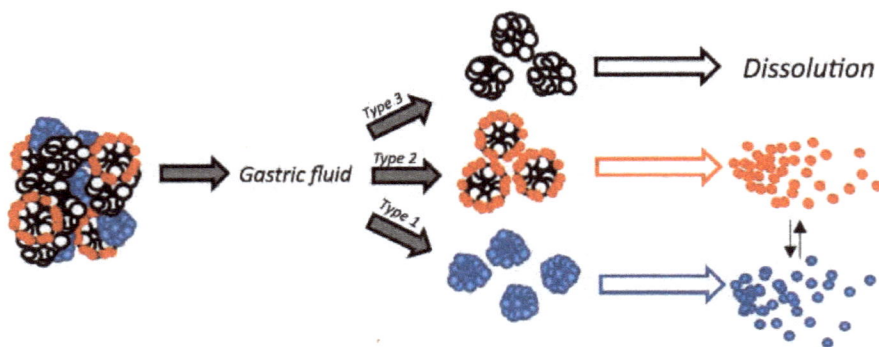

Figure 6. Scheme of hypothetical dissolution events that occur to Resv@MDH powder when it is in contact with simulated stomach fluids. Big powder aggregates divide into three main microparticles named as type 1, 2 and 3. In acidic milieu the type 3 microparticles of magnesium dihydroxide completely dissolves; type 1 microparticles (blue) dissolves in water solution together with type 2 microparticles (red). In this case the limiting step in resveratrol release could be related to acid erosion of dihydroxide core.

The reduced and homogeneous particle size represents a parameter that improves the dissolution rate observed for Resv@MDH is according to Noyes and Whitney law [21]. The comparative dissolution rate of resveratrol displayed in Figure 5 demonstrates that the supersaturating state is not dependent from the particles size of resveratrol. Further studies are needed to clarify the mechanisms of the better solubility of solid dispersion of resveratrol on magnesium dihydroxide. The Resv@MDH represent a new way to uncover the therapeutic potential of resveratrol with possible application as anti-inflammatory, anti-viral, cardio-protective, neuro-protective, anti-cancer and anti-angiogenetic agent [1–3]. As regard the anticancer properties, resveratrol was demonstrated to increase the effect of radio and chemotherapeutic agents [23] in particular against glioblastoma cancer cells [24].

Supplementary Materials: The following are available online at http://www.mdpi.com/2072-6643/10/12/1925/s1, Figure S1: Image of RESV@MDH powder dispersed in glycerol under different eccitation sources. (**A**) Rohdamine fluorescence filter (**B**) brightfield; Note: white arrow indicates the fluorescent shell of resveratrol around the core of magnesium diihydroxide.

Author Contributions: Conceptualization, B.F. and R.S.; validation, L.M. (Laura Menchetti), F.B. and F.R.; formal analysis, F.R. and L.M. (Laura Menchetti); investigation, R.S., M.B., L.M. (Loretta Mancinelli), F.B, I.N., G.B., M.C., and C.A.; resources, R.S. and R.G.I; data curation, R.S and B.F.; writing—original draft preparation, L.M. (Loretta Mancinelli) and B.F.; writing—review and editing, L.M. (Loretta Mancinelli), B.F and R.G.I; visualization, L.M. (Lorenzo Monarca) and F.R.; supervision, B.F.; project administration, B.F.; funding acquisition, B.F.

Funding: This research was funded by Scientific Independent Research (SIR2014) of the Italian MIUR (Ministry of Education, University and Research) to B.F.

Acknowledgments: The authors would like to thank Tommaso Beccari of University of Perugia for his criticism.

Conflicts of Interest: R.S. and B.F. are co-inventors of the patent EPO n EP20130425091; R.G.I is an employee of S&R Farmaceutici S.p.a., whom hold the rights and license of REVIFAST®. All other authors declare no conflict of interest.

References

1. Baur, J.A.; Sinclair, D.A. Therapeutic potential of resveratrol: The in vivo evidence. *Nat. Rev. Drug. Discov.* **2006**, *5*, 493–506. [CrossRef] [PubMed]

2. Smoliga, J.M.; Baur, J.A.; Hausenblas, H.A. Resveratrol and healt—A comprehensive review of human clinical trials. *Mol. Nutr. Food Res.* **2011**, *55*, 1129–1141. [CrossRef] [PubMed]

3. Lombardi, G.; Vannini, S.; Blasi, F.; Marcotullio, M.C.; Dominici, L.; Villarini, M.; Cossignani, L.; Moretti, M. In Vitro Safety/Protection Assessment of Resveratrol and Pterostilbene in a Human Hepatoma Cell Line (HepG2). *Nat. Prod. Commun.* **2015**, *10*, 1403–1408. [PubMed]

4. Timmers, S.; Koning, E.; Bilet, L.; Houtkoopere, R.H.; van de Weijer, T.; Gijs, H.; Goossens, G.H.; Hoeks, J.; van der Krieken, S.; Ryu, D.; et al. Calorie restriction-like effects of 30 days of resveratrol supplementation on energy metabolism and metabolic profile in obese humans. *Cell Metab.* **2011**, *14*, 612–622. [CrossRef] [PubMed]

5. Subramanian, L.; Youssef, S.; Bhattacharya, S.; Kenealey, J.; Polans, A.S.; van Ginkel, P.R.; Polans, A.S. Resveratrol: Challenges in translation to the clinic—A critical discussion. *Clin. Cancer Res.* **2010**, *16*, 5942–5948. [CrossRef] [PubMed]

6. Boocock, D.J.; Faust, G.E.S.; Patel, K.R.; Schinas, A.M.; Brown, V.A.; Ducharme, M.P.; Booth, T.D.; Crowell, J.A.; Perloff, M.; Gescher, A.J.; et al. Phase I dose escalation pharmacokinetic study in healthy volunteers of resveratrol, a potential cancer chemopreventive agent. *Cancer Epidemiol. Biomark. Prev.* **2007**, *16*, 1246–1252. [CrossRef] [PubMed]

7. Almeida, L.; Vaz-da-Silva, M.; Falcão, A.; Soares, E.; Costa, R.; Loureiro, A.I.; Fernandes-Lopes, C.; Rocha, J.F.; Nunes, T.; Wright, L.; et al. Pharmacokinetic and safety profile of trans-resveratrol in a rising multiple-dose study in healthy volunteers. *Mol. Nutr. Food Res.* **2009**, *53*, S7–S15. [CrossRef] [PubMed]

8. Amidon, G.L.; Lennernäs, H.; Shah, V.P.; Crison, J.R. A theoretical basis for a biopharmaceutic drug classification: The correlation of in vitro drug product dissolution and in vivo bioavailability. *Pharm. Res.* **1995**, *12*, 413–420. [CrossRef]

9. Löbenberg, R.; Amidon, G. Modern bioavailability, bioequivalence and biopharmaceutics classification system. New scientific approaches to international regulatory standards. *Eur. J. Pharm. Biopharm.* **2000**, *50*, 3–12. [CrossRef]

10. Amri, A.; Chaumeila, J.C.; Sfarb, S.; Charrueaua, C. Administration of resveratrol: What formulation solutions to bioavailability limitations? *J. Control Release* **2012**, *158*, 182–193. [CrossRef]

11. Amiot, M.J.; Romiera, B.; Dao, T.M.A.; Fanciullino, R.; Ciccolini, J.; Burcelin, R.; Pechere, L.; Emond, C.; Savouret, J.F.; Seree, E. Optimization of trans-Resveratrol bioavailability for human therapy. *Biochimie* **2013**, *95*, 1233–1238. [CrossRef] [PubMed]

12. Das, S.; Lin, H.S.; Ho, P.C.; Ng, K.Y. The impact of aqueous solubility and dose on the pharmacokinetic profiles of resveratrol. *Pharm. Res.* **2008**, *25*, 2593–2600. [CrossRef] [PubMed]

13. Maier-Salamon, A.; Hagenauer, B.; Wirth, M.; Gabor, F.; Szekeres, T.; Jäger, W. Increased transport of resveratrol across monolayers of the human intestinal Caco-2 cells is mediated by inhibition and saturation of metabolites. *Pharm. Res.* **2006**, *23*, 2107–2115. [CrossRef] [PubMed]

14. Hurst, S.; Loi, C.M.; Brodfuehrer, J.; El-Kattan, A. Impact of physiological, physicochemical and biopharmaceutical factors in absorption and metabolism mechanisms on the drug oral bioavailability of rats and humans. *Expert. Opin. Drug. Metab. Toxicol.* **2007**, *3*, 469–489. [CrossRef] [PubMed]

15. Dias, K.; Nikolaou, S. Does the combination of resveratrol with Al (III) and Zn (II) improve its antioxidant activity? *Nat. Prod. Commun.* **2011**, *6*, 1673–1676. [PubMed]

16. Flieger, J.; Tatarczak-Michalewska, M.; Blicharska, E.; Swieboda, R.; Banach, T. HPLCIdentification of Copper (II)-Trans-ResveratrolComplexes in ethanolicAqueousSolution. *J. Chromatogr. Sci.* **2017**, *55*, 445–450. [CrossRef]

17. Biswicka, T.; Jones, W.; Pacula, A.; Serwickab, E. Synthesis, characterisation and anion exchange properties of copper, magnesium, zinc and nickel hydroxy nitrate. *J. Solid State Chem.* **2006**, *179*, 49–55. [CrossRef]

18. Jaisamut, P.; Wiwattanawongsa, K.; Wiwattanapatapee, R. A Novel Self-Microemulsifying System for the Simultaneous Delivery and Enhanced Oral Absorption of Curcumin and Resveratrol. *Planta Med.* **2017**, *83*, 461–467. [CrossRef]

19. Biasutto, L.; Marotta, E.; Carbisa, S.; Zoratti, M.; Paradisi, C. Determination of quercitin and resveratrol in whole blood-implication for bioavalaibility studies. *Molecules* **2010**, *15*, 6570–6579. [CrossRef]

20. Menchetti, L.; Barbato, O.; Filipescu, I.E.; Traina, G.; Leonardi, L.; Polisca, A.; Troisi, A.; Guelfi, G.; Piro, F.; Brecchia, G. Effects of local lipopolysaccharide administration on the expression of Toll-like receptor 4 and pro-inflammatory cytokines in uterus and oviduct of rabbit does. *Theriogenology* **2018**, *107*, 162–174. [CrossRef]

21. Dokoumetzidis, A.; Macheras, P. A century of dissolution research: From Noyes and Whitney to the Biopharmaceutics Classification System. *Int. J. Pharm.* **2006**, *321*, 1–11. [CrossRef] [PubMed]

22. Brouwers, J.; Brewster, M.E.; Augustijns, P. Supersaturating drug delivery systems: The answer to solubility-limited oral bioavailability? *J. Pharm. Sci.* **2009**, *98*, 2549–2572. [CrossRef] [PubMed]

23. Valentovic, M.A. Evaluation of Resveratrol in Cancer Patients and Experimental Models. *Adv Cancer Res.* **2018**, *137*, 171–188. [CrossRef] [PubMed]

24. Yang, H.C.; Wang, J.Y.; Bu, X.Y.; Yang, B.; Wang, B.Q.; Hu, S.; Yan, Z.Y.; Gao, Y.S.; Han, S.Y.; Qu, M.Q. Resveratrol restores sensitivity of glioma cells to temozolamide through inhibiting the activation of Wnt signaling pathway. *J. Cell Physiol.* **2018**. [CrossRef] [PubMed]

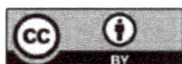

nutrients

MDPI

Article

Protective Effect of Resveratrol against Ischemia-Reperfusion Injury via Enhanced High Energy Compounds and eNOS-SIRT1 Expression in Type 2 Diabetic Female Rat Heart

Natacha Fourny [1,*], Carole Lan [1], Eric Sérée [2], Monique Bernard [1] and Martine Desrois [1]

[1] Aix-Marseille University, CNRS, Centre de Résonance Magnétique Biologique et Médicale (CRMBM), Faculté de Médecine, 27 Boulevard Jean Moulin, 13385 Marseille, CEDEX 05, France; carole.lan@univ-amu.fr (C.L.); monique.bernard@univ-amu.fr (M.B.); martine.desrois@univ-amu.fr (M.D.)
[2] Aix-Marseille University, INSERM, INRA, Centre de Recherche en Cardiovasculaire et Nutrition (C2VN), Faculté de Médecine, 27 Boulevard Jean Moulin, 13385 Marseille, CEDEX 05, France; seree.eric@gmail.com
* Correspondence: natacha.fourny@etu.univ-amu.fr; Tel.: +33-(0)-4-91-32-48-08; Fax: +33-(0)-4-91-25-65-39

Received: 26 November 2018; Accepted: 28 December 2018; Published: 6 January 2019

Abstract: Type 2 diabetic women have a high risk of mortality via myocardial infarction even with anti-diabetic treatments. Resveratrol (RSV) is a natural polyphenol, well-known for its antioxidant property, which has also shown interesting positive effects on mitochondrial function. Therefore, we aim to investigate the potential protective effect of 1 mg/kg/day of RSV on high energy compounds, during myocardial ischemia-reperfusion in type 2 diabetic female Goto-Kakizaki (GK) rats. For this purpose, we used ^{31}P magnetic resonance spectroscopy in isolated perfused heart experiments, with a simultaneous measurement of myocardial function and coronary flow. RSV enhanced adenosine triphosphate (ATP) and phosphocreatine (PCr) contents in type 2 diabetic hearts during reperfusion, in combination with better functional recovery. Complementary biochemical analyses showed that RSV increased creatine, total adenine nucleotide heart contents and citrate synthase activity, which could be involved in better mitochondrial functioning. Moreover, improved coronary flow during reperfusion by RSV was associated with increased eNOS, SIRT1, and P-Akt protein expression in GK rat hearts. In conclusion, RSV induced cardioprotection against ischemia-reperfusion injury in type 2 diabetic female rats via increased high energy compound contents and expression of protein involved in NO pathway. Thus, RSV presents high potential to protect the heart of type 2 diabetic women from myocardial infarction.

Keywords: resveratrol; type 2 diabetes; ischemia-reperfusion; cardiac function; energy metabolism; mitochondria; endothelial function

---

1. Introduction

Cardiovascular (CV) complications are the first causes of morbidity and mortality in type 2 diabetic patients, particularly in women [1]. Cardio-protection is widely recognized in women, and surprisingly, is suppressed with type 2 diabetes, with more serious CV consequences in women than in men [2]. It is known that the risk of myocardial infarction is five times higher in type 2 diabetic women compared with non-diabetic women, while this risk is only multiplied by two in men [3,4]. In addition, mortality due to myocardial infarction is higher in women than in men in type 2 diabetes [5]. Few studies explore female gender and the reasons for higher deterioration of the cardiovascular system are not yet fully understood. Endothelial damage is one likely hypothesis for CV complications in type 2 diabetes. Interestingly, Desrois et al. reported a higher endothelial damage in female GK rat hearts than in males in the absence of ischemic insult, which could explain the higher risk of CV in type 2 diabetic women [6].

Although this is one of the current objectives, most of antidiabetic treatments fail to decrease the CV risk [7]. For this purpose, dietary supplements could be interesting in combination with existing antidiabetic medication to improve CV outcomes in diabetic patients. Resveratrol (RSV), or trans-3,5,4′-trihydroxy stilbene, is a natural polyphenol found in more than 70 plant species like grapes, peanuts, and blackberries [8]. This molecule has shown pleiotropic and beneficial effects on both type 2 diabetes and cardiovascular complications [9]. Various studies, using models of type 2 diabetes or metabolic syndrome, showed that RSV could decrease chronic inflammation [10], improve insulin sensitivity [11], lipid profile [12], and decrease oxidative stress [13]. Other studies also demonstrated the effects of RSV on endothelial function mainly through mechanisms involving nitric oxide (NO) and sirtuin pathways [14–17]. Interestingly, RSV has shown beneficial effects on mitochondrial function by increasing mitochondrial DNA and biogenesis [13]. Consequently, RSV could be an interesting candidate to improve cardiac energy metabolism and CV outcomes of type 2 diabetic women [18–20].

In the literature, the dose of RSV is very different depending on the study. Doses range from 0.1 mg/kg/day [18] to 500 mg/kg/day [21] and even 4g/kg/day [22]. Here we choose a "low-dose" of RSV at 1 mg/kg/day based on Rocha et al. and Lin et al.'s studies. Indeed, Rocha et al. [23] chose a dose of 1 mg/kg based on the actual wine consumption in occidental countries, and the kinetics and bioavailability of resveratrol in the body. Lin et al.'s [18] study showed that a lower dose (0.1 mg/kg) was not sufficient to induce beneficial effects on the heart, while a dose of 1 mg/kg/day improved cardiac function. On the other hand, higher doses (25 mg/kg/day) have shown negative effects on infarct size [24]. Thus, we suppose that the "low-dose" of 1 mg/kg/day of RSV will be sufficient to observe beneficial effects on myocardial energy metabolism.

Here, we aim to determine the effects of a low-dose oral administration of RSV on myocardial sensitivity to ischemia-reperfusion injury in female GK rats, a polygenic model of type 2 diabetes, with the hypothesis that RSV could improve high energy compound contents. We believe this is an original study exploring the effects of RSV on high-energy compounds during an ischemia-reperfusion injury, using ^{31}P magnetic resonance spectroscopy (MRS) and biochemical analysis, combined with measurement of myocardial function and coronary flow. Secondarily, we assessed the effects of RSV on coronary flow and expression of proteins involved in NO pathway, as indicators of endothelial function.

2. Materials and Methods

2.1. Materials and Antibodies

Assay kits were used to determine plasma glucose (Randox Laboratories, Crumlin, Antrim, UK) and free fatty acids (FFAs) (NEFA kit; Roche Diagnostics, Roche Applied Science, Mannheim, Germany). A radioimmunoprecipitation assay buffer (RIPA) lysis buffer was used to extract proteins (sc-24948, Santa Cruz Biotechnology, Santa Cruz, CA, USA). Total protein concentration was determined using the Pierce BCA protein assay kit (ref 23227, Thermo scientific, Rockford, USA). Anti-eNOS (ref 610296, BD Transduction Laboratories, USA), anti-SIRT1 (ref 9475, Cell Signaling Technology), anti-Akt (Cell Signaling Technology, Danvers, MA, USA), anti-PAkt (Ser 473) (Cell Signaling Technology, Danvers, MA, USA), anti-SIRT3 (#2627, Cell Signaling Technology, Danvers, MA, USA), and anti-Actin (sc47 778, Santa Cruz Biotechnology, Santa Cruz, CA, USA) primary antibodies were used for western blots. HRP-conjugated antibodies were used as secondary antibodies (Goat anti-mouse sc2031 or Goat anti-rabbit sc2030, Santa Cruz Biotechnology, Santa Cruz, CA, USA). The immunoblots were developed using an ECL Western Blotting Detection Reagent (GE Healthcare, AmershamTM, Buckinghamshire, U.K.). The protein signals were assessed using the MicroChemi 4.2 System (DNR Bio-Imaging System Ltd., Jerusalem, Israel). Citrate synthase activity was evaluated using the citrate synthase assay kit (CS0720, Sigma-Aldrich, St. Louis, MO, USA). First, protein extraction was performed using the

CelLytic MT extraction buffer (C3228, Sigma, St. Louis, MO, USA). Malondialdehyde (MDA) was assessed with the lipid peroxidation assay kit (MAK085, Sigma-Aldrich, St. Louis, MO, USA).

2.2. Animals

Age-matched (7–8 months) female control Wistar rats (Charles River, France) and type 2 diabetic female Goto-Kakizaki (GK) rats (GK/Par subline; Laboratoire de Biologie et Pathologie du Pancréas Endocrine UMR8251-CNRS—Université Paris Diderot, Paris, France [25]) were used in the experiments. All procedures involving animals were approved by the Animal Experiment Ethics Committee of Aix-Marseille University (n°2017070416019134) and were in conformity with the European Convention for protection of animals used for experimental purpose. The animals were housed in a temperature controlled ventilated cabinet (22–24 °C) and were exposed to light–dark cycles of 12:12 h. Animals had access to food (diet 113, SAFE, Augy, France) and water ad libitum. Four groups were designed for this study: the control group (CTRL; $n = 11$), the type 2 diabetic group (GK; $n = 14$), the type 2 diabetic group under placebo treatment (GK-P; $n = 9$), and the type 2 diabetic group with RSV treatment (GK-RSV; $n = 8$).

2.3. Treatment

RSV was provided for 8 weeks in drinking water at the dose of 1 mg/kg/day as suggested before by Rocha et al. [23,26]. As RSV solubility is higher in ethanol, we first dissolved RSV in ethanol and then in water. The placebo treatment corresponded to 1‰ ethanol in drinking water. Daily water ingestion was evaluated a few weeks before the beginning of the study, to calculate the concentration of RSV solution. During the 8 weeks of RSV treatment, water consumption was also measured to adjust RSV concentration if necessary [23].

2.4. Myocardial Tolerance to Ischemia-Reperfusion Injury

After 8 weeks of RSV treatment, isolated perfused heart experiments were performed to evaluate ex vivo the tolerance to ischemia-reperfusion injury, by measuring energy metabolism, cardiac function and coronary flow during the whole protocol. As previously described, rats were anesthetized by intraperitoneal injection of 90 mg/kg pentobarbital sodium [27]. The hearts were quickly removed from the chest cavity by thoracotomy and arrested in ice-cold Krebs-Henseleit buffer (containing (mM): NaCl (118), KCl (4.7), $MgSO_4$ (1.2), $CaCl_2$ (1.75), $NaHCO_3$ (25), KH_2PO_4 (1.2), EDTA (0.5) and D-glucose (11)). Hearts were weighed and then cannulated via the ascending aorta for retrograde Langendorff-perfusion of coronary arterial network at a constant pressure of 100 mm Hg. A drain was placed at the apex of the heart to evacuate coronary effluents. In the same time, blood samples were immediately taken for glucose and free fatty acids (FFAs) determination in plasma.

2.4.1. Experimental Protocol

After 4 min of stabilization with a Krebs–Henseleit buffer, hearts were perfused for 24 min with a physiological recirculating Krebs–Henseleit buffer (Pa 0.4) containing 0.4 mM palmitate, 3% albumin, 11 mM glucose, 3U/L insulin, 0.8 mM lactate, and 0.2 mM pyruvate. Four minutes before low-flow ischemia, hearts were perfused with a physiological non-recirculating Krebs–Henseleit buffer (Pa 1.2) containing 1.2 mM palmitate, 3% albumin, 11 mM glucose, 3U/L insulin, 0.8 mM lactate, and 0.2 mM pyruvate. Then, the hearts underwent a low-flow ischemia (0.5 mL/min/g wet wt) of 32 min with the same buffer. Finally, flow was restored entirely for 32 min with the physiological Krebs–Henseleit buffer containing 0.4 mM palmitate. The palmitate concentration was increased at the end of the control period and during ischemia to induce a maximum damage [28]. The perfusates were continually gassed with a mixture of 95% O_2 and 5% CO_2 to maintain pH at 7.40. The buffer temperature was maintained at 37 °C during the entire protocol.

2.4.2. Myocardial Function

A water-filled latex balloon was inserted in the left ventricle via the mitral valve and inflated to produce an end diastolic pressure (EDP) of ≈10 mm Hg at the beginning of perfusion. Left ventricular developed pressure (DP) and heart rate (HR) were recorded using a pressure sensor connected to the balloon, as previously described [6]. The product of heart rate and developed pressure was used as an index of cardiac function. During reperfusion, we calculated the percentage recovery between the pre-ischemic and post-ischemic cardiac function. Coronary flow (CF) was measured via collection of coronary effluent before and after ischemia (at 20 min and 80 min), expressed in mL/min/g wet weight.

2.4.3. Myocardial Energy Metabolism

^{31}P Magnetic Resonance Spectroscopy (MRS)

Perfused rat hearts were placed in a 20-mm magnetic resonance sample tube and inserted in a ^{31}P probe that was seated in the bore of a superconducting wide-bore (89-mm) 4.7 Tesla magnet (Oxford instruments, Oxford, U.K.) interfaced with a Bruker-Nicolet Avance WP-200 spectrometer (Bruker, Karlsruhe, Germany). ^{31}P spectra were obtained by accumulating 328 free induction decay signals acquired for 4 min (flip angle 45°, repetition time 0.7 s, spectral width 4500 Hz, 2048 data points) [29]. Prior to Fourier transformation, the free induction decay was multiplied by an exponential function which generated a 20 Hz line broadening. Quantification of the signal integrals was carried out using an external reference containing an aqueous solution of 0.6 mM phenylphosphonic acid. A series of eight ^{31}P spectra were recorded during each period of the experimental protocol to quantify phosphorus metabolites (ATP, PCr, and Pi) and intracellular pH.

Biochemical Analyses in Freeze-Clamped Heart

As a complement to ^{31}P MRS, high performance liquid chromatography (HPLC) analysis, as well as citrate synthase (CS) activity, were performed as indicators of mitochondrial function. First, PCr, creatine, adenine nucleotides, and derivatives were assessed using ion-exchange high performance liquid chromatography (HPLC). A perchloric extraction, adapted from Lazzarino et al., was performed by homogenizing cardiac tissue (50 to 100 mg) with a Polytron homogenizer (Kinematica, Luzern, Switzerland) in ice-cold 0.6 M perchloric acid [30]. Then, homogenates were centrifuged at 5000× g for 10 min at 4 °C and supernatants were preserved for the comparative metabolite determination. Protein concentration calculation was carried out according to Lowry et al. to express the results in µmol/g protein [31]. Separation of adenine nucleotide derivatives, phosphocreatine, and creatine was performed using the ion-pairing reverse phase technique. Qualitative and quantitative analyses were carried out using adenine nucleotide standards and thymine monophosphate (Sigma, Poole, Dorset, UK) as an internal standard. Under these chromatographic conditions, a highly resolved separation of ATP, ADP, AMP, PCr, and creatine was obtained in 40 min. Total adenine nucleotide pool (TAN) was calculated from the sum ATP + ADP + AMP. Energy charge (EC) is equal to ((ATP + 0.5ADP) / (ATP + ADP + AMP)) × 10.

Secondly, CS activity was evaluated using the citrate synthase assay kit. Protein extraction was performed, extracts were centrifuged at 14,000× g for 10 min at 4 °C and total protein concentration in the supernatant was determined using the Pierce BCA protein assay kit. Activity of citrate synthase was assessed at 412 nm in a 96-well plate with a kinetic program. Results are expressed in nmol/g of protein/minute.

2.4.4. Expression of Proteins Involved in NO Pathway

Complementary to coronary flow measurement, we assessed the expression of eNOS, SIRT1, Akt, and P-Akt proteins in freeze-clamped hearts. A piece of left ventricle tissue (≈60 mg) was homogenized in a RIPA lysis buffer and centrifuged at 14,000 rpm for 15 min at 4 °C. Total protein concentration in the supernatant was determined using the Pierce BCA protein assay kit. Equal amounts of proteins (90 µg for eNOS and SIRT1, 50 µg for Akt and P-Akt) were separated by 8% or 10% polyacrylamide gel electrophoresis and transferred onto nitrocellulose membranes. After blocking with 5% skim milk, membranes were incubated overnight at 4 °C with eNOS (1/1000), SIRT1 (1/1000), Akt (1/1000), P-Akt (Ser 473) (1/500), or Actin (1/2000) primary antibodies. Second, membranes were incubated with HRP-conjugated antibodies (1/2000). The immunoblots were developed and the protein signal was quantified using the Quantiscan software (Biosoft, Cambridge, U.K.). The intensity of each protein signal was normalized to the corresponding β-actin stain signal. Data are expressed as ratios between the protein and the corresponding β-actin signal density, except for P-Akt, which was expressed according to Akt.

2.4.5. Oxidative Stress

SIRT3 protein expression, a mitochondrial sirtuin involved in oxidative stress, was assessed in freeze-clamped hearts following the same protocol as described above, with 50 µg of protein separated by 10% polyacrylamide gel. Primary antibody against SIRT3 was used at 1/1000.

MDA was assessed to evaluate lipid peroxidation in freeze-clamped hearts. Lipid peroxidation was determined by the reaction of MDA with thiobarbituric acid (TBA) to form a colorimetric (532 nm)/fluorometric (λex = 532/λem = 553 nm) product, proportional to the MDA present.

2.5. Statistical Analyses

Data are graphically provided as means ± SEM of absolute values. GraphPad Prism software 5.0 (La Jolla, CA, USA) was used for all statistical processing. Significant differences between groups were determined using two-way analysis of variance (ANOVA) with repeated measures over time for the time-dependent variables followed by Bonferroni post-hoc test. An unpaired Student's *t*-test was used for the other parameters. A *p*-value of less than or equal to 0.05 was considered to indicate significant difference.

3. Results

3.1. Effect of Resveratrol on Physiological Parameters

Physiological parameters are shown in Table 1. Plasma glucose was significantly increased in GK, GK-P, and GK-RSV in comparison to CTRL ($p < 0.0001$). RSV treatment did not reduce plasma glucose in GK rats. Plasma-free fatty acids and weight of animals were similar in the four groups. The weight of the heart was significantly higher in the GK group compared to the three other groups ($p < 0.001$). However, the heart weight to body weight ratio was increased in GK ($p < 0.001$), GK-P ($p < 0.01$), and GK-RSV ($p < 0.01$) versus CTRL. The heart weight to body weight ratio was decreased in GK-RSV ($p < 0.05$) and GK-P ($p < 0.01$) in comparison to GK, indicating decreased cardiac hypertrophy by RSV treatment.

Table 1. Physiological parameters of experimental animals.

	CTRL	**GK**	**GK-P**	**GK-RSV**
Glycemia (g/L)	1.64 ± 0.07	2.46 ± 0.09 *	2.52 ± 0.15 *	2.49 ± 0.07 *
Free Fatty Acids (mM)	0.21 ± 0.05	0.18 ± 0.02	0.17 ± 0.04	0.16 ± 0.04
Body Weight (g)	289.4 ± 6.6	284.6 ± 4.4	267.5 ± 5.7	269.7 ± 6.4
Heart Weight (g)	0.85 ± 0.02	1.05 ± 0.03 * † ‡	0.89 ± 0.02	0.91 ± 0.02
(Ratio Heart/Body Weight) × 1000	2.95 ± 0.09	3.69 ± 0.06 * II ¶	3.32 ± 0.06 §	3.38 ± 0.09 §

Data are expressed as means ± SEM. One-way ANOVA test was used for all the parameters. * $p < 0.0001$ vs. CTRL; † $p < 0.0001$ vs. GK-P; ‡ $p < 0.0001$ vs. GK-RSV; § $p < 0.01$ vs. CTRL; II $p < 0.01$ vs. GK-P; ¶ $p < 0.05$ vs. GK-RSV.

3.2. Effect of Resveratrol on Tolerance to Ischemia-Reperfusion Injury

3.2.1. Myocardial Function

Myocardial function (Figure 1A) was impaired in GK, GK-P, and GK-RSV compared with CTRL in baseline conditions ($p < 0.001$ GK and GK-P vs. CTRL; $p < 0.01$ GK-RSV vs. CTRL). RSV did not improve cardiac function in GK-RSV in comparison to CTRL in baseline conditions. After ischemia, GK and GK-P groups presented a higher sensitivity to ischemia-reperfusion injury since myocardial function was significantly impaired compared with CTRL ($p < 0.001$) and the percentage of recovery (Figure 1B) was significantly decreased (respectively $p < 0.001$ and $p < 0.01$ vs. CTRL). Interestingly, GK-RSV rats had a better tolerance to ischemia-reperfusion injury than GK and GK-P rats, with an improvement of cardiac function up to CTRL values.

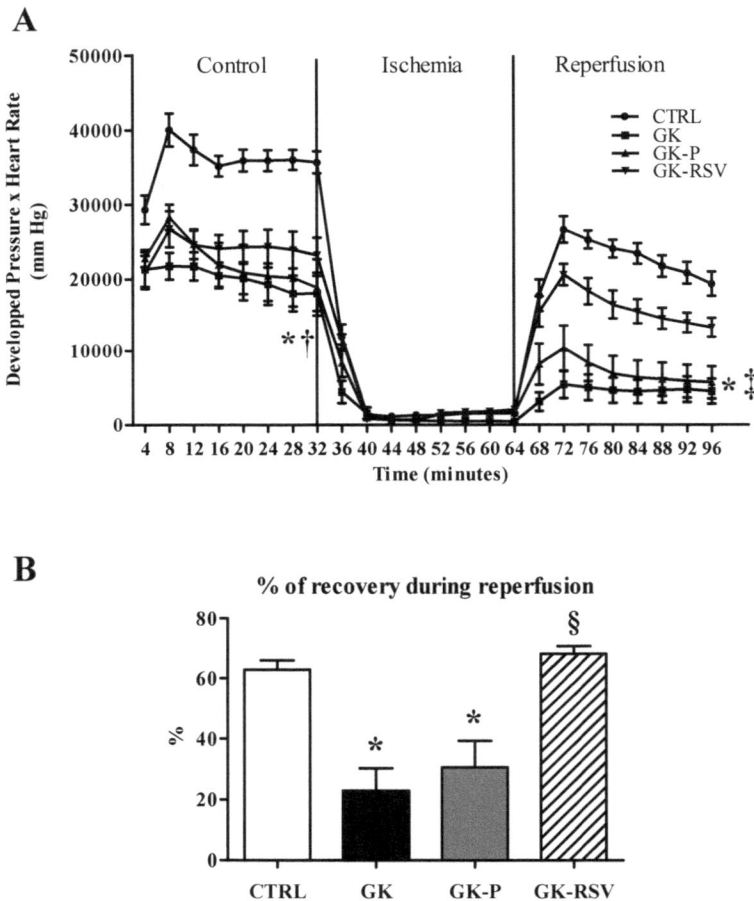

Figure 1. Myocardial function evaluated by the product of developed pressure and heart rate during the experimental time course (**A**) and % of recovery during reperfusion (**B**). Results are expressed as means ± SEM. Two-way ANOVA was performed to observe the effect of group and time. * $p < 0.001$ GK and GK-P vs. CTRL, † $p < 0.01$ GK-RSV vs. CTRL, ‡ $p < 0.01$ GK and GK-P vs. GK-RSV, and § $p < 0.001$ vs. GK and GK-P.

3.2.2. Myocardial Energy Metabolism

^{31}P MRS

Kinetics of PCr, ATP, Pi, and pHi during the experimental time course are shown in Figure 2. No difference was found between groups in baseline conditions and during ischemia for PCr (Figure 2A) and ATP (Figure 2B) heart contents. However, during reperfusion, PCr and ATP heart contents were significantly decreased in GK and GK-P when compared with CTRL ($p < 0.05$). RSV restored PCr and ATP contents to control values during reperfusion. In baseline conditions, Pi (Figure 2C) was not different between groups. During ischemia, Pi was significantly higher in GK and GK-P in comparison with CTRL (respectively $p < 0.001$ and $p < 0.05$). RSV was able to prevent the increase in Pi in GK-RSV rats. No statistical difference was found between CTRL and GK-RSV, and Pi was significantly lower in GK-RSV vs. GK ($p < 0.001$). Finally, pHi (Figure 2D) was identical between groups in baseline conditions. During ischemia, pHi was significantly decreased in GK ($p < 0.01$ vs. CTRL). During reperfusion, pHi was significantly decreased in GK and GK-P compared with GK-RSV (respectively $p < 0.01$ and $p < 0.05$). RSV treatment restored pHi in GK-RSV to control values.

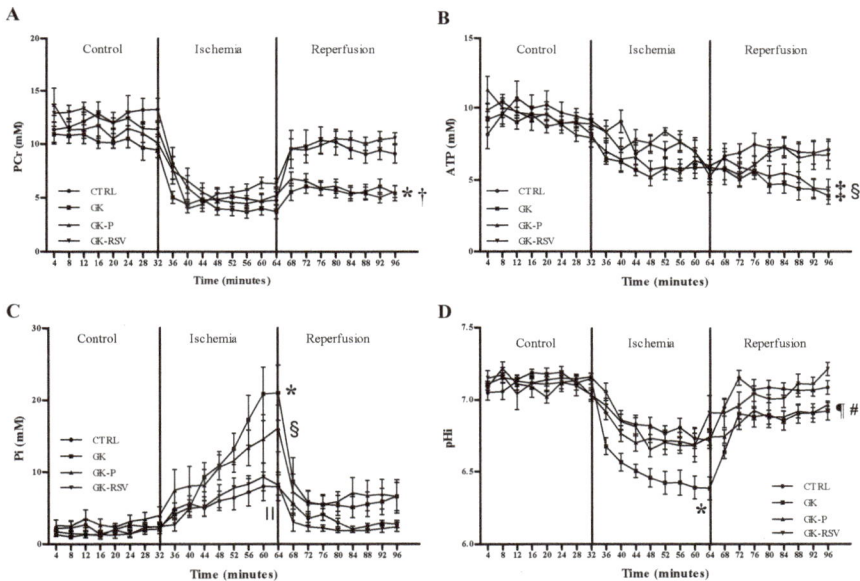

Figure 2. Kinetics of phosphocreatine (PCr) (**A**), ATP (**B**), Pi (**C**), and intracellular pH (pHi) (**D**) during the experimental time course in rat hearts. Data are expressed as means ± SEM. Two-way ANOVA was performed to observe the effect of group and time. * $p < 0.01$ GK vs. CTRL, † $p < 0.01$ GK-P vs. CTRL, ‡ $p < 0.05$ GK vs. CTRL, § $p < 0.05$ GK-P vs. CTRL, II $p < 0.001$ GK-RSV vs. GK, ¶ $p < 0.05$ GK-P vs. GK-RSV, and # $p < 0.01$ GK vs. GK-RSV.

Biochemical Analysis in Freeze-Clamped Hearts

Considering the improvements made by the RSV on high-energy compound contents during ex vivo experiments, we carried out additional biochemical analyses in freeze-clamped hearts. First, a total pool of PCr, creatine, ATP, and total adenine nucleotides (TAN) were assessed using HLPC as shown in Figure 3A. PCr was significantly decreased in GK and GK-P in comparison to CTRL ($p < 0.05$). RSV restored PCr heart content in GK-RSV, which was significantly different compared with GK ($p < 0.01$) and GK-P ($p < 0.05$). Creatine was not different between CTRL, GK, and GK-P groups.

RSV treatment increased creatine heart content in GK-RSV versus GK ($p < 0.001$) and GK-P ($p < 0.05$). The sum of creatine and phosphocreatine was significantly increased in GK-RSV in comparison to GK ($p < 0.001$) and GK-P ($p < 0.01$). ATP was significantly decreased in GK and GK-P in comparison to CTRL ($p < 0.01$). RSV increased ATP content in GK-RSV versus GK and GK-P (respectively $p < 0.01$ and $p < 0.05$). TAN was significantly decreased in GK and GK-P in comparison to CTRL ($p < 0.01$). RSV restored TAN in GK-RSV, which was increased in comparison to GK ($p < 0.01$) and GK-P ($p < 0.05$). These results are in line with energy metabolism measured by ^{31}P MRS. AMP, ADP, and energy charge results are shown in the supplementary material (Figure S1). No statistical difference was found between groups for AMP content. ADP content was significantly decreased only in GK versus CTRL ($p < 0.05$). RSV increased ADP content but it did not reach statistical difference. No difference was found between groups for energy charge. Second, citrate synthase activity (Figure 3B) was also assessed in freeze-clamped hearts. Citrate synthase activity was significantly increased by RSV treatment in GK-RSV in comparison to the other groups ($p < 0.0001$). Together these results indicate that RSV could improve cardiac mitochondrial function in type 2 diabetic female rats.

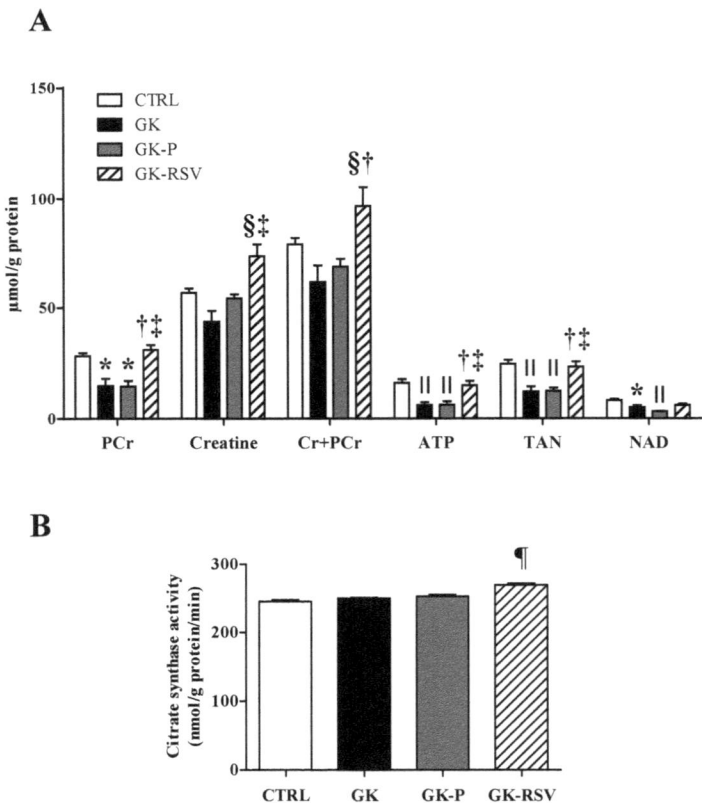

Figure 3. Total pool of phosphocreatine, creatine, PCr + Cr, ATP, total adenine nucleotides (TAN) (**A**) and citrate synthase activity (**B**) in rat hearts. Data are expressed as means ± SEM and one-way ANOVA was used to compare the groups. * $p < 0.05$ vs. CTRL, † $p < 0.01$ vs. GK, ‡ $p < 0.05$ vs. GK-P, § $p < 0.001$ vs. GK; II $p < 0.01$ vs. CTRL; and ¶ $p < 0.0001$ vs. CTRL, GK, and GK-P.

3.2.3. Coronary Flow and Expression of Proteins Involved in NO Pathway

Before ischemia (Figure 4A), CF was significantly decreased in GK-P in comparison to GK-RSV ($p < 0.05$). During reperfusion (Figure 4B), CF was significantly impaired in GK and GK-P in comparison to CTRL ($p < 0.01$). Treatment with RSV maintained CF during reperfusion to control values in GK-RSV.

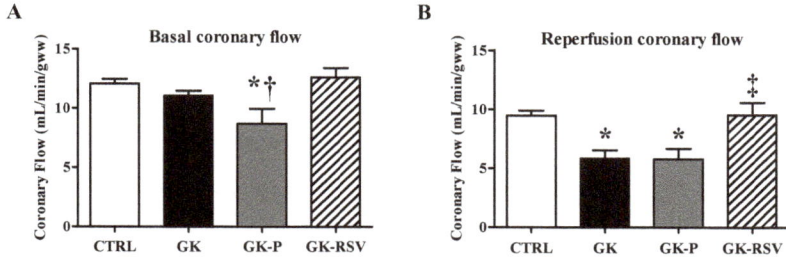

Figure 4. Baseline coronary flow evaluated at 20 min (**A**) and reperfusion coronary flow evaluated at 80 min (**B**). Data are expressed as means ± SEM and one-way ANOVA was used to compare the groups. * $p < 0.05$ vs. CTRL, † $p < 0.01$ vs. GK-RSV, and ‡ $p < 0.05$ vs. GK and GK-P.

Complementary to the coronary flow measurement, we assessed the expression of eNOS, SIRT1, Akt and P-Akt proteins involved in the NO pathway in freeze-clamped hearts. Expression of eNOS, Akt, PAkt (Ser 473), and SIRT1 protein is shown in Figure 5. eNOS protein expression was significantly increased in GK-RSV in comparison to the three other groups ($p < 0.05$ vs. CTRL and GK-P; $p < 0.01$ vs. GK). Akt protein was similarly expressed in the four groups. The phosphorylated form of Akt was significantly increased in GK-RSV vs. CTRL and GK-P ($p < 0.05$). SIRT1 was increased in GK-RSV compared to the other groups ($p < 0.05$). These results suggest an improvement of NO pathway by RSV leading to higher coronary flow during reperfusion. iNOS was not expressed in the four groups (data not shown).

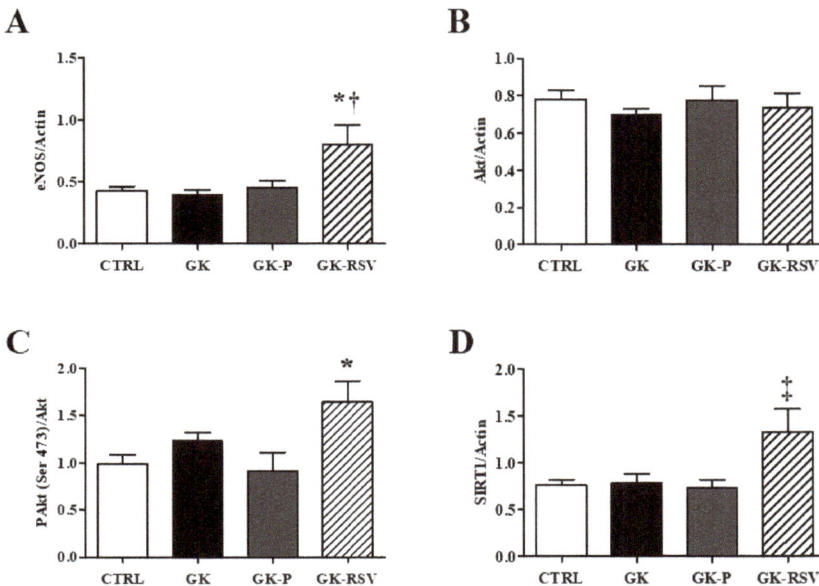

Figure 5. *Cont.*

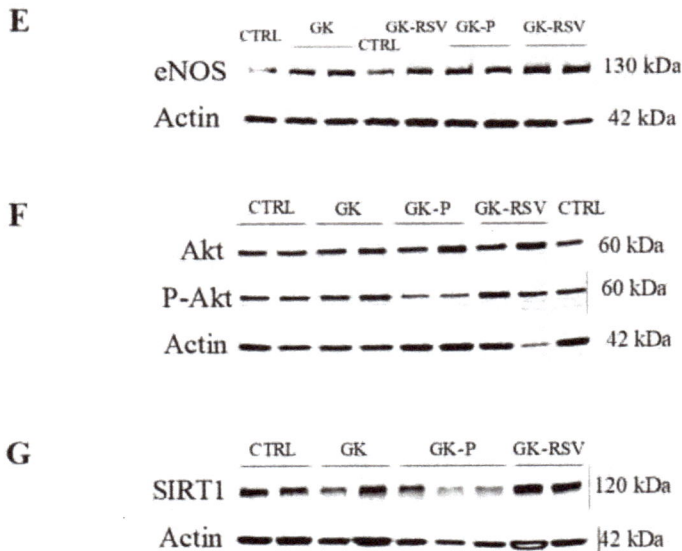

Figure 5. Protein expression of eNOS (**A**), Akt (**B**), PAkt (Ser 473) (**C**), and SIRT1 (**D**). Representative western blot of eNOS (**E**), Akt and its phosphorylated form (**F**), and SIRT1 (**G**). Data are expressed as means ± SEM and one-way ANOVA to compare the groups. * $p < 0.05$ vs. CTRL and GK-P; † $p < 0.01$ vs. GK; and ‡ $p < 0.05$ vs. CTRL, GK, and GK-P.

Oxidative Stress

SIRT3 protein expression and MDA heart content were not different between groups, with no effect of RSV (Supplementary Material, Figures S2 and S3).

4. Discussion

The main objective of this study was to investigate the potential protective effects of RSV on high-energy compounds during ischemia-reperfusion injury in type 2 diabetic female rat hearts. We found in GK rat hearts a lower tolerance to ischemia-reperfusion injury, characterized by impaired energy metabolism and associated with a decrease in functional recovery and coronary flow. Eight-week treatment with a low dose of RSV was able to protect the heart from the loss of energetic compounds during reperfusion and to improve cardiac function and coronary flow. Biochemical analyses confirmed the positive effects of RSV on ATP and PCr, as well as TAN, creatine, and citrate synthase activity, which are indicators of mitochondrial function. Moreover, the improvement of coronary flow during reperfusion by RSV was associated to increased eNOS, SIRT1, and P-Akt protein expression in GK rat hearts.

RSV has been associated to the French paradox, which reflects the lower incidence and mortality by CV disease in the French population, as a link with daily consumption of red wine [32]. As specified in the introduction, a dose of less than 1 mg/kg/day may not have cardiovascular effects [18], while a high dose may damage the heart during an ischemia-reperfusion injury [24]. Thus, the dose used in our study seems to be a good compromise.

The Goto-Kakizaki rat is one of the best characterized animal models of spontaneous type 2 diabetes [33] presenting cardiac insulin resistance and CV complications [34]. Here we found cardiac hypertrophy and basal cardiac dysfunction in GK vs. CTRL due to the decrease of both developed pressure and heart rate. The modification of high energy compounds does not explain the impaired cardiac function found in baseline conditions. Interestingly, the alteration of excitation–contraction coupling [35] and the downregulation and upregulation of multiple genes, such as Trpc6 or Ryr2, involved in the activity of the sinoatrial node [36] have been previously reported in GK rats and could explain the impairment in myocardial function shown here. RSV had no effect on cardiac function prior to ischemic insult, as previously reported by Robich et al. [37]. However, 1 mg/kg/day of RSV decreased cardiac hypertrophy and improved the myocardial tolerance to ischemia-reperfusion injury. Recently, Bagul et al. showed cardiac hypertrophy with increased cardiac cell size in rats under a high-fat diet, with a reverse effect of RSV administered in the food at 10 mg/kg/day for 8 weeks [19]. Lin et al. pointed out the decrease of atrial natriuretic peptide and TGF1β related to reduced infarct size in animals treated with RSV by intraperitoneal injection for 4 weeks [18]. RSV has also been shown to reduce pro-hypertrophic markers such as ANP, BNP, and β-MHC, and improve redox balance by increasing SOD [13] in streptozotocin (STZ) and high-fat model of type 2 diabetes. Interestingly, placebo treatment also showed a decrease in cardiac hypertrophy in type 2 diabetic rats. Placebo treatment (ethanol 1‰) may have an effect on cardiac hypertrophy, as suggested by Ninh et al. in a rodent model of pressure overload with cardiac hypertrophy [38]. Moreover, Miyamae et al. also showed a higher myocardial tolerance to ischemia-reperfusion injury in animals treated with ethanol [39]. Nonetheless, the authors used up to 20% of ethanol in the drinking water, which might explain why we did not see an effect on the tolerance to ischemia-reperfusion injury in our study.

Myocardial tolerance to ischemia-reperfusion injury was impaired in type 2 diabetic GK rats and was associated with altered energy metabolism, characterized by a decrease in high energy compound contents. Indeed, mitochondrial dysfunction has been widely suggested to explain the mechanisms involved in heart failure of diabetic patients [40]. Studies on type 2 diabetic animals also showed decreased expression of mitochondrial respiratory chain complexes, and mitochondrial biogenesis through PGC1α [41]. Interestingly, a previous study on the GK model showed impaired cardiac function during ischemia-reperfusion injury, without alteration of energy metabolism in male gender [27]. In addition, Billimoria et al. showed a decrease of mitochondrial respiration in diabetic STZ rat hearts with a higher impairment in female than in male [42], unlike female GK here. Remarkably, RSV improved high energy compounds during reperfusion in GK-RSV rats and this observation may explain the better myocardial functional recovery. ATP and PCr were significantly increased in GK-RSV rats, up to control values. In parallel RSV prevented the high increase in Pi during ischemia and decrease in pHi during reperfusion. Consistent with these results, HPLC analysis in the cardiac tissue highlighted the restoration in ATP and PCr heart contents in GK-RSV at the end of reperfusion. In addition, we showed a preservation in the pool of creatine and TAN, crucial for ATP and PCr synthesis, in type 2 diabetic animals under RSV after ischemic insult. Here, RSV treatment also increased CS activity in GK rat hearts, as recently reported by Lagouge et al. in mice treated orally with a dose of 400 mg/kg/day RSV, indicating enhanced mitochondrial enzymatic activity [43]. Consequently, taken together, our results suggest that the RSV-induced cardioprotection against ischemia-reperfusion injury in type 2 diabetes could be associated to better mitochondrial functioning. In the literature, mitochondrial function has been shown to be improved by RSV via increase in mitochondrial DNA, biogenesis mitochondrial factor PGC1α [13], Nrf-1, and Tfam mRNA expression [44], and decrease in the opening of mitochondrial transition pore [21]. Further studies need to be performed to elucidate the molecular mechanisms involved in the RSV-induced mitochondrial protection.

On the other hand, the expression of the SIRT3 protein, a mitochondrial sirtuin involved in mitochondrial function and oxidative stress [45], was the same in all groups. This result is consistent with MDA heart content which was also similar in all groups. Thus, the improvement of energy metabolism by RSV was independent from SIRT3 and oxidative stress.

Multiple studies have shown the effect of RSV, a well-known SIRT1 activator, on endothelial function [14–17]. Here, we assessed coronary flow and expression of proteins involved in NO pathway as indicators of endothelial function. During reperfusion, coronary flow was altered in both GK and GK-P versus CTRL. No difference was shown in eNOS, Akt, P-Akt, and SIRT1 expression, between CTRL and GK rats, although previous studies reported decreased eNOS expression in type 2 diabetes. The literature is still inconclusive concerning the expression of eNOS in type 2 diabetes. Indeed, some studies reported a decrease [46] while others showed an increase [27] in eNOS expression. Interestingly, RSV was able to fully restore the coronary flow during reperfusion and to significantly increase the expression of eNOS, P-Akt, and SIRT1 proteins in GK rat hearts. Previously, Huang et al. showed that RSV increased the expression of P-Akt and eNOS in the thoracic aorta of rats under high-fat diet [47]. In type 2 diabetic db/db mice, RSV also enhance cardiac NO production and eNOS protein expression [48]. More generally, RSV has also been shown to enhance NO production, increase NOS expression and activity, prevent eNOS uncoupling and increase NO bioavailability [9]. In fact, increasing NO production and bioavailability via eNOS is one of the mechanisms involved in cardioprotection against ischemia-reperfusion [49]. Then, exploring the phosphorylated form of eNOS, eNOS uncoupling or NO availability could help us understand the higher coronary flow reported in GK-RSV rats during reperfusion. Remarkably, RSV increased tolerance to ischemia-reperfusion injury independently from glycemic improvements. Indeed, we did not observe any effect on glycemia with a low-dose of 1 mg/kg/day. Some studies present RSV as a new potential anti-diabetic treatment when used at high dose [13,50]. The mechanisms involved might go through the increase in GLP-1 secretion [50], beta cell insulin secretion, beta cell gene expression, or improvement of insulin sensitivity [51]. At this point, it is important to remind that the GK model presents mild hyperglycemia, which could explain why effects of RSV might go unnoticed. Therefore, we may suppose an estrogen-like effect of RSV on mitochondrial and endothelial pathways, which could improve tolerance to ischemia-reperfusion injury, independently from glycemic control. Estrogens have positive effects on vessels by improving vasorelaxation [52] and on key regulators of energy metabolism and mitochondrial biogenesis (PGC1α) [13]. Moreover, RSV has an estrogen-like effect by activating estrogen receptors at nuclear and extracellular levels [53]. Recently, RSV has shown better effects on metabolic parameters in female controls than in ovariectomized female rats [54]. It would, therefore, be interesting to assess the effects of RSV on ovariectomized female GK rats to better understand the involvement of hormones in cardiovascular RSV effects.

In conclusion, RSV had a protective effect against ischemia-reperfusion injury via increased high energy compound contents and eNOS-SIRT1 expression in type 2 diabetic female rat heart. We believe our results could contribute to a better understanding of the mechanisms involved in RSV-induced cardioprotection. As type 2 diabetic women present a high risk of mortality by myocardial infarction, low dose of RSV supplementation could be an interesting way to improve myocardial infarction survival. Indeed, mitochondrial and endothelial dysfunctions have been reported in the type 2 diabetic patients, with a decrease in PCr/ATP ratio in the heart and a high rate of coronary artery diseases. Thus, RSV presents high potential for preventing and treating cardiovascular complications of type 2 diabetic women.

Supplementary Materials: The following are available online at http://www.mdpi.com/2072-6643/11/1/105/s1. Figure S1: AMP (A), ADP (B) and EC*10 (C) in rat hearts, Figure S2: Protein expression of SIRT3 in rat hearts, Figure S3: MDA heart content in rat hearts.

Author Contributions: All the authors participated substantially in the investigations reported here as indicated: N.F. contributed to design, performed the experiments, data analysis, and wrote the paper; C.L. contributed to experiments; E.S. contributed to the design of the study; M.B. and M.D. contributed to design, interpretation of the overall study, and manuscript writing. All authors read and approved the final manuscript.

Funding: This work was supported by Aix-Marseille Université, CNRS (UMR 7339), and France Life Imaging (ANR-11-INBS-0006). We further acknowledge funding from Agence Nationale de la Recherche (ANR-14-CE17-0016–COFLORES) and Fondation pour la Recherche Médicale (FRM DBS20140930772).

Acknowledgments: We thank Laurent Pechere from YVERY for providing RSV treatment. We also would like to thank Jamileh Movassat and Danielle Bailbé who contributed to animal supply.

Conflicts of Interest: The authors declare no conflict of interest. The providing funding were not involved in the study design; in collection, analysis and interpretation of data; in the writing of the report; or in the decision to submit the article for publication.

References

1. Peters, S.A.; Huxley, R.R.; Woodward, M. Diabetes as risk factor for incident coronary heart disease in women compared with men: A systematic review and meta-analysis of 64 cohorts including 858,507 individuals and 28,203 coronary events. *Diabetologia* **2014**, *57*, 1542–1551. [CrossRef] [PubMed]
2. Regensteiner, J.G.; Golden, S.; Huebschmann, A.G.; Barrett-Connor, E.; Chang, A.Y.; Chyun, D.; Fox, C.S.; Kim, C.; Mehta, N.; Reckelhoff, J.F.; et al. Sex Differences in the Cardiovascular Consequences of Diabetes Mellitus: A Scientific Statement From the American Heart Association. *Circulation* **2015**, *132*, 2424–2447. [CrossRef] [PubMed]
3. Kannel, W.B.; Hjortland, M.; Castelli, W.P. Role of diabetes in congestive heart failure: The Framingham study. *Am. J. Cardiol.* **1974**, *34*, 29–34. [CrossRef]
4. Wannamethee, S.G.; Papacosta, O.; Lawlor, D.A.; Whincup, P.H.; Lowe, G.D.; Ebrahim, S.; Sattar, N. Do women exhibit greater differences in established and novel risk factors between diabetes and non-diabetes than men? The British Regional Heart Study and British Women's Heart Health Study. *Diabetologia* **2012**, *55*, 80–87. [CrossRef] [PubMed]
5. Hu, G.; Jousilahti, P.; Qiao, Q.; Katoh, S.; Tuomilehto, J. Sex differences in cardiovascular and total mortality among diabetic and non-diabetic individuals with or without history of myocardial infarction. *Diabetologia* **2005**, *48*, 856–861. [CrossRef] [PubMed]
6. Desrois, M.; Lan, C.; Movassat, J.; Bernard, M. Reduced up-regulation of the nitric oxide pathway and impaired endothelial and smooth muscle functions in the female type 2 diabetic goto-kakizaki rat heart. *Nutr. Metab.* **2017**, *14*, 6. [CrossRef] [PubMed]
7. Cefalu, W.T.; Kaul, S.; Gerstein, H.C.; Holman, R.R.; Zinman, B.; Skyler, J.S.; Green, J.B.; Buse, J.B.; Inzucchi, S.E.; Leiter, L.A.; et al. Cardiovascular Outcomes Trials in Type 2 Diabetes: Where Do We Go From Here? Reflections From a Diabetes Care Editors' Expert Forum. *Diabetes Care* **2018**, *41*, 14–31. [CrossRef]
8. Selvaraju, V.; Joshi, M.; Kotha, S.R.; Parinandi, N.L.; Maulik, N. Resveratrol Emerges as a Miracle Cardioprotective Phytochemical Polyphenol and Nutraceutical. In *Cardiovascular Diseases: Nutritional and Therapeutic Interventions*; CRC Press: Boca Raton, FL, USA, 2013; pp. 401–420.
9. Xia, N.; Forstermann, U.; Li, H. Resveratrol and endothelial nitric oxide. *Molecules* **2014**, *19*, 16102–16121. [CrossRef]
10. Luciano, T.F.; Marques, S.D.O.; Pieri, B.L.D.S.; Souza, D.R.D.; Lira, F.S.D.; Souza, C.T.D. Resveratrol reduces chronic inflammation and improves insulin action in the myocardium of high-fat diet-induced obese rats. *Rev. Nutr.* **2014**, *27*, 151–159. [CrossRef]
11. Su, H.C.; Hung, L.M.; Chen, J.K. Resveratrol, a red wine antioxidant, possesses an insulin-like effect in streptozotocin-induced diabetic rats. *Am. J. Physiol. Endocrinol. Metab.* **2006**, *290*, E1339–E1346. [CrossRef]
12. Do, G.M.; Kwon, E.Y.; Kim, H.J.; Jeon, S.M.; Ha, T.Y.; Park, T.; Choi, M.S. Long-term effects of resveratrol supplementation on suppression of atherogenic lesion formation and cholesterol synthesis in apo E-deficient mice. *Biochem. Biophys. Res. Commun.* **2008**, *374*, 55–59. [CrossRef] [PubMed]
13. Fang, W.J.; Wang, C.J.; He, Y.; Zhou, Y.L.; Peng, X.D.; Liu, S.K. Resveratrol alleviates diabetic cardiomyopathy in rats by improving mitochondrial function through PGC-1alpha deacetylation. *Acta Pharmacol. Sin.* **2018**, *39*, 59–73. [CrossRef] [PubMed]
14. Li, H.; Forstermann, U. Pharmacological prevention of eNOS uncoupling. *Curr. Pharm. Des.* **2014**, *20*, 3595–3606. [CrossRef] [PubMed]
15. Silan, C. The effects of chronic resveratrol treatment on vascular responsiveness of streptozotocin-induced diabetic rats. *Biol. Pharm. Bull.* **2008**, *31*, 897–902. [CrossRef] [PubMed]
16. Bhatt, S.R.; Lokhandwala, M.F.; Banday, A.A. Resveratrol prevents endothelial nitric oxide synthase uncoupling and attenuates development of hypertension in spontaneously hypertensive rats. *Eur. J. Pharmacol.* **2011**, *667*, 258–264. [CrossRef] [PubMed]
17. Fukuda, S.; Kaga, S.; Zhan, L.; Bagchi, D.; Das, D.K.; Bertelli, A.; Maulik, N. Resveratrol ameliorates myocardial damage by inducing vascular endothelial growth factor-angiogenesis and tyrosine kinase receptor Flk-1. *Cell. Biochem. Biophys.* **2006**, *44*, 43–49. [CrossRef]

18. Lin, J.F.; Lin, S.M.; Chih, C.L.; Nien, M.W.; Su, H.H.; Hu, B.R.; Huang, S.S.; Tsai, S.K. Resveratrol reduces infarct size and improves ventricular function after myocardial ischemia in rats. *Life Sci.* **2008**, *83*, 313–317. [CrossRef]

19. Bagul, P.K.; Banerjee, S.K. Application of resveratrol in diabetes: Rationale, strategies and challenges. *Curr. Mol. Med.* **2015**, *15*, 312–330. [CrossRef]

20. Chen, T.; Li, J.; Liu, J.; Li, N.; Wang, S.; Liu, H.; Zeng, M.; Zhang, Y.; Bu, P. Activation of SIRT3 by resveratrol ameliorates cardiac fibrosis and improves cardiac function via the TGF-beta/Smad3 pathway. *Am. J. Physiol. Heart Circ. Physiol.* **2015**, *308*, H424–H434. [CrossRef]

21. Meng, Z.; Jing, H.; Gan, L.; Li, H.; Luo, B. Resveratrol attenuated estrogen-deficient-induced cardiac dysfunction: Role of AMPK, SIRT1, and mitochondrial function. *Am. J. Transl. Res.* **2016**, *8*, 2641–2649.

22. Shah, A.; Reyes, L.M.; Morton, J.S.; Fung, D.; Schneider, J.; Davidge, S.T. Effect of resveratrol on metabolic and cardiovascular function in male and female adult offspring exposed to prenatal hypoxia and a high-fat diet. *J. Physiol.* **2016**, *594*, 1465–1482. [CrossRef]

23. Rocha, K.K.; Souza, G.A.; Ebaid, G.X.; Seiva, F.R.; Cataneo, A.C.; Novelli, E.L. Resveratrol toxicity: Effects on risk factors for atherosclerosis and hepatic oxidative stress in standard and high-fat diets. *Food Chem. Toxicol.* **2009**, *47*, 1362–1367. [CrossRef] [PubMed]

24. Dudley, J.I.; Lekli, I.; Mukherjee, S.; Das, M.; Bertelli, A.A.A.; Das, D.K. Does White Wine Qualify for French Paradox? Comparison of the Cardioprotective Effects of Red and White Wines and Their Constituents: Resveratrol, Tyrosol, and Hydroxytyrosol (Retraction of vol 56, pg 9362, 2008). *J. Agric. Food Chem.* **2012**, *60*, 2767. [CrossRef] [PubMed]

25. Portha, B. Programmed disorders of beta-cell development and function as one cause for type 2 diabetes? The GK rat paradigm. *Diabetes Metab. Res. Rev.* **2005**, *21*, 495–504. [CrossRef] [PubMed]

26. Ferreira, M.P.; Willoughby, D. Alcohol consumption: The good, the bad, and the indifferent. *Appl. Physiol. Nutr. Metab.* **2008**, *33*, 12–20. [CrossRef] [PubMed]

27. Desrois, M.; Clarke, K.; Lan, C.; Dalmasso, C.; Cole, M.; Portha, B.; Cozzone, P.J.; Bernard, M. Upregulation of eNOS and unchanged energy metabolism in increased susceptibility of the aging type 2 diabetic GK rat heart to ischemic injury. *Am. J. Physiol. Heart Circ. Physiol.* **2010**, *299*, H1679–H1686. [CrossRef] [PubMed]

28. Oliver, M.F. Fatty acids and the risk of death during acute myocardial ischaemia. *Clin. Sci.* **2015**, *128*, 349–355. [CrossRef]

29. Desrois, M.; Sciaky, M.; Lan, C.; Cozzone, P.J.; Bernard, M. L-arginine during long-term ischemia: Effects on cardiac function, energetic metabolism and endothelial damage. *J. Heart Lung Transpl.* **2000**, *19*, 367–376. [CrossRef]

30. Lazzarino, G.; Nuutinen, M.; Tavazzi, B.; Di Pierro, D.; Giardina, B. A method for preparing freeze-clamped tissue samples for metabolite analyses. *Anal. Biochem.* **1989**, *181*, 239–241. [CrossRef]

31. Lowry, O.H.; Rosebrough, N.J.; Farr, A.L.; Randall, R.J. Protein measurement with the Folin phenol reagent. *J. Biol. Chem.* **1951**, *193*, 265–275.

32. Renaud, S.; de Lorgeril, M. Wine, alcohol, platelets, and the French paradox for coronary heart disease. *Lancet* **1992**, *339*, 1523–1526. [CrossRef]

33. Portha, B.; Giroix, M.H.; Tourrel-Cuzin, C.; Le-Stunff, H.; Movassat, J. The GK rat: A prototype for the study of non-overweight type 2 diabetes. *Methods Mol. Biol.* **2012**, *933*, 125–159. [CrossRef] [PubMed]

34. Desrois, M.; Sidell, R.J.; Gauguier, D.; King, L.M.; Radda, G.K.; Clarke, K. Initial steps of insulin signaling and glucose transport are defective in the type 2 diabetic rat heart. *Cardiovasc. Res.* **2004**, *61*, 288–296. [CrossRef] [PubMed]

35. Salem, K.A.; Qureshi, M.A.; Sydorenko, V.; Parekh, K.; Jayaprakash, P.; Iqbal, T.; Singh, J.; Oz, M.; Adrian, T.E.; Howarth, F.C. Effects of exercise training on excitation-contraction coupling and related mRNA expression in hearts of Goto-Kakizaki type 2 diabetic rats. *Mol. Cell. Biochem.* **2013**, *380*, 83–96. [CrossRef] [PubMed]

36. Howarth, F.C.; Qureshi, M.A.; Jayaprakash, P.; Parekh, K.; Oz, M.; Dobrzynski, H.; Adrian, T.E. The Pattern of mRNA Expression Is Changed in Sinoatrial Node from Goto-Kakizaki Type 2 Diabetic Rat Heart. *J. Diabetes Res.* **2018**, *2018*, 8454078. [CrossRef] [PubMed]

37. Robich, M.P.; Chu, L.M.; Burgess, T.A.; Feng, J.; Han, Y.; Nezafat, R.P.; Leber, M.P.; Laham, R.J.; Manning, W.J.; Sellke, F.W. Resveratrol Preserves Myocardial Function and Perfusion in Remote Nonischemic Myocardium in a Swine Model of Metabolic Syndrome. *J. Am. College Surg.* **2012**, *215*, 681–689. [CrossRef] [PubMed]

38. Ninh, V.K.; El Hajj, E.C.; Mouton, A.J.; El Hajj, M.C.; Gilpin, N.W.; Gardner, J.D. Chronic Ethanol Administration Prevents Compensatory Cardiac Hypertrophy in Pressure Overload. *Alcohol. Clin. Exp. Res.* **2018**. [CrossRef] [PubMed]
39. Miyamae, M.; Diamond, I.; Weiner, M.W.; Camacho, S.A.; Figueredo, V.M. Regular alcohol consumption mimics cardiac preconditioning by protecting against ischemia-reperfusion injury. *Proc. Natl. Acad. Sci. USA* **1997**, *94*, 3235–3239. [CrossRef]
40. Montaigne, D.; Marechal, X.; Coisne, A.; Debry, N.; Modine, T.; Fayad, G.; Potelle, C.; El Arid, J.M.; Mouton, S.; Sebti, Y.; et al. Myocardial contractile dysfunction is associated with impaired mitochondrial function and dynamics in type 2 diabetic but not in obese patients. *Circulation* **2014**, *130*, 554–564. [CrossRef]
41. Rovira-Llopis, S.; Banuls, C.; Diaz-Morales, N.; Hernandez-Mijares, A.; Rocha, M.; Victor, V.M. Mitochondrial dynamics in type 2 diabetes: Pathophysiological implications. *Redox Biol.* **2017**, *11*, 637–645. [CrossRef]
42. Billimoria, F.R.; Katyare, S.S.; Patel, S.P. Insulin status differentially affects energy transduction in cardiac mitochondria from male and female rats. *Diabetes Obes. Metab.* **2006**, *8*, 67–74. [CrossRef] [PubMed]
43. Lagouge, M.; Argmann, C.; Gerhart-Hines, Z.; Meziane, H.; Lerin, C.; Daussin, F.; Messadeq, N.; Milne, J.; Lambert, P.; Elliott, P.; Geny, B.; Laakso, M.; Puigserver, P.; Auwerx, J. Resveratrol Improves Mitochondrial Function and Protects against Metabolic Disease by Activating SIRT1 and PGC-1α. *Cell.* **2006**, *127*, 1109–1122. [CrossRef] [PubMed]
44. Csiszar, A.; Labinskyy, N.; Pinto, J.T.; Ballabh, P.; Zhang, H.; Losonczy, G.; Pearson, K.; de Cabo, R.; Pacher, P.; Zhang, C.; et al. Resveratrol induces mitochondrial biogenesis in endothelial cells. *Am. J. Physiol. Heart Circ. Physiol.* **2009**, *297*, H13–H20. [CrossRef] [PubMed]
45. Osborne, B.; Bentley, N.L.; Montgomery, M.K.; Turner, N. The role of mitochondrial sirtuins in health and disease. *Free Radic. Biol. Med.* **2016**, *100*, 164–174. [CrossRef] [PubMed]
46. Zhang, R.; Thor, D.; Han, X.; Anderson, L.; Rahimian, R. Sex differences in mesenteric endothelial function of streptozotocin-induced diabetic rats: A shift in the relative importance of EDRFs. *Am. J. Physiol. Heart Circ. Physiol.* **2012**, *303*, H1183–H1198. [CrossRef] [PubMed]
47. Huang, J.P.; Hsu, S.C.; Li, D.E.; Chen, K.H.; Kuo, C.Y.; Hung, L.M. Resveratrol Mitigates High-Fat Diet-Induced Vascular Dysfunction by Activating the Akt/eNOS/NO and Sirt1/ER Pathway. *J. Cardiovasc. Pharmacol.* **2018**, *72*, 231–241. [CrossRef] [PubMed]
48. Zhang, H.; Morgan, B.; Potter, B.J.; Ma, L.; Dellsperger, K.C.; Ungvari, Z.; Zhang, C. Resveratrol improves left ventricular diastolic relaxation in type 2 diabetes by inhibiting oxidative/nitrative stress: In vivo demonstration with magnetic resonance imaging. *Am. J. Physiol. Heart Circ. Physiol.* **2010**, *299*, H985–H994. [CrossRef]
49. Brunner, F.; Maier, R.; Andrew, P.; Wolkart, G.; Zechner, R.; Mayer, B. Attenuation of myocardial ischemia/reperfusion injury in mice with myocyte-specific overexpression of endothelial nitric oxide synthase. *Cardiovasc. Res.* **2003**, *57*, 55–62. [CrossRef]
50. Dao, T.M.; Waget, A.; Klopp, P.; Serino, M.; Vachoux, C.; Pechere, L.; Drucker, D.J.; Champion, S.; Barthelemy, S.; Barra, Y.; et al. Resveratrol increases glucose induced GLP-1 secretion in mice: A mechanism which contributes to the glycemic control. *PLoS ONE* **2011**, *6*, e20700. [CrossRef]
51. Kong, W.; Chen, L.L.; Zheng, J.; Zhang, H.H.; Hu, X.; Zeng, T.S.; Hu, D. Resveratrol supplementation restores high-fat diet-induced insulin secretion dysfunction by increasing mitochondrial function in islet. *Exp. Biol. Med.* **2015**, *240*, 220–229. [CrossRef]
52. Ventura-Clapier, R.; Moulin, M.; Piquereau, J.; Lemaire, C.; Mericskay, M.; Veksler, V.; Garnier, A. Mitochondria: A central target for sex differences in pathologies. *Clin. Sci.* **2017**, *131*, 803–822. [CrossRef] [PubMed]
53. Turan, B.; Tuncay, E.; Vassort, G. Resveratrol and diabetic cardiac function: Focus on recent in vitro and in vivo studies. *J. Bioenerg. Biomembr.* **2012**, *44*, 281–296. [CrossRef] [PubMed]
54. Sharma, R.; Sharma, N.K.; Thungapathra, M. Resveratrol regulates body weight in healthy and ovariectomized rats. *Nutr. Metab.* **2017**, *14*, 30. [CrossRef] [PubMed]

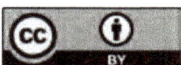

nutrients

MDPI

Review

Resveratrol and Its Human Metabolites—Effects on Metabolic Health and Obesity

Margherita Springer [1,2] and Sofia Moco [1,*]

[1]   Nestle Institute of Health Sciences, Nestle Research, EPFL Innovation Park, Building H, 1015 Lausanne, Switzerland; margherita.springer@rd.nestle.com
[2]   TUM Graduate School, Technical University of Munich, 85748 Munich, Germany
*   Correspondence: sofia.moco@rd.nestle.com; Tel.: +41-21-632-6165

Received: 22 November 2018; Accepted: 8 January 2019; Published: 11 January 2019

Abstract: Resveratrol is one of the most widely studied polyphenols and it has been assigned a plethora of metabolic effects with potential health benefits. Given its low bioavailability and extensive metabolism, clinical studies using resveratrol have not always replicated in vitro observations. In this review, we discuss human metabolism and biotransformation of resveratrol, and reported molecular mechanisms of action, within the context of metabolic health and obesity. Resveratrol has been described as mimicking caloric restriction, leading to improved exercise performance and insulin sensitivity (increasing energy expenditure), as well as having a body fat-lowering effect by inhibiting adipogenesis, and increasing lipid mobilization in adipose tissue. These multi-organ effects place resveratrol as an anti-obesity bioactive of potential therapeutic use.

Keywords: resveratrol; polyphenols; metabolism; obesity; diabetes; metabolic pathways

1. Introduction

Resveratrol (3,5,4'-trihydroxy-*trans*-stilbene, RSV, Figure 1.1) is one of the most widely studied polyphenols with over ten thousand reports in the literature. This stilbene has attracted interest in popular culture over the years for its potential, yet often controversial, health benefits. RSV was first discovered in the roots of the white hellebore (*Veratrum grandiflorum* Loes. fil.) in 1939 [1], even though it is mostly recognized as the phytoalexin present in red wine [2]. When epidemiological studies showed the cardioprotective benefits of wine [3,4], the association with RSV followed [5], opening the field to a wealth of scientific research. RSV has since been identified as: being cancer chemoprotective [6], being anti-inflammatory [7], improving vascular function [8], extending the lifespan and ameliorating aging-related phenotypes [9,10], opposing the effects of a high calorie diet [11], mimicking the effects of calorie restriction [12], and improving cellular function and metabolic health in general [13].

Even though RSV has been widely studied both in vitro and in vivo, its mechanism of action across conditions and doses remains elusive. From the many effects elucidated in in vitro studies, most have failed to reproduce in vivo [14,15]. Reasons for such non-reproducibility among studies are diverse. One reason is its pharmacokinetics, as in humans RSV is highly absorbed orally (~70%), yet has poor systemic bioavailability (~0.5%) [16]. Rapid metabolism into RSV sulfate and glucuronide conjugates occurs, in addition to accumulation in tissues, as detected in radioactive trials and other studies [16–18]. Furthermore, a wide range of inter-individual responses upon oral ingestion of RSV is known in humans and is a common feature of many food bioactives [19,20]. Gut microbiota [20,21] and genetic background [22,23], including enzyme regioselectivity [24], are some of the possible known sources of the variation in responses. In contrast, in vitro studies have described an array of mechanistic effects that generate controversy given the likely non-physiological concentrations used, as well as the omission of the contribution of RSV metabolites [25].

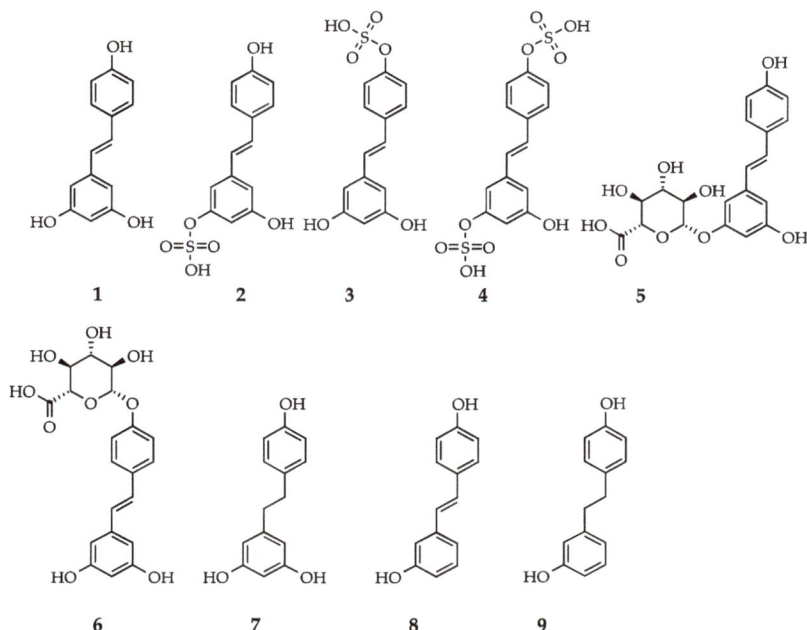

Figure 1. Resveratrol and reported human metabolites: (**1**) *trans*-resveratrol (RSV); (**2**) *trans*-resveratrol-3-*O*-sulfate; (**3**) *trans*-resveratrol-4′-*O*-sulfate; (**4**) *trans*-resveratrol-3,4′-*O*-disulfate; (**5**) *trans*-resveratrol-3-*O*-glucuronide; (**6**) *trans*-resveratrol-4′-*O*-glucuronide; (**7**) dihydroresveratrol (DHR); (**8**) 3,4′-*O*-dihydroxy-*trans*-stilbene; and (**9**) lunularin (also see Table 1).

Obesity is rising worldwide and is mainly attributed to changes in lifestyle, including overconsumption of food and decreased physical activity [26]. When energy intake exceeds energy expenditure over prolonged periods, then an obesity phenotype can develop [27]. Obesity has major health effects, and increased BMI (body mass index) is a risk factor in the development of type 2 diabetes, cardiovascular disease, dyslipidemias, non-alcoholic fatty liver disease, gallstones, Alzheimer's disease and even certain cancers [26,27]. To reduce obesity, lifestyle changes and therapies are aimed at reducing energy consumption or increasing energy expenditure, or both, and/or by managing its side effects. This can be achieved by altering diet and increasing exercise. However not all individuals respond to these lifestyle changes, leading to surgery or drug therapies. For instance, RSV was shown to improve exercise endurance by significantly increasing aerobic capacity and consumption of oxygen in the gastrocnemius muscle in mice. RSV treatment induced oxidative phosphorylation and mitochondrial biogenesis by activating the peroxisome proliferator-activated receptor γ coactivator (PGC1α) through nicotinamide dinucleotide (NAD)-dependent deacetylase sirtuin-1 (SIRT1) leading to improved insulin sensitivity [13]. In addition, RSV has body fat-lowering effects as demonstrated by its anti-lipolytic affect in human adipocytes [28], as well as by decreasing adipocyte size, increasing SIRT1 expression, lowering nuclear factor kappa-light-chain-enhancer of activated B cells (NF-kB) activation and improving insulin sensitivity in visceral white adipose tissue in mice [29].

Even though RSV has been widely studied and associated with many benefits, many open questions remain, such as: (i) the activity of RSV at the nanomolar range, or of its human metabolites at the low micromolar range; (ii) levels of accumulation of these in target tissues able to elicit a biological effect; (iii) given an oral dose which preferred organs will be target sites of activity in which conditions or diseases; (iv) in physiological conditions which and how many protein targets are modulated; (v) how do these effects reproduce among individuals and populations; and (vi) how can one modulate RSV therapeutically. In this review we specifically discuss the role of RSV metabolism to better understand the mechanism of action, with particular emphasis on its potential effects in managing metabolic health and obesity.

2. Human Metabolism of Resveratrol

Being a phytoalexin, RSV levels vary greatly among food sources, seasons and batches. Certain foods are naturally rich in RSV, such as wine, peanuts and selected teas; however, RSV content in dietary sources remains at the lower milligram range [30]. To dose higher levels of RSV, dietary supplements are available in the open market at recommended daily doses between high milligram and gram levels [31]. Once RSV enters the gastro-intestinal tract, it suffers rapid and extensive biotransformation, with distribution into various organs (Figure 2), leading to consequences for its bioavailability and activity.

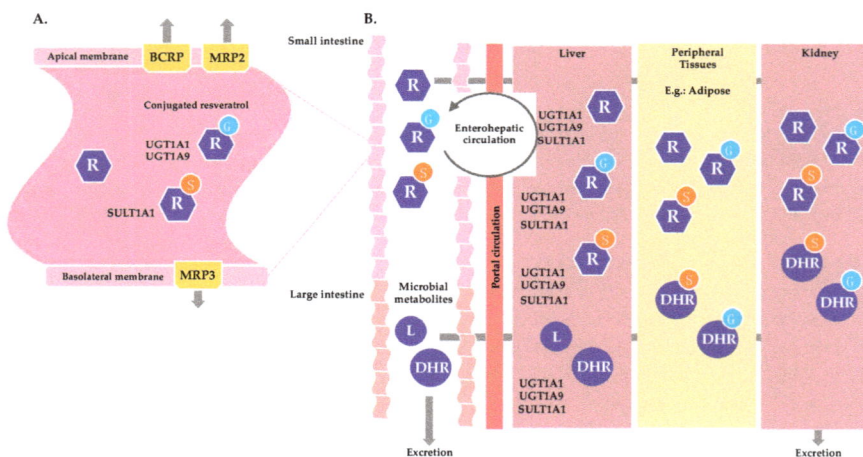

Figure 2. Metabolic fate and biotransformation of resveratrol in the human gastro-intestinal tract, and metabolism in different organs. (**A**) Metabolism of resveratrol (R) in the small intestine's enterocyte. Resveratrol is absorbed into the enterocyte and undergoes sulfation (S) by SULT1A1 and glucuronidation (G) by UGT1A1 and UGTA9. Conjugated resveratrol exits the cell via BRCP and MRP2 transporters on the apical membrane and MRP3 on the basolateral membrane. A small faction of resveratrol escapes conjugation and exits the enterocyte via the basolateral membrane. (**B**) Integrated human metabolism of resveratrol. Resveratrol and conjugated metabolites exit the apical membrane of the small intestine and move towards the large intestine where they can be metabolized by the gut microbiota to generate dihydroresveratrol (DHR), lunularin (L) and 3,4′-dihydroxy-*trans*-stilbene (not shown). Resveratrol and metabolites that exit the enterocyte enter portal circulation. The liver expresses SULT1A1, UGT1A1 and UGTA9, which can further conjugate resveratrol. In addition, conjugated resveratrol and metabolites undergo enterohepatic circulation, leaving the liver to be reabsorbed in the intestine after hydrolysis, and entering portal circulation to reach the liver again for further metabolism. From the liver, resveratrol and metabolites enter systemic circulation and are absorbed by peripheral tissues, such as adipose tissue. The kidneys also participate in the metabolism of resveratrol, leading to excretion of polar resveratrol metabolites.

2.1. RSV is Absorbed and Metabolized in Target Tissues

The major function of the intestine is to digest food, making nutrients available for energy, while preventing the uptake of potentially harmful compounds. Bioactive compounds such as RSV can be perceived by the intestine as xenobiotics and therefore cross the intestinal epithelium to the blood via a transcellular pathway [32]. This route takes place through the enterocytes in the small intestine. Enterocytes, also known as absorptive epithelial cells, are the first site of reported RSV metabolism after being internalized by either passive diffusion [33] or carrier-mediated transport [32]. Once RSV is absorbed into the enterocyte, like other xenobiotics, it undergoes phase II of drug metabolism, producing polar metabolites, with easier excretion in the body. Specifically, RSV undergoes conjugation with sulfate (mediated by sulfotransferases, SULTs) and with glucuronate (mediated by uridine 5'-diphospho-glucuronosyltransferases, UGTs).

Drug metabolism takes place in multiple organs and cell types, and the observed biotransformation differs in metabolite levels [18], enzyme expression [34] and selectivity [24]. The superfamily of SULTs sulfates a broad spectrum of diverse endogenous and exogenous substrates. SULT1A1 is the main enzyme responsible for the transfer of a sulfate group to a hydroxyl group in phenolic compounds [35]. Biochemical studies have shown that, SULT1A1 is the main SULT responsible for the sulfation of RSV into RSV-3-O-sulfate (Figure 1.2), and to a minor extent SULT1A2, SULT1A3 and SULT1E1, whilst RSV-4'O-sulfate (Figure 1.3) is mainly produced by SULT1A2, and RSV-3,4'-O-disulfate (Figure 1.4) is mainly catalyzed by SULT1A2 and SULT1A3 [18,36], Table 1. Similar to the SULT family, UGT is also a large family of related enzymes involved in detoxification, which glucuronidate various substrates [37]. The glucuronidation of RSV is mainly catalyzed by UGT1A1 and UGT1A9, and to a minor extent by UGT1A6, UGT1A7, and UGT1A10 leading to RSV-3-O-glucuronide (Figure 1.5) and/or RSV-4'-O-glucuronide (Figure 1.6) [18], Table 1. In human tissues, the small intestine contains the highest amount of SULT proteins of any tissue, yet preferably expresses SULT1B1, followed by SULT1A3 and then SULT1A1 [34]. In the liver and kidney, however, SULT1A1 is the main SULT protein isoform expressed [34]. SULT1A1 was also recently found in adipocytes, and modulates RSV sulfation in the SGBS (Simpson-Golabi-Behmel syndrome) human adipocyte [28]. Again, the intestine is the human tissue with higher UGT1A content, largely expressing UGT1A10 and 1A1, while the kidney preferably expresses UGT1A9, and the liver expresses UGT1A4, 1A1, 1A6 and 1A9 at the protein level [38]. Of note is the inter-species variation of phase II metabolism in which RSV sulfates are the main conjugates in humans, while glucuronides are the preferred conjugates in pigs and rats [32]. More importantly, drug metabolism is a known cause of inter-individual variability, as both SULTs and UGTs have genetic polymorphisms [22,35]. From animal and human studies, RSV and metabolites thereof have been reported to reach many tissues and biofluids, Table 1.

After absorption and conjugation, RSV sulfates and glucuronides have two fates: they can either be transported through the apical membrane and reach the intestinal lumen or they can pass through the basolateral membrane and enter the bloodstream (Figure 2A). On both membranes, the enterocyte contains ABC (ATP-binding cassette) transporters, which are part of a large family of transport proteins and are considered to be instrumental in drug absorption and response [39]. On the apical side, breast cancer resistance protein (BCRP/ABCG2), multidrug resistance-associated protein 2 (MRP2/ABCC2), and P-glycoprotein (P-gp/MDR1/ABCB1) transporters are expressed, while on the basolateral side, MRP3 (ABCC3) is expressed instead. BCRP and MRP2 play a major role in the efflux of conjugated RSV, while P-gp plays a minor role. On the basolateral membrane, conjugated RSV is transported into blood capillaries by the ABC transporter MRP3 [32]. Transporters are not limited to playing a role in the absorption and distribution of RSV and metabolites in the small intestine, as they are also expressed in other tissues, such as the liver and kidneys [40]. When RSV and metabolites reach the bloodstream, they can be transported by binding to blood proteins such as lipoproteins [5], hemoglobin, and albumin, before reaching other tissues, such as liver, kidney and other peripheral tissues.

Table 1. Human, rat, and mouse resveratrol metabolites after oral administration in different biofluids and tissues (see structures in Figure 1).

Metabolite	Species and Tissue or Biofluid [Reference]
trans-resveratrol	Human: serum [41], plasma [15,16,42], urine [16,20] Rat: plasma [43–45], liver [44], lung [44], brain [44], kidney [44] Mouse: plasma [18,44,46], liver [18,44,46], lung [18,44], brain [44,46], kidney [18,44], heart [18,46], stomach [18], duodenum [18], intestine [18], muscle [18], spleen [18], thymus [18], urine [18], feces [18]
trans-resveratrol-4'-*O*-glucuronide	Human: serum [41], plasma [42], urine [42] Mouse: plasma [46]
trans-resveratrol-3-*O*-glucuronide	Human: serum [41], plasma [42], *urine* [16,42] Rat: plasma [43], liver [47], adipose tissue [47,48], skeletal muscle [47] Mouse: plasma [18,46], liver [18,46], lung [18], brain [46], kidney [18], heart [18,46], stomach [18], duodenum [18], intestine [18], muscle [18], spleen [18], thymus [18], urine [18], feces [18]
trans-resveratrol-diglucuronide	Human: plasma [49], urine [49] Mouse: plasma [46], liver [46]
trans-resveratrol-3-*O*-sulfate	Human: plasma [42], *plasma* [16], *urine* [16] Rat: adipose tissue [47,48] Mouse: plasma [18,46], liver [18,46], lung [18], brain [46], kidney [18], heart [18,46], stomach [18], duodenum [18], intestine [18], muscle [18], spleen [18], thymus [18], urine [18], feces [18]
trans-resveratrol-4'-*O*-sulfate	Human: plasma [42], *plasma* [16], *urine* [16,42] Rat: liver [47], adipose tissue [47,48]
cis-resveratrol-3-*O*-sulfate	Rat: adipose tissue [47,48]
trans-resveratrol-3,4'-disulfate	Human: *plasma* [42] Rat: adipose tissue [48] Mouse: plasma [18], liver [18], lung [18], kidney [18], heart [18], stomach [18], duodenum [18], intestine [18], muscle [18], urine [18], feces [18]
trans-resveratrol-glucuronide-sulfate	Mouse: plasma [46], liver [46]
dihydroresveratrol	Human: urine [20], plasma [15] Rat: liver [47], skeletal muscle [47]
dihydroresveratrol-glucuronide	Human: urine [16] Rat: liver [47] Mouse: plasma [46], liver [46]
dihydroresveratrol-sulfate	Human: urine [16] Rat: liver [47], adipose tissue [47] Mouse: plasma [46], liver [46]
dihydroresveratrol-glucuronide-sulfate	Mouse: plasma [46]
3,4'-dihydroxy-*trans*-stilbene	Human: urine [20]
lunularin	Human: urine [20]

italic: likely identification.

2.2. The Gut Microbiome Metabolizes RSV and RSV Influences Gut Microbial Composition

RSV and the metabolites thereof can be further metabolized in the colon by the gut microbiota (Figure 2B). Here, RSV metabolites may be hydrolyzed, regenerating RSV, and additional reduction reactions may take place. The most described microbial metabolite of RSV is dihydroresveratrol (DHR, Figure 1.7, Table 1). Intestinal bacteria are able to metabolize RSV into DHR by reduction of the double bond between the two phenol rings. DHR produced by the intestinal bacteria can then be absorbed, conjugated and excreted in the urine. In addition to DHR, 3,4'-dihydroxy-*trans*-stilbene (Figure 1.8, Table 1) and lunularin (Figure 1.9, Table 1) have also been identified as gut metabolites of RSV in human urine. A large inter-individual variation between subjects was observed, in which some proved to be lunularin producers, DHR producers or mixed producers, according to levels of these metabolites [20]. Using 16s rRNA sequencing of fecal samples, lunularin producers were associated with a higher abundance of *Bacteroidetes, Actinobacteria, Verrucomicrobia,* and *Cyanobacteria* and a lower abundance of *Firmicutes* than either the DHR or mixed producers. The bacterial strains *Slackia equolifaciens* and *Adlercreutzia equolifaciens*, species not previously known to metabolize RSV, were found to metabolize RSV to DHR [20].

From the gut, RSV microbial metabolites may be absorbed and reach the liver as well as other tissues for further metabolism or excretion. A common feature of certain xenobiotics, including RSV, is the enterohepatic circulation, in which RSV metabolites may go from the liver to the bile and re-enter the intestine. From the small intestine, RSV and metabolites may suffer hydrolysis before reaching the portal circulation and being re-transported into the liver. The extensive presence of RSV and metabolites in the bloodstream can be attributed to enterohepatic circulation [16], Figure 2B.

Beyond the metabolic capacity of the gut microbiota to convert polyphenols such as RSV into often smaller and simpler molecules, the gut microbiota has been associated with other functions. The influence of gut microbiota on the metabolism of polyphenols, and conversely the modulation of the gut microbial composition due to polyphenol intake, are significant topics for understanding the metabolism and activity of these bioactives in humans [19,50]. RSV supplementation is known to alter the microbiome in at least two ways, by acting as an antimicrobial agent and through modulating gut microbial composition. Dao et al. reported that RSV-treated mice lacked three gut bacteria compared to controls: *Parabacteroides jonsonii, Alistipes putredinis* and *Bacteroides vulgatus* [51]. RSV increased levels of *Bifidobacterium* and *Lactobacillus*, while decreasing levels of *Escherichia coli* and Enterobacteria in RSV-treated rats [52]. The antimicrobial activity of RSV against *E. coli* lies in the inhibition of bacterial cell growth by suppressing FtsZ (filamenting temperature-sensitive mutant Z) expression and Z-ring formation, essential for cell division [53]. RSV has a wide range of antimicrobial activity, as it seems to be effective against both gram-positive and gram-negative pathogenic bacteria [54].

RSV supplementation can alter the gut microbial composition and some suggest this may be an essential mechanism of action of RSV [55]. RSV leads to functional changes in the gut microbiome of obese mice, including: decreased relative abundance of *Turicibacteraceae, Moryella, Lachnospiraceae,* and *Akkermansia* and increased relative abundance of *Bacteroides* and *Parabacteroides*. Glucose homeostasis in obese mice was improved by faecal transplantation from healthy RSV-fed donor mice [55]. Obese gut microbiota has been associated with a reduced *Bacteroidetes/Firmicutes* ratio in mice and humans [56] and RSV was found to increase this ratio in rodent studies [55,57]. *Firmicutes*, more prevalent in the obese, produce greater amounts of energy from dietary fiber than other major gut bacterial phyla, such as *Bacteroidetes*, by increasing the production of short chain fatty acids (SCFAs) [58]. Furthermore, an increase in the *Bacteriodetes* population in the gut was also observed in overweight men, upon RSV and epigallocatechin-3-gallate supplementation [59]. *Bacteroidetes* is also associated with postprandial fat oxidation [58]. In addition to SCFAs production, the gut microbiota produces many other small molecules. Dietary choline, L-carnitine and lecithin can be converted into trimethylamine in the gut, which is converted to trimethylamine-*N*-oxide (TMAO) in the liver. TMAO production is associated with chronic diseases like cardiovascular disease, type II diabetes, and obesity [58,60]. RSV supplementation was shown to reduce TMAO production by increasing the *Bacteroidetes* population in the gut of mice [61].

2.3. Biotransformation of RSV Limits Plasma Bioavailability

The metabolic fate of RSV in the body is therefore widespread into different tissues, and its metabolism is rapid and extensive. A preclinical study in rats demonstrated that only a small fraction of RSV (1.5%) is able to escape conjugation and enter the bloodstream unmodified. About 75% enters the enterocyte while the remaining 25% is directly excreted. Once inside the cell, 60% is glucuronidated and 13.5% sulfated. These conjugates partially return to the intestine (42% glucuronides and 12% sulfates), leaving 17% glucuronides and 1.5% sulfates in the bloodstream [32,62]. Administering the metabolites RSV-3-*O*-sulfate (Figure 1.2) and RSV-4'-*O*-sulfate (Figure 1.3) to mice has shown that these metabolites are absorbed yet at low bioavailability (14% and 3%, respectively). Interestingly, regeneration of free RSV (2%) into the bloodstream was observed, indicating in vivo hydrolysis of sulfates, depending on membrane transporter activities [63].

Many studies, both preclinical and clinical, have detected RSV metabolites in plasma (Table 1). Plasma concentration is an indicator of RSV bioavailability and determines the amount of RSV and metabolites available to peripheral target tissues. Regarding human studies, plasma concentration of RSV after single (Table 2) and repeated dosing (Table 3) was measured for studies from 2010 to 2018. Earlier studies have been reviewed already by Cottart et al. [64]. Administered in either single or repeated dosing, the peak levels of RSV in plasma were very low, given its poor bioavailability.

Table 2. Reported resveratrol plasma concentration in humans after a single dose of resveratrol (studies after 2010).

Number of Participants, Characteristics	Dose (mg)	Administration	Peak Plasma Concentration (ng/mL)	Reference
15, healthy	500	Tablet	71.18	[65]
6, low BMI 6, high BMI	2125	Tablet and drink	634.32 498.56	[66]
7, healthy	500	Capsule [1]	1598	[67]
8-9/dose, healthy	250 500	Capsule	5.65 14.4	[68]
2, healthy	146	Lozenge	328.5	[69]

body mass index (BMI); [1] Capsule also contained 10 mg of piperine.

Table 3. Reported resveratrol plasma concentration in humans after repeated doses of resveratrol (studies after 2010).

Number of Participants, Characteristics, Study Type	Dose (mg/day)	Days	Administration	Peak Plasma Concentration (ng/mL)	Reference
6, low BMI 6, high BMI	2125	11	Tablet and drink	903.0 245.0	[66]
35, healthy males, cross-over study	800	5	Capsule Dairy drink Soy drink Protein-free drink	Capsule: 0.56 Dairy drink: 0.61 Soy drink: 0.58 Protein free drink: 0.70	[70]
7, healthy	500	28	Capsule [1]	2967.25	[67]
40, healthy, repeated sequential dosing	500 1000 2500 5000	29	Caplet	43.8 141 331 967	[71]
6, patients with hepatic metastases, randomized double-blind clinical trial	5000	14	Micronized resveratrol mixed in liquid	1942	[72]
8, healthy subjects	2000	7	Capsule	1274	[73]
19, overweight or obese, randomized, double-blind, placebo-controlled, crossover intervention	30 90 270	6	Capsule	181.31 532.00 1232.16	[74]

body mass index (BMI); [1] Capsule also contained 10 mg of piperine.

3. Molecular Action of Resveratrol and Metabolites

3.1. RSV Modulates a Panoply of Protein Targets

Many and diverse effects have been described for RSV, indicating an array of possible protein targets that can be (in)directly modulated by this compound [75–80]. Recently, a computational approach was used to map all publically available polyphenol-protein interactions [81]. Among all polyphenols and human metabolites, RSV was found to be one of the polyphenols with the most known interactions with proteins (738 RSV-protein interactions). Only five protein interactions were reported with RSV metabolites, specifically interacting with DHR, highlighting the lack of studies on RSV metabolites. Taken together, the protein interactome of RSV and DHR led to 743 interactions (Figure 3). The interacting proteins can be classified in terms of diseases, using DAVID's [82] genetic association database (GAD) [83] disease classification system. RSV showed low coverage for most diseases (<50%), yet a widespread representation, highlighting its potential pleotropic effect. RSV modulates genes within pathways of cancer, metabolic and cardiovascular diseases, and to lesser extent other disease classes (Figure 3A). Taking the same list of RSV-interacting proteins, these could be classified in terms of protein super-families, using the InterPro [84] protein classification in DAVID. This analysis highlighted an enrichment in many protein super-families modulated by RSV (Figure 3B), of relevance in metabolic diseases and obesity, such as nuclear hormone receptor-type (e.g., PPARγ), insulin related, NF-κB, enolases, sirtuins, and nitric oxide related proteins. Using STITCH [85], a protein-metabolite database, proteins of experimental evidence were further selected to interact with RSV (Figure 3C). This obtained network highlighted, with substantial overlap, the enrichment of RSV-interacting proteins previously identified by InterPro classification (Figure 3B).

While RSV may establish a large number of possible interactions, some of these proteins are already established direct targets of RSV, at least in vitro [77]. The structure of some of these protein-RSV complexes can be found in the Protein Databank (PDB) [86], accounting for 24 RSV-protein complexes, and even a handful of RSV metabolite protein complexes.

3.2. RSV Increases Energy Expenditure and Vascular Function

One of the most studied mechanisms of RSV is its capacity to increase energy expenditure by modulating protein targets within central energy pathways and signaling, specifically by inducing mitochondrial biogenesis. RSV can directly activate SIRT1 and SIRT5. Because sirtuins are NAD-dependent deacetylases, they directly depend on NAD^+ and therefore are quite sensitive to cellular energy via imbalances of the redox pair $NAD^+/NADH$. Sirtuins act as caloric restriction mimetics, with potential benefits in longevity and preventing age-related complications, as well as type II diabetes and obesity. By activating SIRT1, RSV elicits deacetylation of PGC1α, a key regulator of energy metabolism, leading to decreased glycolysis in muscle and the liver, and increased lipid use [13,87]. In addition, RSV inhibits ATP production by interfering with mitochondrial function, leading to an increase of AMP/ATP ratio, which activates AMP-activated protein kinase (AMPK) [75]. AMPK is a pivotal protein in governing energy homeostasis and its activation takes place in cases of nutrient starvation or in the presence of agonists, such as certain drugs (e.g., metformin) or natural compounds such as RSV. Furthermore, AMPK may inhibit mTOR signaling, that in certain species has been associated with an extended lifespan, given its anti-ageing effects. The signaling pathway of AMPK crosstalks with Akt (protein kinase B). Akt are kinases involved in metabolism and cell proliferation and are part of the PI3K/AKT/mTOR pathway that governs the cell cycle. Activation of Akt reduces the activity of AMPK through direct phosphorylation [79].

Interestingly, AMPK and Akt have been shown to directly phosphorylate the endothelial nitric oxide synthase (eNOS). eNOS, responsible for the production of nitric oxide (NO), is activated by shear stress and agonists, and has a protective function in the cardiovascular system. RSV has been shown to be such an agonist, by improving vascular function and vasoprotective effects, including vascular

NO production and bioavailability, and perivascular adipose tissue function [88]. Akt and AMPK may contribute to the stimulation of NO production by eNOS in response to RSV treatment [79].

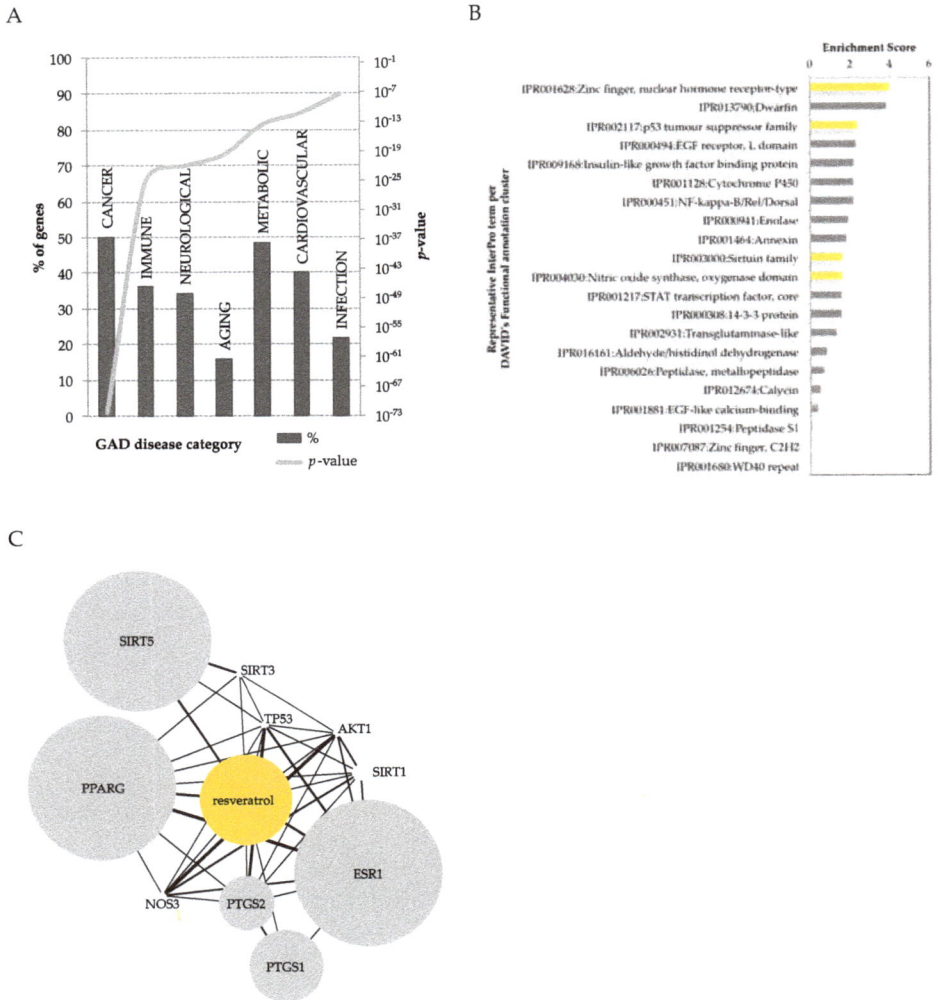

Figure 3. Using Lacroix et al.'s [81] human polyphenol-protein interactome, proteins (743) interacting with resveratrol and dihydroresveratrol were functionally analyzed in DAVID [82]. (**A**) Resveratrol interacting genes annotated according to the genetic association database (GAD) [83] disease categories, according to percentage of genes and *p*-value. (**B**) Clustering of protein super-families according to the InterPro [84] protein classification, at the highest stringency (in yellow, protein classes represented in (**C**). (**C**), Human resveratrol-protein interactome using experimental evidence obtained from STITCH [89]. The size of the node reflects the strength of the resveratrol-protein interaction. Depicted proteins: peroxisome proliferator-activated receptor gamma (PPARG), NAD-dependent deacetylase sirtuin-1 (SIRT1), 3 (SIRT3) and 5 (SIRT5), nitric oxide synthase 3 (NOS3), prostaglandin-endoperoxide synthase 1 (PTGS1) and 2 (PTGS2), estrogen receptor 1 (ESR1), tumor protein p53 (TP53), and AKT serine/threonine kinase 1 (AKT1).

Beyond central metabolism and bioenergetics, RSV also impacts lipid metabolism. RSV can directly inhibit PPARγ, a nuclear receptor expressed in adipose tissue, or do so indirectly via SIRT1, leading to decreased adipogenesis and increased lipolysis [87]. SIRT1 is also known to repress NF-κB activity, and thereby reduce inflammation. RSV modulates inflammation by directly interacting with cyclooxygenases (COX), which catalyze the formation of prostaglandins, bioactive lipids with hormone-like effects [77].

3.3. Effect of RSV on Epigenietics

While RSV has an impact on metabolism, some of its mechanisms are a consequence of epigenetic modifications. In fact, RSV can induce epigenetic modifications to the DNA sequence. Epigenetic modifications include DNA methylation, histone modifications and nucleosome positioning. These modifications can interact with each other to influence gene expression [90]. RSV supplementation can influence DNA methylation and histone modification, with the latter being most relevant in the context of obesity and energy balance. Histones are subject to post-transcriptional modification like methylation, phosphorylation, ubiquitination, SUMOylation and ADP-ribosylation. These modifications can be reversed by methyltransferases, histone demethylases, kinases, histone acetyltransferases and histone deacetylases. For instance, RSV can influence histone deacetylation via sirtuins, and sirtuins activated by RSV can deacetylate sites on PGC1α [13]. The nuclear bile acid receptor farnesoid X receptor (FXR) is a target a SIRT1 that plays a critical role in the regulation of lipid and glucose metabolism. RSV treatment reduced acetylated FXR levels, with benefits for metabolic health [91].

3.4. RSV Influences Redox Metabolism

RSV has 16-times lower antioxidant capacity than alpha-tocopherol [92], nature's ubiquitous antioxidant, and therefore will be inefficient per se for radical scavenging in physiological conditions. However RSV, in addition to other polyphenols, has been described as undergoing redox cycling, being able to adopt a quinone-like structure and generate reactive oxygen species (ROS). ROS production leads to the activation of the nuclear factor-erythroid 2-related factor-2 (Nrf2), a transcription factor that regulates redox status, and reacts against stresses. In addition, Nrf2 improves cellular recycling and cross-talks with central and lipid metabolism, as well as modulates phase I and II metabolism enzymes and transporters [93,94]. One of these phase II detoxifying enzymes, quinone reductase 2 (QR2) has been shown to interact directly with RSV. The inhibition of QR2 by RSV may induce other cellular antioxidant enzymes and increase cellular resistance to oxidative stress [77]. Oxidative stress contributes to type II diabetes, and RSV showed antioxidant effects after eight weeks of supplementation with 800 mg/day in the blood and PBMCs (peripheral blood mononuclear cells) of diabetic patients. After RSV consumption, the expression of Nrf2 and superoxide dismutase (SOD) was significantly increased, along with reductions in body weight, BMI and blood pressure [95].

3.5. RSV Metabolites Exhibit Activity

RSV metabolites have been examined for their potential activity only recently. A biochemical study compared the action of RSV, and RSV-3- and 4'-O-sulfates (Figure 1.2,3) on three direct targets: COX, SIRT1 and QR2. RSV and metabolites can inhibit both COX and QR2 enzymes. SIRT1 is activated by RSV and metabolites, but the activation seems to be a substrate-dependent phenomenon questioning in vivo relevance [96]. Comparable in vitro activities were also found for RSV glucuronides [97]. The ability to bind to human serum albumin was found to be comparable between RSV, RSV-4'-glucuronide (Figure 1.6) and DHR (Figure 1.7), while RSV-3-O-glucuronide (Figure 1.5) showed a slightly lower affinity. RSV-4'-glucuronide was able to inhibit COX-2 and DHR presented comparable activity in inhibiting NO production [97]. The metabolites RSV-3- and 4'-O-sulfates were also studied in vivo, by dosing these conjugates directly to mice. Both compounds led to low bioavailability, but hydrolysis of sulfate moieties was identified, contributing to the recirculation of free RSV. In human cancer cells, RSV metabolites partially regenerated free RSV and prompted autophagy and senescence [63]. Thus, these studies lead to the suggestion of a metabolic interplay between RSV and phase II metabolites in the body. According to the cell's specific conditions, RSV metabolites function as a pool of RSV, actively contributing to a wide variety of actions, previously solely attributed to RSV.

4. Resveratrol, Metabolic Health and Obesity

Obesity is characterized by an excess accumulation of adipose tissue which is a risk factor for the development of chronic diseases [26,98]. Adipose tissue is composed of specialized cells, adipocytes, which store and release energy. To store energy, adipocytes convert free fatty acids to triglycerides through lipogenesis, and to release energy triglycerides are metabolized through a process called lipolysis. Adipocytes also produce hormones, adipokines, which relay information from the adipose tissue to the central nervous system [99]. Reduction of adipose tissue through increased physical activity and decreased energy intake can reduce the risk of adverse health outcomes. Though increased exercise and reduced calorie intake are effective methods to reduce adiposity, compliance is low and genetic factors may be unfavorable; therefore, alternative treatments are needed. RSV has been shown to influence adipose tissue function [100].

RSV was found to have an anti-lipolytic effect at low physiological concentration in a human adipocyte model [28]. A decreased sulfation of RSV, by knock-down of SULT1A1, resulted in an increased anti-lipolytic effect, as demonstrated by lower glycerol accumulation, probably attributed to lower activity of the lipolytic protein perilipin, suggesting the role of phase II enzymes in RSV bioavailability in adipose tissue. A comprehensive review on effects of RSV on adipose tissue [101] detailed effects on how RSV can modulate adipogenesis, apoptosis, de novo lipogenesis and lipoprotein lipase functions, lipolysis, thermogenesis, and fatty acid oxidation, in vitro and in rodent models.

Although adipose tissue is an attractive target site of RSV, only a few human studies have so far been conducted to consider RSV-treatment in this tissue. A recent human clinical trial investigated the effect of RSV supplementation on the adipose tissue metabolome [102]. In this study, male subjects with metabolic syndrome (characterized by elevations in at least three of the following: abdominal obesity, blood lipids, blood pressure and fasting blood glucose) were treated for four months with 1 g of resveratrol. The metabolome of these biological samples were characterized using untargeted metabolomics. This approach identified 282 metabolites in adipose tissue, of which 45 changed significantly in response to RSV treatment. RSV supplementation was associated with increased long chain-fatty acids, increased polyunsaturated fatty acids and decreased steroids [102]. Another study in obese men, supplemented for 30 days with 150 mg of RSV, observed changes in adipose tissue morphology. RSV decreased abdominal subcutaneous adipocyte size. Transcriptome profiling on the adipose tissue samples and subsequent pathway analysis identified an enrichment of genes involved in cell cycle regulation pathways, suggesting enhanced adipogenesis [103].

In terms of obesity and the sphere of weight management, RSV has demonstrated significant improvement of glucose control and insulin sensitivity in diabetics [104]. A few studies indicate potential in enhancing adipogenesis as well as lipid markers in adipose tissue [102,103], therefore this is an application area worth further exploring. Even though clinical interventions can be particularly challenging, perhaps it is in the preventive health space that RSV can offer its full potential [31,78].

5. Outlook

With over 140 human clinical trials using RSV (clinicaltrials.gov), and more than 10,000 scientific publications describing the uses and effects of RSV, much research has been conducted on this small molecule. Due to varying doses, disparate experimental setups, low statistical power, and a myriad of biological or other types of confounders, the ultimate fate and effect of RSV in humans remains elusive. Mechanisms of action are varied and of potential benefit for cardiovascular health, obesity, metabolic health, inflammation, and cancer management, therefore, RSV is of wide pleiotropy. Systems-driven approaches [81] aid in mapping effects of multi-targeted compounds such as RSV and highlight links between bioenergetics [27], phase II metabolism [38] and redox pathways [93], linked by protein targets modulated by RSV.

The bioavailability of RSV is often mentioned as a limitation and is subject to controversy. Nevertheless, studies on RSV metabolites seem to be encouraging, as these either have similar effects or can act as a RSV pool in the body, fostering the metabolic effects previously solely attributed to free RSV [63]. On the note of enhancing knowledge on RSV metabolites and its potential actions, the use of untargeted metabolomics analysis [105] can widen the spectrum of RSV metabolites known so far, and also map metabolic sub-network effects induced by RSV [102]. Stable isotopes are an elegant tool to unravel metabolic fate of specific compounds [106] and offer advantages compared to radioactive labeling strategies.

Inter-individual variability [19] upon RSV intake can be attributed to various factors such as: (i) gut microbiota composition; (ii) genetic polymorphisms in phase II metabolism enzymes (e.g., UGTs, SULTs) and transporters, including tissue specificity and/or enzymatic regioselectivity; (iii) variability inherent in specific ethnicities or geographic subpopulations; (iv) specific lifestyles and diets; or (v) simply part of natural human variation. As bioactive-intervention studies often rely on small human studies, the variability can be overpowering. These factors need to be taken into account in future studies. Efforts to conduct larger and more deeply characterized studies could be an aim of the research community in order to bridge the current gaps in knowledge on RSV metabolism and beneficial effects.

Author Contributions: Both authors (M.S. and S.M.) conceptualized, wrote and approved the final version of this manuscript.

Funding: This research received no external funding.

Acknowledgments: S.M. is a participant in the EU-funded COST Action FA1403 POSITIVe (interindividual variation in response to consumption of plant food bioactives and determinants involved).

Conflicts of Interest: The authors are employees of Nestle Research.

References

1. Takaoka, M. The Phenolic Substances of White Hellebore (*Veratrum Grandiflorum* Hoes. Fil.) I. *Nippon Kagaku Kaishi* **1939**, *60*, 1090–1100. [CrossRef]
2. Siemann, E.H.; Creasy, L.L. Concentration Of The Phytoalexin Resveratrol In Wine. *Am. J. Enol. Vitic.* **1992**, *43*, 49–52.
3. St Leger, A.S.; Cochrane, A.; Moore, F. Factors Associated With Cardiac Mortality In Developed Countries With Particular Reference To The Consumption Of Wine. *Lancet* **1979**, *313*, 1017–1020. [CrossRef]
4. Renaud, S.; De Lorgeril, M. Wine, Alcohol, Platelets, And The French Paradox For Coronary Heart Disease. *Lancet* **1992**, *339*, 1523–1526. [CrossRef]
5. Frankel, E.N.; Waterhouse, A.L.; Kinsella, J.E. Inhibition Of Human Ldl Oxidation By Resveratrol. *Lancet* **1993**, *341*, 1103–1104. [CrossRef]
6. Jang, M.; Cai, L.; Udeani, G.O.; Slowing, K.V.; Thomas, C.F.; Beecher, C.W.W.; Fong, H.H.S.; Farnsworth, N.R.; Kinghorn, A.D.; Mehta, R.G.; et al. Cancer Chemopreventive Activity Of Resveratrol, A Natural Product Derived From Grapes. *Science* **1997**, *275*, 218–220. [CrossRef]
7. Subbaramaiah, K.; Chung, W.J.; Michaluart, P.; Telang, N.; Tanabe, T.; Inoue, H.; Jang, M.; Pezzuto, J.M.; Dannenberg, A.J. Resveratrol Inhibits Cyclooxygenase-2 Transcription And Activity In Phorbol Ester-Treated Human Mammary Epithelial Cells. *J. Biol. Chem.* **1998**, *273*, 21875–21882. [CrossRef]
8. Wallerath, T.; Deckert, G.; Ternes, T.; Anderson, H.; Li, H.; Witte, K.; Förstermann, U. Resveratrol, A Polyphenolic Phytoalexin Present In Red Wine, Enhances Expression And Activity Of Endothelial Nitric Oxide Synthase. *Circulation* **2002**, *106*, 1652–1658. [CrossRef]
9. Park, S.-J.; Ahmad, F.; Philp, A.; Baar, K.; Williams, T.; Luo, H.; Ke, H.; Rehmann, H.; Taussig, R.; Brown, A.L.; et al. Resveratrol Ameliorates Aging-Related Metabolic Phenotypes By Inhibiting Camp Phosphodiesterases. *Cell* **2012**, *148*, 421–433. [CrossRef]

10. Howitz, K.T.; Bitterman, K.J.; Cohen, H.Y.; Lamming, D.W.; Lavu, S.; Wood, J.G.; Zipkin, R.E.; Chung, P.; Kisielewski, A.; Zhang, L.-L.; et al. Small Molecule Activators Of Sirtuins Extend Saccharomyces Cerevisiae Lifespan. *Nature* **2014**, *19*, 191–196. [CrossRef]

11. Baur, J.A.; Pearson, K.J.; Price, N.L.; Jamieson, H.A.; Lerin, C.; Kalra, A.; Prabhu, V.V.; Allard, J.S.; Lopez-Lluch, G.; Lewis, K.; et al. Resveratrol Improves Health And Survival Of Mice On A High-Calorie Diet. *Nature* **2006**, *444*, 337–342. [CrossRef] [PubMed]

12. Timmers, S.; Konings, E.; Bilet, L.; Houtkooper, R.H.; Van De Weijer, T.; Goossens, G.H.; Hoeks, J.; Van Der Krieken, S.; Ryu, D.; Kersten, S.; et al. Calorie Restriction-Like Effects Of 30 Days Of Resveratrol Supplementation On Energy Metabolism And Metabolic Profile In Obese Humans. *Cell Metab.* **2011**, *14*, 612–622. [CrossRef] [PubMed]

13. Lagouge, M.; Argmann, C.; Gerhart-Hines, Z.; Meziane, H.; Lerin, C.; Daussin, F.; Messadeq, N.; Milne, J.; Lambert, P.; Elliott, P.; et al. Resveratrol Improves Mitochondrial Function And Protects Against Metabolic Disease By Activating Sirt1 And Pgc-1α. *Cell* **2006**, *127*, 1109–1122. [CrossRef] [PubMed]

14. Baur, J.A.; Sinclair, D.A. Therapeutic Potential Of Resveratrol: The In Vivo Evidence. *Nat. Rev. Drug Discov.* **2006**, *5*, 493–506. [CrossRef]

15. Timmers, S.; De Ligt, M.; Phielix, E.; Van De Weijer, T.; Hansen, J.; Moonen-Kornips, E.; Schaart, G.; Kunz, I.; Hesselink, M.K.C.; Schrauwen-Hinderling, V.B.; et al. Resveratrol As Add-On Therapy In Subjects With Well-Controlled Type 2 Diabetes: A Randomized Controlled Trial. *Diabetes Care* **2016**, *39*, 2211–2217. [CrossRef] [PubMed]

16. Walle, T.; Hsieh, F.; Delegge, M.H.; John, E.; Oatis, J.; Walle, U.K. High Absorption But Very Low Bioavailability Of Oral Resveratrol In Humans. *Drug Metab. Dispos.* **2004**, *32*, 1377–1382. [CrossRef] [PubMed]

17. Yu, C.; Geun Shin, Y.; Chow, A.; Li, Y.; Kosmeder, J.W.; Sup Lee, Y.; Hirschelman, W.H.; Pezzuto, J.M.; Mehta, R.G.; Van Breemen, R.B. Human, Rat, And Mouse Metabolism Of Resveratrol. *Pharm. Res.* **2002**, *19*, 1907–1914. [CrossRef]

18. Böhmdorfer, M.; Szakmary, A.; Schiestl, R.; Vaquero, J.; Riha, J.; Brenner, S.; Thalhammer, T.; Szekeres, T.; Jäger, W. Involvement Of Udp-Glucuronosyltransferases And Sulfotransferases In The Excretion And Tissue Distribution Of Resveratrol In Mice. *Nutrients* **2017**, *9*, 1347. [CrossRef]

19. Manach, C.; Milenkovic, D.; Van De Wiele, T.; Rodriguez-Mateos, A.; De Roos, B.; Garcia-Conesa, M.T.; Landberg, R.; Gibney, E.R.; Heinonen, M.; Tomás-Barberán, F.; et al. Addressing The Inter-Individual Variation In Response To Consumption Of Plant Food Bioactives: Towards A Better Understanding Of Their Role In Healthy Aging And Cardiometabolic Risk Reduction. *Mol. Nutr. Food Res.* **2017**, *61*, 1600557. [CrossRef]

20. Bode, L.M.; Bunzel, D.; Huch, M.; Cho, G.; Ruhland, D.; Bunzel, M.; Bub, A.; Franz, C.M.; Kulling, S.E. In Vivo And In Vitro Metabolism Of Trans-Resveratrol By Human Gut Microbiota. *Am. J. Clin. Nutr.* **2013**, *97*, 295–309. [CrossRef]

21. Tomás-Barberán, F.A.; Selma, M.V.; Espín, J.C. Interactions Of Gut Microbiota With Dietary Polyphenols And Consequences To Human Health. *Curr. Opin. Clin. Nutr. Metab. Care* **2016**, *19*, 471–476. [CrossRef] [PubMed]

22. Ritter, J.K. Intestinal Ugts As Potential Modifiers Of Pharmacokinetics And Biological Responses To Drugs And Xenobiotics. *Expert Opin. Drug Metab. Toxicol.* **2007**, *3*, 93–107. [CrossRef] [PubMed]

23. Chen, B.-H.; Wang, C.-C.; Hou, Y.-H.; Mao, Y.-C.; Yang, Y.-S. Mechanism Of Sulfotransferase Pharmacogenetics In Altered Xenobiotic Metabolism. *Expert Opin. Drug Metab. Toxicol.* **2015**, *11*, 1053–1071. [CrossRef] [PubMed]

24. Lamba, J.K.; Lin, Y.S.; Schuetz, E.G.; Thummel, K.E. Genetic Contribution To Variable Human Cyp3a-Mediated Metabolism. *Adv. Drug Deliv. Rev.* **2012**, *64*, 256–269. [CrossRef]

25. Mena, P.; Del Rio, D. Gold Standards For Realistic (Poly)Phenol Research. *J. Agric. Food Chem.* **2018**, *66*, 8221–8223. [CrossRef] [PubMed]

26. Swinburn, B.A.; Sacks, G.; Hall, K.D.; Mcpherson, K.; Finegood, D.T.; Moodie, M.L.; Gortmaker, S.L. The Global Obesity Pandemic: Shaped By Global Drivers And Local Environments. *Lancet* **2011**, *378*, 804–814. [CrossRef]

27. Tseng, Y.H.; Cypess, A.M.; Kahn, C.R. Cellular Bioenergetics As A Target For Obesity Therapy. *Nat. Rev. Drug Discov.* **2010**, *9*, 465–481. [CrossRef] [PubMed]

28. Gheldof, N.; Moco, S.; Chabert, C.; Teav, T.; Barron, D.; Hager, J. Role Of Sulfotransferases In Resveratrol Metabolism In Human Adipocytes. *Mol. Nutr. Food Res.* **2017**, *61*, 1700020. [CrossRef]

29. Jimenez-Gomez, Y.; Mattison, J.A.; Pearson, K.J.; Martin-Montalvo, A.; Palacios, H.H.; Sossong, A.M.; Ward, T.M.; Younts, C.M.; Lewis, K.; Allard, J.S.; et al. Resveratrol Improves Adipose Insulin Signaling And Reduces The Inflammatory Response In Adipose Tissue Of Rhesus Monkeys On High-Fat, High-Sugar Diet. *Cell Metab.* **2013**, *18*, 533–545. [CrossRef]

30. Burns, J.; Yokota, T.; Ashihara, H.; Lean, M.E.J.; Crozier, A. Plant Foods And Herbal Sources Of Resveratrol. *J. Agric. Food Chem.* **2002**, *50*, 3337–3340. [CrossRef]

31. Pezzuto, J.M. Resveratrol: Twenty Years Of Growth, Development And Controversy. *Biomol. Ther.* **2018**, *14*, 1–14. [CrossRef] [PubMed]

32. Planas, J.M.; Alfaras, I.; Colom, H.; Juan, M.E. The Bioavailability And Distribution Of Trans-Resveratrol Are Constrained By Abc Transporters. *Arch. Biochem. Biophys.* **2012**, *527*, 67–73. [CrossRef] [PubMed]

33. Henry, C.; Vitrac, X.; Decendit, A.; Ennamany, R.; Krisa, S.; Mérillon, J.-M. Cellular Uptake And Efflux Of Trans -Piceid And Its Aglycone Trans -Resveratrol On The Apical Membrane Of Human Intestinal Caco-2 Cells. *J. Agric. Food Chem.* **2005**, *53*, 798–803. [CrossRef] [PubMed]

34. Riches, Z.; Stanley, E.L.; Bloomer, J.C.; Coughtrie, M.W.H. Quantitative Evaluation Of The Expression And Activity Of Five Major Sulfotransferases (Sults) In Human Tissues: The Sult "Pie". *Drug Metab. Dispos.* **2009**, *37*, 2255–2261. [CrossRef] [PubMed]

35. Ung, D.; Nagar, S. Variable Sulfation Of Dietary Polyphenols By Recombinant Human Sulfotransferase (Sult) 1a1 Genetic Variants And Sult1e1. *Drug Metab. Dispos.* **2007**, *35*, 740–746. [CrossRef] [PubMed]

36. Miksits, M.; Maier-Salamon, A.; Aust, S.; Thalhammer, T.; Reznicek, G.; Kunert, O.; Haslinger, E.; Szekeres, T.; Jaeger, W. Sulfation Of Resveratrol In Human Liver: Evidence Of A Major Role For The Sulfotransferases Sult1a1 And Sult1e1. *Xenobiotica* **2005**, *35*, 1101–1119. [CrossRef] [PubMed]

37. Oda, S.; Fukami, T.; Yokoi, T.; Nakajima, M. A Comprehensive Review Of Udp-Glucuronosyltransferase And Esterases For Drug Development. *Drug Metab. Pharmacokinet.* **2015**, *30*, 30–51. [CrossRef]

38. Rouleau, M.M.; Audet-Delage, Y.; Desjardins, S.; Rouleau, M.M.; Girard-Bock, C.; Guillemette, C. Endogenous Protein Interactome Of Human Udp-Glucuronosyltransferases Exposed By Untargeted Proteomics. *Front. Pharmacol.* **2017**, *8*, 23. [CrossRef]

39. Dietrich, C.G.; Geier, A.; Oude Elferink, R.P.J. Abc Of Oral Bioavailability: Transporters As Gatekeepers In The Gut. *Gut* **2003**, *52*, 1788–1795. [CrossRef]

40. Maier-Salamon, A.; Böhmdorfer, M.; Riha, J.; Thalhammer, T.; Szekeres, T.; Jaeger, W. Interplay Between Metabolism And Transport Of Resveratrol. *Ann. N. Y. Acad. Sci.* **2013**, *1290*, 98–106. [CrossRef]

41. Vitaglione, P.; Sforza, S.; Galaverna, G.; Ghidini, C.; Caporaso, N.; Vescovi, P.P.; Fogliano, V.; Marchelli, R. Bioavailability Of Trans-Resveratrol From Red Wine In Humans. *Mol. Nutr. Food Res.* **2005**, *49*, 495–504. [CrossRef] [PubMed]

42. Patel, K.R.; Scott, E.; Brown, V.A.; Gescher, A.J.; Steward, W.P.; Brown, K. Clinical Trials Of Resveratrol. *Ann. N. Y. Acad. Sci.* **2011**, *1215*, 161–169. [CrossRef] [PubMed]

43. Marier, J.-F. Metabolism And Disposition Of Resveratrol In Rats: Extent Of Absorption, Glucuronidation, And Enterohepatic Recirculation Evidenced By A Linked-Rat Model. *J. Pharmacol. Exp. Ther.* **2002**, *302*, 369–373. [CrossRef] [PubMed]

44. Asensi, M.; Medina, I.; Ortega, A.; Carretero, J.; Baño, M.C.; Obrador, E.; Estrela, J.M. Inhibition Of Cancer Growth By Resveratrol Is Related To Its Low Bioavailability. *Free Radic. Biol. Med.* **2002**, *33*, 387–398. [CrossRef]

45. Emília Juan, M.; Buenafuente, J.; Casals, I.; Planas, J.M. Plasmatic Levels Of Trans-Resveratrol In Rats. *Food Res. Int.* **2002**, *35*, 195–199. [CrossRef]

46. Menet, M.-C.; Baron, S.; Taghi, M.; Diestra, R.; Dargère, D.; Laprévote, O.; Nivet-Antoine, V.; Beaudeux, J.-L.; Bédarida, T.; Cottart, C.-H. Distribution Of Trans -Resveratrol And Its Metabolites After Acute Or Sustained Administration In Mouse Heart, Brain, And Liver. *Mol. Nutr. Food Res.* **2017**, *61*, 1600686. [CrossRef] [PubMed]

47. Andres-Lacueva, C.; Macarulla, M.T.; Rotches-Ribalta, M.; Boto-Ordóñez, M.; Urpi-Sarda, M.; Rodríguez, V.M.; Portillo, M.P. Distribution Of Resveratrol Metabolites In Liver, Adipose Tissue, And Skeletal Muscle In Rats Fed Different Doses Of This Polyphenol. *J. Agric. Food Chem.* **2012**, *60*, 4833–4840. [CrossRef]

48. Alberdi, G.; Rodríguez, V.M.; Miranda, J.; Macarulla, M.T.; Arias, N.; Andrés-Lacueva, C.; Portillo, M.P. Changes In White Adipose Tissue Metabolism Induced By Resveratrol In Rats. *Nutr. Metab.* **2011**, *8*, 29. [CrossRef]

49. Burkon, A.; Somoza, V. Quantification Of Free And Protein-Boundtrans-Resveratrol Metabolites And Identification Oftrans-Resveratrol-C/O-Conjugated Diglucuronides—Two Novel Resveratrol Metabolites In Human Plasma. *Mol. Nutr. Food Res.* **2008**, *52*, 549–557. [CrossRef]

50. Selma, M.V.; Espín, J.C.; Tomás-Barberán, F.A. Interaction Between Phenolics And Gut Microbiota: Role In Human Health. *J. Agric. Food Chem.* **2009**, *57*, 6485–6501. [CrossRef]

51. Dao, T.-M.A.; Waget, A.; Klopp, P.; Serino, M.; Vachoux, C.; Pechere, L.; Drucker, D.J.; Champion, S.; Barthélemy, S.; Barra, Y.; et al. Resveratrol Increases Glucose Induced Glp-1 Secretion In Mice: A Mechanism Which Contributes To The Glycemic Control. *PLoS ONE* **2011**, *6*, E20700. [CrossRef]

52. Larrosa, M.; Gonza, A.; Toti, S.; Joaqui, J.; Yañéz-Gascón, M.J.; Selma, M.V.; González-Sarrías, A.; Toti, S.; Cerón, J.J.; Tomás-Barberán, F.; et al. Effect Of A Low Dose Of Dietary Resveratrol On Colon Microbiota, Inflammation And Tissue Damage In A Dss-Induced Colitis Rat Model. *J. Agric. Food Chem.* **2009**, *57*, 2211–2220. [CrossRef] [PubMed]

53. Hwang, D.; Lim, Y.-H. Resveratrol Antibacterial Activity Against Escherichia Coli Is Mediated By Z-Ring Formation Inhibition Via Suppression Of Ftsz Expression. *Sci. Rep.* **2015**, *5*, 10029. [CrossRef]

54. Paulo, L.; Ferreira, S.; Gallardo, E.; Queiroz, J.A.; Domingues, F. Antimicrobial Activity And Effects Of Resveratrol On Human Pathogenic Bacteria. *World J. Microbiol. Biotechnol.* **2010**, *26*, 1533–1538. [CrossRef]

55. Sung, M.M.; Kim, T.T.; Denou, E.; Soltys, C.-L.M.; Hamza, S.M.; Byrne, N.J.; Masson, G.; Park, H.; Wishart, D.S.; Madsen, K.L.; et al. Improved Glucose Homeostasis In Obese Mice Treated With Resveratrol Is Associated With Alterations In The Gut Microbiome. *Diabetes* **2017**, *66*, 418–425. [CrossRef] [PubMed]

56. Ley, R.E.; Bäckhed, F.; Turnbaugh, P.; Lozupone, C.A.; Knight, R.D.; Gordon, J.I. Obesity Alters Gut Microbial Ecology. *Proc. Natl. Acad. Sci. USA* **2005**, *102*, 11070–11075. [CrossRef]

57. Etxeberria, U.; Arias, N.; Boqué, N.; Macarulla, M.T.; Portillo, M.P.; Martínez, J.A.; Milagro, F.I. Reshaping Faecal Gut Microbiota Composition By The Intake Of. *J. Nutr. Biochem.* **2015**, *26*, 1–26. [CrossRef]

58. Bird, J.K.; Raederstorff, D.; Weber, P.; Steinert, R.E. Cardiovascular And Antiobesity Effects Of Resveratrol Mediated Through The Gut Microbiota. *Adv. Nutr.* **2017**, *8*, 839–849. [CrossRef]

59. Most, J.; Penders, J.; Lucchesi, M.; Goossens, G.H.; Blaak, E.E. Gut Microbiota Composition In Relation To The Metabolic Response To 12-Week Combined Polyphenol Supplementation In Overweight Men And Women. *Eur. J. Clin. Nutr.* **2017**, *71*, 1040–1045. [CrossRef]

60. Koeth, R.A.; Wang, Z.; Levison, B.S.; Buffa, J.A.; Org, E.; Sheehy, B.T.; Britt, E.B.; Fu, X.; Wu, Y.; Li, L.; et al. Intestinal Microbiota Metabolism Of L-Carnitine, A Nutrient In Red Meat, Promotes Atherosclerosis. *Nat. Med.* **2013**, *19*, 576–585. [CrossRef]

61. Chen, M.; Yi, L.; Zhang, Y.; Zhou, X.; Ran, L.; Yang, J.; Zhu, J.; Zhang, Q.; Mi, M. Atherosclerosis By Regulating Tmao Synthesis And Bile Acid Metabolism Via Remodeling Of The Gut Microbiota. *Mbio* **2016**, *7*, E02210–E02215. [CrossRef] [PubMed]

62. Juan, M.E.; González-Pons, E.; Planas, J.M. Multidrug Resistance Proteins Restrain The Intestinal Absorption Of Trans-Resveratrol In Rats. *J. Nutr.* **2010**, *140*, 489–495. [CrossRef] [PubMed]

63. Patel, K.R.; Andreadi, C.; Britton, R.G.; Horner-Glister, E.; Karmokar, A.; Sale, S.; Brown, V.A.; Brenner, D.E.; Singh, R.; Steward, W.P.; et al. Sulfate Metabolites Provide An Intracellular Pool For Resveratrol Generation And Induce Autophagy With Senescence. *Sci. Transl. Med.* **2013**, *5*. [CrossRef] [PubMed]

64. Cottart, C.; Nivet-Antoine, V.; Laguillier-Morizot, C.; Beaudeux, J. Resveratrol Bioavailability And Toxicity In Humans. *Mol. Nutr. Food Res.* **2010**, *54*, 7–16. [CrossRef] [PubMed]

65. Sergides, C.; Chirilă, M.; Silvestro, L.; Pitta, D.; Pittas, A. Bioavailability And Safety Study Of Resveratrol 500 Mg Tablets In Healthy Male And Female Volunteers. *Exp. Ther. Med.* **2016**, *11*, 164–170. [CrossRef] [PubMed]

66. Novotny, J.A.; Chen, T.-Y.; Terekhov, A.I.; Gebauer, S.K.; Baer, D.J.; Ho, L.; Pasinetti, G.M.; Ferruzzi, M.G. The Effect Of Obesity And Repeated Exposure On Pharmacokinetic Response To Grape Polyphenols In Humans. *Mol. Nutr. Food Res.* **2017**, *61*, 1700043. [CrossRef] [PubMed]

67. Wightman, E.L.; Haskell-Ramsay, C.F.; Reay, J.L.; Williamson, G.; Dew, T.; Zhang, W.; Kennedy, D.O. The Effects Of Chronic Trans-Resveratrol Supplementation On Aspects Of Cognitive Function, Mood, Sleep, Health And Cerebral Blood Flow In Healthy, Young Humans. *Br. J. Nutr.* **2015**, *114*, 1427–1437. [CrossRef]

68. Kennedy, D.O.; Wightman, E.L.; Reay, J.L.; Lietz, G.; Okello, E.J.; Wilde, A.; Haskell, C.F. Effects Of Resveratrol On Cerebral Blood Flow Variables And Cognitive Performance In Humans: A Double-Blind, Placebo-Controlled, Crossover Investigation. *Am. J. Clin. Nutr.* **2010**, *91*, 1590–1597. [CrossRef]

69. Blanchard, O.L.; Friesenhahn, G.; Javors, M.A.; Smoliga, J.M. Development Of A Lozenge For Oral Transmucosal Delivery Of Trans-Resveratrol In Humans: Proof Of Concept. *PLoS ONE* **2014**, *9*. [CrossRef]

70. Draijer, R.; Van Dorsten, F.A.; Zebregs, Y.E.; Hollebrands, B.; Peters, S.; Duchateau, G.S.; Grün, C.H. Impact Of Proteins On The Uptake, Distribution, And Excretion Of Phenolics In The Human Body. *Nutrients* **2016**, *8*, 814. [CrossRef]

71. Brown, V.A.; Patel, K.R.; Viskaduraki, M.; Crowell, J.A.; Perloff, M.; Booth, T.D.; Vasilinin, G.; Sen, A.; Schinas, A.M.; Piccirilli, G.; et al. Repeat Dose Study Of The Cancer Chemopreventive Agent Resveratrol In Healthy Volunteers: Safety, Pharmacokinetics, And Effect On The Insulin-Like Growth Factor Axis. *Cancer Res.* **2010**, *70*, 9003–9011. [CrossRef] [PubMed]

72. Howells, L.M.; Berry, D.P.; Elliott, P.J.; Jacobson, E.W.; Hoffmann, E.; Hegarty, B.; Brown, K.; Steward, W.P.; Gescher, A.J. Phase I Randomized, Double-Blind Pilot Study Of Micronized Resveratrol (Srt501) In Patients With Hepatic Metastases—Safety, Pharmacokinetics, And Pharmacodynamics. *Cancer Prev. Res.* **2011**, *4*, 1419–1425. [CrossRef] [PubMed]

73. La Porte, C.; Voduc, N.; Zhang, G.; Seguin, I.; Tardiff, D.; Singhal, N.; Cameron, D.W. Steady-State Pharmacokinetics And Tolerability Of Trans-Resveratrol 2000mg Twice Daily With Food, Quercetin And Alcohol (Ethanol) In Healthy Human Subjects. *Clin. Pharmacokinet.* **2010**, *49*, 449–454. [CrossRef] [PubMed]

74. Wong, R.H.X.; Howe, P.R.C.; Buckley, J.D.; Coates, A.M.; Kunz, I.; Berry, N.M. Acute Resveratrol Supplementation Improves Flow-Mediated Dilatation In Overweight/Obese Individuals With Mildly Elevated Blood Pressure. *Nutr. Metab. Cardiovasc. Dis.* **2011**, *21*, 851–856. [CrossRef] [PubMed]

75. Kulkarni, S.S.; Cantó, C. The Molecular Targets Of Resveratrol. *Biochim. Biophys. Acta Mol. Basis Dis.* **2015**, *1852*, 1114–1123. [CrossRef] [PubMed]

76. Pervaiz, S.; Holme, A.L. Resveratrol: Its Biologic Targets And Functional Activity. *Antioxid. Redox Signal.* **2009**, *11*, 2851–2897. [CrossRef] [PubMed]

77. Britton, R.G.; Kovoor, C.; Brown, K. Direct Molecular Targets Of Resveratrol: Identifying Key Interactions To Unlock Complex Mechanisms. *Ann. N. Y. Acad. Sci.* **2015**, *1348*, 124–133. [CrossRef]

78. Vang, O. Resveratrol: Challenges In Analyzing Its Biological Effects. *Ann. N. Y. Acad. Sci.* **2015**, *1348*, 161–170. [CrossRef]

79. Dolinsky, V.W.; Dyck, J.R.B. Calorie Restriction And Resveratrol In Cardiovascular Health And Disease. *Biochim. Biophys. Acta Mol. Basis Dis.* **2011**, *1812*, 1477–1489. [CrossRef]

80. Tomé-Carneiro, J.; Larrosa, M.; González-Sarrías, A.; Tomás-Barberán, F.; García-Conesa, M.; Espín, J. Resveratrol And Clinical Trials: The Crossroad From In Vitro Studies To Human Evidence. *Curr. Pharm. Des.* **2013**, *19*, 6064–6093. [CrossRef]

81. Lacroix, S.; Klicic Badoux, J.; Scott-Boyer, M.-P.; Parolo, S.; Matone, A.; Priami, C.; Morine, M.J.; Kaput, J.; Moco, S. A Computationally Driven Analysis Of The Polyphenol-Protein Interactome. *Sci. Rep.* **2018**, *8*, 2232. [CrossRef] [PubMed]

82. Huang, D.W.; Sherman, B.T.; Tan, Q.; Kir, J.; Liu, D.; Bryant, D.; Guo, Y.; Stephens, R.; Baseler, M.W.; Lane, H.C.; Lempicki, R.A. David Bioinformatics Resources: Expanded Annotation Database And Novel Algorithms To Better Extract Biology From Large Gene Lists. *Nucleic Acids Res.* **2007**, *35*, 169–175. [CrossRef] [PubMed]

83. Becker, K.G.; Barnes, K.C.; Bright, T.J.; Wang, S.A. The Genetic Association Database. *Nat. Genet.* **2004**, *36*, 431–432. [CrossRef]

84. Finn, R.D.; Attwood, T.K.; Babbitt, P.C.; Bateman, A.; Bork, P.; Bridge, A.J.; Chang, H.-Y.; Dosztányi, Z.; El-Gebali, S.; Fraser, M.; et al. Interpro In 2017—Beyond Protein Family And Domain Annotations. *Nucleic Acids Res.* **2017**, *45*, D190–D199. [CrossRef] [PubMed]

85. Kuhn, M.; Von Mering, C.; Campillos, M.; Jensen, L.J.; Bork, P. Stitch: Interaction Networks Of Chemicals And Proteins. *Nucleic Acids Res.* **2008**, *36*, 684–688. [CrossRef] [PubMed]

86. Berman, H.M.; Westbrook, J.; Feng, Z.; Gilliland, G.; Bhat, T.N.; Weissig, H.; Shindyalov, I.N.; Bourne, P.E. The Protein Data Bank. *Nucleic Acids Res.* **2000**, *28*, 235–242. [CrossRef] [PubMed]

87. Houtkooper, R.H.; Pirinen, E.; Auwerx, J. Sirtuins As Regulators Of Metabolism And Healthspan. *Nat. Rev. Mol. Cell Biol.* **2012**, *13*, 225–238. [CrossRef]

88. Xia, N.; Förstermann, U.; Li, H. Effects Of Resveratrol On Enos In The Endothelium And The Perivascular Adipose Tissue. *Ann. N. Y. Acad. Sci.* **2017**, *1403*, 132–141. [CrossRef]

89. Szklarczyk, D.; Santos, A.; Von Mering, C.; Jensen, L.J.; Bork, P.; Kuhn, M. Stitch 5: Augmenting Protein-Chemical Interaction Networks With Tissue And Affinity Data. *Nucleic Acids Res.* **2016**, *44*, D380–D384. [CrossRef]

90. Portela, A.; Esteller, M. Epigenetic Modifications And Human Disease. *Nat. Biotechnol.* **2010**, *28*, 1057. [CrossRef]

91. Kemper, J.K.; Xiao, Z.; Ponugoti, B.; Miao, J.; Fang, S.; Kanamaluru, D.; Tsang, S.; Wu, S.; Chiang, C.; Veenstra, T.D. Fxr Acetylation Is Normally Dynamically Regulated By P300 And Sirt1 But Constitutively Elevated In Metabolic Disease States. *Cell Metab.* **2009**, *10*, 392–404. [CrossRef] [PubMed]

92. Keylor, M.H.; Matsuura, B.S.; Stephenson, C.R.J. Chemistry And Biology Of Resveratrol-Derived Natural Products. *Chem. Rev.* **2015**, *115*, 8976–9027. [CrossRef] [PubMed]

93. Hayes, J.D.; Dinkova-Kostova, A.T. The Nrf2 Regulatory Network Provides An Interface Between Redox And Intermediary Metabolism. *Trends Biochem. Sci.* **2014**, *39*, 199–218. [CrossRef] [PubMed]

94. Erlank, H.; Elmann, A.; Kohen, R.; Kanner, J. Polyphenols Activate Nrf2 In Astrocytes Via H2o2, Semiquinones, And Quinones. *Free Radic. Biol. Med.* **2011**, *51*, 2319–2327. [CrossRef]

95. Seyyedebrahimi, S.; Khodabandehloo, H.; Nasli Esfahani, E.; Meshkani, R. The Effects Of Resveratrol On Markers Of Oxidative Stress In Patients With Type 2 Diabetes: A Randomized, Double-Blind, Placebo-Controlled Clinical Trial. *Acta Diabetol.* **2018**, *55*, 341–353. [CrossRef] [PubMed]

96. Calamini, B.; Ratia, K.; Malkowski, M.G.; Cuendet, M.; Pezzuto, J.M.; Santarsiero, B.D.; Mesecar, A.D. Pleiotropic Mechanisms Facilitated By Resveratrol And Its Metabolites. *Biochem. J.* **2010**, *429*, 273–282. [CrossRef] [PubMed]

97. Lu, D.L.; Ding, D.J.; Yan, W.J.; Li, R.R.; Dai, F.; Wang, Q.; Yu, S.S.; Li, Y.; Jin, X.L.; Zhou, B. Influence Of Glucuronidation And Reduction Modifications Of Resveratrol On Its Biological Activities. *Chembiochem* **2013**, *14*, 1094–1104. [CrossRef] [PubMed]

98. Hruby, A.; Hu, F.B. The Epidemiology Of Obesity: A Big Picture. *Pharmacoeconomics* **2015**, *33*, 673–689. [CrossRef]

99. Sethi, J.K.; Vidal-Puig, A.J. Thematic Review Series: Adipocyte Biology. Adipose Tissue Function And Plasticity Orchestrate Nutritional Adaptation. *J. Lipid Res.* **2007**, *48*, 1253–1262. [CrossRef]

100. Maclean, P.S.; Higgins, J.A.; Giles, E.D.; Sherk, V.D.; Jackman, M.R. The Role For Adipose Tissue In Weight Regain After Weight Loss. *Obes. Rev.* **2015**, *16*, 45–54. [CrossRef]

101. Aguirre, L.; Fernández-Quintela, A.; Arias, N.; Portillo, M. Resveratrol: Anti-Obesity Mechanisms Of Action. *Molecules* **2014**, *19*, 18632–18655. [CrossRef]

102. Korsholm, A.; Kjær, T.; Ornstrup, M.; Pedersen, S. Comprehensive Metabolomic Analysis In Blood, Urine, Fat, And Muscle In Men With Metabolic Syndrome: A Randomized, Placebo-Controlled Clinical Trial On The Effects Of Resveratrol After Four Months' Treatment. *Int. J. Mol. Sci.* **2017**, *18*, 554. [CrossRef]

103. Konings, E.; Timmers, S.; Boekschoten, M.V.; Goossens, G.H.; Jocken, J.W.; Afman, L.A.; Müller, M.; Schrauwen, P.; Mariman, E.C.; Blaak, E.E. The Effects Of 30 Days Resveratrol Supplementation On Adipose Tissue Morphology And Gene Expression Patterns In Obese Men. *Int. J. Obes.* **2014**, *38*, 470–473. [CrossRef]

104. Liu, K.; Zhou, R.; Wang, B.; Mi, M. Effect Of Resveratrol On Glucose Control And Insulin Sensitivity: A Meta-Analysis Of 11 Randomized Controlled Trials. *Am. J. Clin. Nutr.* **2014**, *99*, 1510–1519. [CrossRef]

105. Moco, S.; Bino, R.J.; De Vos, R.C.H.; Vervoort, J. Metabolomics Technologies And Metabolite Identification. *Trends Analaytical Chem.* **2007**, *26*, 1694–1703. [CrossRef]

106. Naranjo Pinta, M.; Montoliu, I.; Aura, A.-M.; Seppänen-Laakso, T.; Barron, D.; Moco, S. In Vitro Gut Metabolism Of [U-^{13}C]-Quinic Acid, The Other Hydrolysis Product Of Chlorogenic Acid. *Mol. Nutr. Food Res.* **2018**, 1800396. [CrossRef]

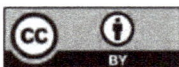

MDPI

St. Alban-Anlage 66

4052 Basel

Switzerland

Tel. +41 61 683 77 34

Fax +41 61 302 89 18

www.mdpi.com

Nutrients Editorial Office

E-mail: nutrients@mdpi.com

www.mdpi.com/journal/nutrients

www.ingramcontent.com/pod-product-compliance
Lightning Source LLC
Chambersburg PA
CBHW051725210326
41597CB00032B/5612